PRISONS AFTER WOOLF

For the past few years prisons have attracted much media attention, due to substantial increases in the prison population, deteriorations in regimes and conditions and a substantial expansion of the prison estate. In addition there has been widespread industrial action by prison officers, and a series of disturbances and riots by prisoners.

Following the riot at Strangeways prison in Manchester, and subsequent disturbances in thirty other establishments across England and Wales, Lord Justice Woolf was appointed to conduct an inquiry into the six most serious riots and their causes. *Prisons after Woolf* serves as a basic source of information on prison issues, reviewing major areas of penal practice in the light of Lord Justice Woolf's recommendations and proposals, and the Government's response in the White Paper, *Custody, Care and Justice.* In so doing, the contributors, who comprise both academics and practitioners in criminal justice, present an important and broad perspective on the major questions in penology today.

They consider the practical and theoretical issues which need to be addressed if Woolf's vision of a proper balance between security, control and justice in prisons is to be realised. This includes such issues as prisoners' rights, disciplinary procedures and prison medicine. In addition, the book examines the impact of the recommendations on particular groups of prisoners such as those on remand, the mentally disordered, long-termers and women. Finally, *Prisons after Woolf* examines the relationship between prisons and the community. It will be required reading for students in criminology, criminal justice and social policy, as well as everyone working in the criminal justice system.

Elaine Player is Lecturer in Law at King's College, London. She has written a number of articles on prisons and female crime, and is the author (with Elaine Genders) of *Race Relations in Prisons.* **Mike Jenkins** retired as an area Manager of the Prison Service in 1992. During his career he was Deputy Chief Inspector of Prisons from 1987 to 1990.

Also available from Routledge:

RACISM AND ANTI-RACISM IN PROBATION
David Denney

PRISONERS' CHILDREN
What are the Issues?
Edited by Roger Shaw

CRIME, CRIMINAL JUSTICE AND THE PROBATION SERVICE
Robert Harris

MAKING AMENDS
Mediation and Reparation in Criminal Justice
Gwynn Davis, with Heinz Messmer, Mark Umbreit and Robert Coates

CRIME, POLICING AND PLACE
Essays in Environmental Criminology
Edited by David Evans, Nicholas Fyfe and David Herbert

CRIME IN EUROPE
Edited by Frances Heidensohn and Martin Farrell

THE STATE OF THE PRISONS – 200 YEARS ON
Edited by Dick Whitfield for the Howard League

PRISONS AFTER WOOLF

Reform through riot

Edited by
Elaine Player
and
Michael Jenkins

ROUTLEDGE

London and New York

First published 1994
by Routledge
11 New Fetter Lane, London EC4P 4EE

Simultaneously published in the USA and Canada
by Routledge
29 West 35th Street, New York, NY 10001

Typeset in Baskerville by LaserScript, Mitcham, Surrey
Printed and bound in Great Britain by
T.J. Press (Padstow) Ltd, Padstow Cornwall

British Library Cataloguing in Publication Data
A catalogue record for this book is available from the British Library.

Library of Congress Cataloging in Publication Data

Prisons after Woolf: reform through riot/edited by Elaine Player
and Michael Jenkins.
p. cm.
Includes bibliographical references and index.
1. Prisons – Great Britain. I. Player, Elaine. II. Jenkins, Michael.
HV9646.P75 1993
365′.7′0941 – dc20 93-14816
CIP

ISBN 0-415-07956-X

CONTENTS

FOREWORD

The idea for this book emerged in 1991 when we were both commuting to London and regularly meeting at 6.00am, courtesy of the Oxford Bus Company. Whilst our fellow passengers sensibly went back to sleep we discussed the Woolf Report and planned this book. Dark mornings are notoriously disorientating and perhaps all that can be said in retrospect is that it seemed like a good idea at the time.

Both of us had been involved in the Perrie Lecturers since they began in 1986. They were designed to be annual events which would focus on current issues concerned with prisons and would aim to bring together prison staff, policy makers, academics and others concerned with prison affairs. In 1991 the Lectures were entitled *Prisons After Woolf* and were given by Silvia Casale, Joe Pilling and Lord Harris (see Prison Service Journal 85, pp 21–44). We were aware, however, that a single day conference could hardly do justice to the broad canvas of the Woolf Report. A book could provide a more comprehensive examination and would be more accessible. We therefore invited academics and practitioners to reflect on the application of the principles and proposals in the Woolf Report.

It is now two years since the Woolf Report and the Government's response were published. At a time when political attention is focused on agency status, new management and 'privatisation', it is an appropriate moment to reinforce Woolf's agenda. We are most grateful to all our contributors for enabling us to do that.

We would like to thank all the authors for their hard work and for their patience during the inevitable delays in completing the manuscript. A special word of thanks is also owed to Laura Masters who undertook the secretarial duties. We appreciate too the helpfulness of staff at the Home Office Library. Others who have provided invaluable support and assistance along the way include Andrew Ashworth, Jack Wright and our colleagues on the Perrie Lectures Committee: Colin Archer, Janet Harber, John Thomas-Ferrand, Mike Walker, Trevor Williams, David Wilson and Jackie Worrall. Finally, we thank our families and close friends for their patience with us during the protracted period of this project.

E.P. M.J.

CONTRIBUTORS

A. Keith Bottomley is Professor of Criminology and Director of the Centre for Criminology and Criminal Justice, University of Hull. He is the author of several books on criminology and the penal system, including *Decisions in the Penal Process* (Rothman, 1973), *Criminology in Focus* (Martin Robertson, 1979) and *Crime and Punishment, Interpreting the Data* (Open University Press, 1986) and has carried out research into various aspects of the treatment of young offenders and adults in custody and in the community. Most recently he has acted as consultant for the Home Office and Scottish Office in evaluations of the special units for difficult prisoners. He is a former member of the Parole Board for England and Wales and was a Specialist Advisor to the House of Lords' Select Committee on Murder and Life Imprisonment (1988–9).

Silvia Casale is an independent consultant in criminology, studied at Oxford and Yale, and has worked in Sweden and the USA. Her books include *Minimum Standards for Prison Establishments* (NACRO, 1984), *Women Inside* (Civil Liberties Trust, 1989) and *Regimes for Remand Prisoners* (co-authored with Joyce Plotnikoff, Prison Reform Trust, 1990); she assisted Ian Dunbar on *A Sense of Direction* (Home Office, 1986) and with Judge Eric Stockdale has co-edited *Criminal Justice under Stress* (Blackstone Press Ltd., 1992). She served as a member of the Parole Board from 1987 to 1990 and currently works as a guest inspector with HM Inspectorate of Prisons, as policy advisor on the National AIDs and Prisons Forum and as a member of the Home Office Steering Group on Prison Standards.

Adrian Grounds qualified in medicine at the University of Nottingham in 1977. He then trained in psychiatry and forensic psychiatry at the Maudsley Hospital, Broadmoor Hospital and the Institute of Psychiatry. Since April 1987 he has been a university lecturer in Forensic Psychiatry at the Institute of Criminology, Cambridge and Honorary Consultant Forensic Psychiatrist for Cambridge Health Authority and East Anglian Regional Health Authority.

Mike Jenkins joined the Prison Service in 1958 after reading law at Cambridge. He worked in borstals and prisons and governed Oxford and Long Lartin Prisons. He was Deputy Chief Inspector of Prisons, 1987–90, and retired as an Area Manager in 1992. He was awarded his MA in Applied Social Studies at Bradford University and edited the *Prison Service Journal.* He contributed 'Prison: its reform and its alternative' to *Crime And The Responsible Community* (J. Stott and N. Miller (eds), Hodder & Stoughton, 1979) and 'Control problems in dispersals' to *Problems of Long-Term Imprisonment* (A.E. Bottoms and R. Light (eds), Gower, 1987). He has been Chairman of the Perrie Lectures Committee since the lectures began in 1986.

Roy D. King is Professor of Social Theory and Institutions at the University of Wales, Bangor. He has previously been Research Fellow at the Medical Research Council, and at the University of London; Ford Foundation Research Fellow at Yale Law School and Visiting Professor at the University of Wisconsin, Madison; and Lecturer and Senior Lecturer at the University of Southampton. He has authored and co-authored several books and numerous articles on prisons – including *Albany: Birth of a Prison – End of an Era* (with Ken Elliott, Routledge, 1977) and *A Taste of Prison* (Routledge, 1976) and *The Future of the Prison System* (Gower, 1980) (both with Rod Morgan).

Stephen Livingstone is a lecturer in Law in the School of Law, Queen's University of Belfast and is Director of the School's Centre for International and Comparative Human Rights Law. He has been a Visiting Professor at the University of Detroit School of Law and is a former chairperson of the Committee on the Administration of Justice (Northern Ireland Civil Liberties Council). He has written a number of articles on issues of prison law and human rights law and is currently working on a book on prisoners' rights with Tim Owen which is to be published by Oxford University Press towards the end of 1993.

Rod Morgan is Professor of Criminal Justice and Dean of the Faculty of Law, University of Bristol. He was an Assessor to Lord Justice Woolf's Inquiry into the disturbances at Strangeways Prison, Manchester and elsewhere in April 1990. He has published widely on aspects of criminal justice policy (particularly prisons policy and policing) and is currently working on the international regulation of conditions of custody; sentencing policy reform; and the treatment of sexual offenders. He is an expert advisor to Amnesty International and the Council of Europe Committee for the Prevention of Torture and Inhuman and Degrading Treatment or Punishment.

Elaine Player is a lecturer in the School of Law, King's College, London. Between 1980 and 1990 she was a Research Fellow at the Centre for Criminological Research, University of Oxford. She co-authored *Race Relations in Prisons* (with Elaine Genders, Oxford University Press, 1989) and has published a number of articles on prisons and female crime. She is currently completing a book (with Elaine Genders) on the therapeutic regime at Grendon prison. She is a member of the editorial board of the British Journal of Sociology and has been a member of the Perrie Lectures Committee since its inception in 1986.

Roger A. Ralli is a Principal Medical Officer in the Prison Department, Directorate of Health Care. He qualified in medicine at the University of Dundee, working in General Practice and Psychiatry before joining the Prison Service. His current responsibilities include oversight of health-care services in prisons in East Anglia and Southeast England and he is a central policy advisor in the fields of Drugs and HIV. Currently he is serving as the United Kingdom representative on a Council of Europe Committee concerning Drugs, HIV/AIDS and Prisons. He has presented papers at national and international forums on Prison Health Care and Prison HIV issues.

Genevra Richardson is a Reader in Law in the University of London at Queen Mary and Westfield College. She has been a member of the Mental Health Act Commission since 1987. She has published widely in the area of prison law and is author of *Law, Process and Custody: Prisoners and Patients* (Weidenfeld and Nicolson, 1993).

Jenny Roberts trained as a probation officer at Nottingham and worked in Nottinghamshire and Staffordshire before becoming Chief Probation Officer of Hereford and Worcester in January 1983. From 1970 to 1972 she worked as a Research Assistant on the Nottingham Prisoners' Families project. She is the current Chair of the Association of Chief Officers of Probation and was previously a member of the committee which reviewed the parole system in England and Wales under the chairmanship of Lord Carlisle.

Adam Sampson has been Deputy Director of the Prison Reform Trust since 1989. He was previously a probation officer in Tottenham specialising in work with long-term prisoners. Before that he was Junior Dean of Brasenose College, Oxford. His book on the penal response to sexual crime will be published in 1993.

Joe Sim is Professor of Sociology at the Institute of Crime, Justice and Welfare Studies, School of Social Science, Liverpool John Moore's University. He is the author of *Medical Power in Prisons* (Open University Press, 1990) and co-author of *British Prisons* (with Mike Fitzgerald, Basil Blackwell,

1979) and *Prisons Under Protest* (with Phil Scraton and Paula Skidmore, Open University Press, 1991).

Vivien Stern is Director of the National Association for the Care and Resettlement of Offenders (NACRO). She is a member of a number of other organisations concerned with the welfare of offenders and the prevention of crime, and has visited prisons in Canada, Australia, Germany, France, Belgium, Sweden and Poland. She is a member of a Council of Europe Committee drafting basic rules for non-custodial penalities. In November 1989 she became the first Secretary General of 'Penal Reform International', a non-governmental organisation dedicated to promoting penal reform throughout the world. Her publications include *Imprisoned by our Prisons* (Unwin Paperbacks, 1989) and *Bricks of Shame, Britain's Prisons* (Penguin, 1987) which won the Oddfellows Social Concern Book Awards in 1988. She is also the author of *Deprived of their Liberty,* (report for *Caribbean Rights,* 1990).

J. E. Thomas is Professor of Adult Education and Pro-Vice Chancellor in the University of Nottingham. He is also Senior Academic Advisor on Staff Training to the Prison Department. He has been consultant on administration and training to the governments of Western Australia, South Australia and Victoria. He is author of many books and articles on prisons, including *The English Prison Officer Since 1850: A Study in Conflict* (Routledge and Kegan Paul, 1972) and *House of Care: Prisons and Prisoners in England 1500–1800* (University of Nottingham, 1988).

INTRODUCTION

> Were these proposals to be followed, then we believe that they would substantially influence the way prisoners come to view the prison system. While not preventing all disruptions, they could marginalise those who claim they must resort to deeply damaging and costly disturbances on the grounds that there is no other way to have their voices heard.
>
> (Woolf 1991, para. 14.438)

The Woolf Report represents the culmination of an unprecedentedly wide-ranging and open inquiry into the prison disturbances of April 1990. Its recommendations, which were framed for implementation without a new Act of Parliament, have been broadly accepted by the Government as providing an agenda for change for the next quarter of a century. Such a landmark in the penal history of England and Wales requires academic criminologists and criminal justice practitioners to examine closely the implications of the Woolf Report for particular areas of penal practice and to assess its recommendations in the light of other significant and contemporary developments. *Prisons after Woolf* thus focuses attention upon some of the major issues that have emerged over the last two decades or more, following such influential publications as the Mountbatten Report (Home Office 1966) on prison security, the Radzinowicz Report (Advisory Council on the Penal System 1968) on long-term imprisonment and the Butler Report (Home Office/Department of Health 1975) on mentally abnormal offenders. Throughout this period prisoners have sought to have their voices heard through a series of major disturbances. The purpose of this eclectic collection of essays is to examine the development of specific strands of prisons policy, to consider the fundamental questions and dilemmas which besiege these areas and to provide a critical review of the viability and relevance of both the Woolf Report and the subsequent White Paper *Custody, Care and Justice* (Home Office 1991a). The primary question is whether the riots of 1990 and the subsequent burst of official activity can generate change which reforms the day-to-day experiences of prisoners and prison staff and can thus realise Lord Justice Woolf's 'legitimate expectation' of a secure, safe and just prison system.

BACKGROUND TO THE WOOLF REPORT

On 1 April 1990 prisoners at HMP Strangeways began the longest and most devastating riot in British penal history. During the twenty-five days of the siege serious riots broke out in five other prisons and various forms of disruption occurred in more than thirty establishments across England and Wales. As a result of the events at Strangeways one prisoner lost his life and 147 prison officers and 47 inmates were injured. The cost of repairing the damage to the fabric of the institution is in the order of £30 million. The level of media coverage was as unprecedented as the scale of the disruption. Early reports spread sensational accounts of killings and torture on a massive scale. Every night news programmes relayed explicit evidence of the much vaunted prisons' 'crisis' into the nation's living-rooms. One of the messages consistently broadcast on national and international news networks was that the Prison Department had lost control and was in disarray. Disorder and discontent was thus dramatised not only in the daily episodes of the roof-top antics of the protesters, but in the accumulated reports of conflict between the governor and senior managers in headquarters.

Events in Manchester quickly overtook the explosive poll-tax riot in London which had occurred one day earlier on 31 March. On 2 April the then Home Secretary, Mr David Waddington, reported both events to Parliament. He was pressed by such veteran Labour politicians as Mr Roy Hattersley and Mr Tony Benn, to mount a full public inquiry into the poll-tax riot, but he refused. Instead, he informed Parliament that criminal investigations would be carried out and that the Commissioner of the Metropolitan Police would conduct an inquiry to discover 'what lessons [could] be learnt from what occurred'. In relation to Strangeways he immediately pledged 'a thorough inquiry into this extremely serious incident'.[1] After due consideration he announced on 6 April, the fifth day of the uprising, that an independent public inquiry would be carried out under the direction of a high court judge, Lord Justice Woolf. This decision marked a departure from previous Home Office responses to prisoner unrest. On this occasion the inquiry was not to be an in-house investigation, without the publication of a full report, as had happened after the disturbances in 1988, at Haverigg and Lindholme, and again in 1989 at Risley. Nor was the task to be delegated exclusively to the Prison Inspectorate, as it had in 1986, following a wave of prison disturbances between 29 April and 2 May. In April 1990 there were new and compelling reasons to establish a full and open public inquiry which would be *manifestly* independent of the Home Office. The scale of the violence and devastation, together with the doubts raised about the managerial competence of senior Prison Department officials, undoubtedly influenced the decision. But arguably of crucial importance was the fact that the events at Strangeways had become so public that only a high-profile response on the part of ministers could hope to assuage public anxiety and restore the Government's credibility as an administration committed to law and order.

THE METHODS OF INQUIRY

The task given to Lord Justice Woolf was to examine what had happened during the six most serious riots which had occurred across a spectrum of different types of establishment: Strangeways, Cardiff and Bristol which are local prisons; Dartmoor, which is a Category B training prison; and Glen Parva and Pucklechurch where the disturbances took place in remand accommodation and involved young offenders under the age of 21. The Home Secretary had made clear that Lord Justice Woolf was free to interpret his terms of reference as he saw fit. Woolf's response was to adopt what he described as a 'broad canvas approach', addressing questions concerned not only with what happened during the course of the riots and how they were handled, but with their underlying causes and how disturbances of this kind might be prevented in the future. The 600-page Report of the Inquiry, published only nine months after the riots, was thus divided into two parts (Woolf 1991). In Part I Woolf concentrates on the circumstances of the riots, their management by the Prison Department and on proposing a number of technical and managerial strategies to improve security and control. In Part II he collaborates with Judge Stephen Tumim, Her Majesty's Chief Inspector of Prisons, to provide a wide-ranging review of prison conditions. There followed 12 key recommendations, and 204 supplementary proposals.

A key feature of the Inquiry was that it was not a *committee* of inquiry with joint or shared responsibility amongst an inquiry team, but a *judicial* inquiry for which Lord Justice Woolf was singly responsible and the sole signatory to the final report (together with Judge Tumim for Part II). Although Woolf was assisted by three assessors, each with specialist knowledge of the Prison Service, their role was essentially advisory. The way in which the Inquiry was conducted has been described in the Report (paras. 2.1–2.59) and elaborated and commented upon in papers written by two of the Assessors (Morgan 1991; Tuck 1991). All of these accounts make clear that, from the outset, efforts were made to establish a methodology which, 'to the greatest possible extent', would be open to the public, would promote wide consultation and participation and would facilitate fairness between parties. Six major strategies were employed to achieve these ends and arguably they combine to create an innovative approach to a public inquiry.

First, public hearings were held in London, Manchester and Taunton in Somerset, with the purpose of examining evidence pertaining to the six major disturbances. The public hearings assumed the appearance of formal tribunals, although the Inquiry had not been established under the Tribunals and Inquiries Act 1921 and, therefore, did not have powers to compel evidence or attach privilege to any evidence submitted, unless it had been specifically granted by the Attorney General. The parties to appear were representatives of the Home Office, the Prison Officers' Association (POA) and the Prison Governors' Association, all of whom were legally represented by senior counsel (instructed by solicitors). Inmates were also invited to give evidence but, at this point, a major structural inequality emerged. No request for legal representation had been made by any organisation on behalf of the prisoners and, as a result, the inmates who appeared at the hearings were advised only by the duty solicitor. Furthermore, no prisoner alleged to have played a major role in the Strangeways riots was invited to testify, although each had been interviewed by the assessors and the statements they made during the course of these interviews were apparently taken into account. The political content of this decision has been described by Rod Morgan in his account of the Inquiry's *modus operandi*, as reflecting the 'balance which has to be struck between procedural fairness and establishing broad public legitimacy for the Inquiry' (Morgan 1991, p. 720). It was justified by Lord Justice Woolf on the grounds that future criminal proceedings could be prejudiced; that the prisoners, rather than assist the Inquiry, might seize the opportunity for self-publicity, and that any examination, which because of the pending criminal proceedings would have to be in private, would be likely to be inconclusive.[2]

The second method adopted by the Inquiry may be seen as an attempt to increase the opportunities for prisoners' participation in the consultative process. Lord Justice Woolf wrote personally to every prisoner and member of staff believed to have been located in one of the six target prisons at the time of the disturbances, as well as a general letter to staff and prisoners in all other establishments, inviting them to contribute any comments they thought would be of use to the Inquiry. The Report notes that 'not all of these letters were delivered; and some of them arrived late' (para. 2.26). However, these efforts resulted in replies being received from just over 600 inmates and about 260 members of staff in the target establishments and from around 700 inmates and 170 staff located elsewhere in the system.

A third and rather more conventional strategy utilised by the Inquiry was to seek written submissions from organisations and individuals with particular knowledge or experience of prisons. Requests for evidence were sent out and personal networks of communication were activated by the Assessors who contacted researchers known to them in the field. This produced just over 170 written submissions, more than double the total received by the May Committee which had undertaken the last major inquiry into prisons (Morgan 1991, p. 721).

Reputedly the most innovative technique employed by Woolf was the holding of public seminars. These were conducted in London, jointly chaired by Lord Justice Woolf and Judge Tumim, and were designed to facilitate round-table discussions between invited experts on specific policy matters. Five seminars were organised, each one lasting for either a day, or a day and a half, the press and members of the public were free to attend and free to contribute when the debate was opened to the floor. One of the Assessors records that the Home Office had 'substantial misgivings' about the public nature of these seminars, fearing that the Prison Officers' Association would misappropriate the opportunity to air old industrial relations grievances, and believing that it would place civil servants in an invidious position if they were called upon 'to defend policies which were not their own but ministers' in a 'potentially hostile public arena' (Morgan 1991, p. 722). The latter objection appears to have been overcome by establishing an agreement that all participants would be speaking in a personal capacity unless they chose to do otherwise. Home Office anxieties about the POA hijacking the proceedings proved unfounded and Morgan reports that a considerable consensus emerged and genuine dialogue occurred. In total 145 people attended the seminars as participants or contributed to the discussions. Woolf records that he and Judge Tumim found the seminars valuable in helping to test out the strength of particular ideas and in enabling them to vary or discard provisional views.

The public seminars, however, like the public hearings, noticeably lacked the participation of prisoners. Woolf and Tumim decided that a direct 'opportunity should be provided to hear the contributions of prison inmates and prison service staff within the same format' (para. 2.55). Two half-day seminars were duly held in Lincoln Prison. One in the morning for the prisoners and one in the afternoon for the staff, who were joined by colleagues from neighbouring Stocken Prison.

Finally, Lord Justice Woolf and members of the inquiry team personally engaged in a programme of fieldwork, visiting prisons in the United Kingdom and in seven other countries. Woolf reports that he had visited a total of 43 prisons and had consulted inmates, prison staff at all levels, Boards of Visitors and representatives of the local POA. The three Assessors were also given specific tasks in accordance with their fields of expertise. These included organising a team of ex-prison governors to investigate the incidents which took place in the six target establishments; analysing the many hundreds of letters sent to the Inquiry from prisoners and prison officers; and interviewing prisoners who had been in the establishments when the disturbances had broken out.

THE WOOLF REPORT

Prison riots are not new phenomena, but the ways in which they have been defined and responded to in this country have undoubtedly changed over time. Robert Adams (1992) has argued that after the Second World War and up until the early 1970s, the Home Office tended to ignore or deny the existence of prison riots. The defensiveness and secrecy with which the prison authorities worked during this period enabled protests by prisoners to remain firmly out of public view. Lord Justice Woolf describes briefly the main disturbances which have occurred in English prisons since 1969 (paras. 9.7–9.18). In the late 1960s there was serious unrest in prisons in the United States and in Scandinavia, so serious that it featured in the British press. In 1972 there were extensive, collective demonstrations in English prisons. After a summer of 'sit-down protests', which were largely peaceful and in pursuit of specific improvements, there were violent disturbances at Albany and Gartree, both dispersal prisons. By this time the Prison Department had little alternative but to acknowledge openly that prisoner unrest was now a problem in English prisons too. Chapter 10 of its Annual Report for 1972 began:

> The potential of unrest is inherent in an organisation which has the complex aims of both containing and rehabilitating.
>
> (Home Office 1973, para. 147)

This seems to reflect the views of Gresham Sykes who described prison riots not as 'accidents' or 'an inexplicable, momentary flurry', but as an integral part of the nature of confinement – 'a logical step in a pattern of repeated social change' (1958, p.110). The Prison Department, however, went on to distinguish passive demonstrations, which involved large numbers of prisoners, from riots which were blamed on a 'minority of exceptionally difficult prisoners' (Home Office 1973, para. 153). Such statements effectively denied the relevance of systemic factors arising from the ways in which prisons are organised and prisoners treated. This perspective was bolstered by the fact that prisoner unrest was concentrated in the high-security, dispersal prisons, holding men serving long sentences for serious offences, including terrorism. The predominant strategies for dealing with prison riots were consequently focused upon punitive measures designed to control and suppress angry demonstrations by inmates. Control units were introduced to provide intentionally harsh and punitive regimes 'for the small hard core of really persistent and serious troublemakers who are reckoned to be capable of mending their ways' (quoted in Adams 1992, p. 154). After the major disturbance at Hull in 1976 military methods of riot control were introduced in 1978. Specially trained teams of prison officers known as MUFTI (minimum use of force – tactical intervention) squads were set up to intervene forcibly to quash protests by prisoners. The Prison

Department also devised methods to prevent disruptive situations occurring. A routine tactic has been to segregate and disperse disruptive inmates, or those suspected of being trouble-makers, by sudden transfers or 'ghostings' to other, usually local, prisons.

The 'rotten apple' theory became more difficult to sustain after the riots of 1986, because these disturbances occurred in more than 20 establishments and involved prisoners in low-security categories. Sir James Hennessy, the then Chief Inspector of Prisons, who had undertaken the official inquiry, described the events as 'the worst night of violence the English prison system has ever known' (Home Office 1987a, p. 101). Serious riots occurred again in June and July 1988 in Haverigg and Lindholme, both Category C establishments, where the official inquiry was undertaken by Mr Gordon Lakes, the then Deputy Director General of the Prison Service. Less than a year later a major disturbance broke out in Risley Remand Centre and was investigated by Mr Ian Dunbar, then a Regional Director. The report by Gordon Lakes was never made public. However, the report by Sir James Hennessy was published and a summary was produced from Ian Dunbar's report on Risley (1989). Both of these publications gave some consideration to the contribution which the prison system itself makes to the occurrence of riots. Inadequate regimes and strained relationships between inmates and staff were, for the first time, explicitly examined as contributory factors.

This shift of emphasis accords with what Adams (1992) has described as a typical liberal view of riots. Such a perspective, he claims, acknowledges the need for prisoners' grievances to be taken seriously and for reforms to be made, but takes for granted, or assumes the continuance of, 'the structures and principles' of imprisonment which form the broader context of the debates: 'responses at the inquiry stage tend to be framed in terms of how riots can be curbed or prevented in future, rather than examining discourse about the riots themselves, how they are understood and how imprisonment itself may be questioned' (p. 185). In consequence, Adams argues that liberal reports typically fail to take a sufficiently critical and independent stance and become trapped in administrative questions which result in only minor adjustments and revisions and which ultimately serve to reinforce existing penal policy.

The Woolf Report falls squarely within the liberal tradition of official reports in so far as it accepts the parameters of a continuing prison estate and excludes fundamental questions about the purpose or legitimacy of imprisonment. Although the methodology of the Inquiry was wide ranging and Woolf had avowed a 'broad-canvas approach', he excluded from his remit any review of sentencing decisions. It is evident too, throughout the Report, that he did not see his task as providing a blueprint for a 'new world order' in prisons, but aimed instead to find answers to specific policy questions relating to issues of order and control in prisons. In so doing he accepted the Prison Department's own statement of purpose and defined the aim of the Inquiry as being to build and continue the programme of change which had already been initiated by the Prison Department before the riots struck (paras. 1.6–1.7). The priority which Woolf attached to providing the Home Secretary with a response in the shortest possible time, 'consistent with fairness and thoroughness', also determined that the final portrait would be painted with a broad brush and that the Report would have to concentrate on erecting a series of signposts, indicating the direction in which penal policy should move, rather than a detailed operational plan. Woolf explains that the 12 key recommendations of his Report represent these signposts, and that the 204 accompanying proposals are 'the steps which, over a period of time, the Prison Service should take' in order to reach these destinations (para. 1.15). The 12 recommendations are as follows:

1. Closer cooperation between the different parts of the Criminal Justice System. For this purpose a national forum and local committees should be established;
2. More visible leadership of the Prison Service by a Director General who is and is seen to be the operational head and in day to day charge of the Service. To achieve this there should be a published 'compact' or 'contract' given by Ministers to the Director General of the Prison Service, who should be responsible for the performance of that 'contract' and publicly answerable for the day to day operations of the Prison Service;
3. Increased delegation of responsibility to Governors of establishments;
4. An enhanced role for prison officers;
5. A 'compact' or 'contract' for each prisoner setting out the prisoner's expectations and responsibilities in the prison in which he or she is held;
6. A national system of Accredited Standards, with which, in time, each prison establishment would be required to comply;
7. A new Prison Rule that no establishment should hold more prisoners than is provided for in its certified normal level of accommodation, with provisions for Parliament to be informed if exceptionally there is to be a material departure from that rule;
8. A public commitment from Ministers setting a timetable to provide access to sanitation for all inmates at the earliest practical date, not later than February 1996;
9. Better prospects for prisoners to maintain their links with families and the community through more visits and home leaves and through being located in community prisons as near to their homes as possible;
10. A division of prison establishments into small and more manageable and secure units;

11. A separate statement of purpose, separate conditions and generally a lower security categorisation for remand prisoners;
12. Improved standards of justice within prisons involving the giving of reasons to a prisoner for any decision which materially and adversely affects him; a grievance procedure and disciplinary proceedings which ensure that the Governor deals with most matters under his present powers; relieving Boards of Visitors of their adjudicatory role; and providing for final access to an independent Complaints Adjudicator.

(para. 15.5)

This agenda indicates a more radical approach to prisons policy than has hitherto been advanced in official reports. Three important examples illustrate the major departure which the Woolf Report has made. First, Woolf recognises that the balance of power in prisons has to be adjusted so that the authorities' demands for security and control do not impinge upon or violate a prisoner's access to justice. A central conclusion of the Report is that stability in prisons rests upon there being a proper balance between three elements of prison regimes: *security* arrangements, to prevent prisoners escaping; *control* measures, to prevent disruption and disorder within establishments; and procedures for *justice*, to ensure that all prisoners are treated with humanity and fairness. A recurrent theme in the evidence received from prisoners involved in the riots was that their actions represented a protest against the ways in which they were treated in prison. Woolf concludes that the failure of the Prison Service to convince prisoners that they were being treated fairly created serious difficulties for the maintenance of security and control. He emphasises the need to improve communication between prisoners and staff and for prisoners to be given a greater degree of responsibility for the conduct of their lives in prisons. However, the specific measures which are proposed to facilitate this shift of power may be less radical than the principle they espouse. Prisoners may have 'contracts', they may challenge an adjudication, or pursue a grievance to the independent Complaints Adjudicator and ultimately seek judicial review. However, unless sufficient judges and court time are made available, judicial delays can only compound injustice and foster unrest. Judge Tumim has recently pressed again for the 'sensible involvement of inmates in running their own lives' but has recognised the twin dangers of 'the abandonment of the initiative to prisoners, with particularly unhappy consequences for the weaker amongst them, or a return to the authoritarianism on the part of staff' (Home Office 1992c, para. 5.21). Inevitably the balance requires a negotiation between prisoners and prison staff. The literature on bargaining in prisons indicates that prisons 'work' because accommodations have to be reached between inmates and officers and that these are then preserved by the leaders on both sides to their mutual advantage (Reich 1972; Bottoms and Light 1987). Reich argues that prison managers may recognise the need for balance but seldom communicate to staff or inmates how the process of accommodation is to be achieved. He recommends that such bargaining should be formalised to ensure that the adverse circumstances referred to by Judge Tumim are avoided. Such a proposal would require governors to take an active role in the process of achieving a just stability in their establishments, working with staff and prisoners in an open process of negotiation. 'Contracts' would then have real meaning.

Second, Woolf marks a radical departure from earlier official reports by explicitly rejecting superficial or cosmetic changes which ignore the underlying causes of the problems. The Report states that its recommendations and proposals have to be seen as a package and not subjected to selective and piecemeal implementation:

> the full significance of each recommendation or proposal can only be appreciated if they are considered collectively. A number of the recommendations and proposals are dependent upon the implementation of others. In other words, the picture must be looked at as a whole.
>
> (para. 1.12)

Finally, the Woolf Report demonstrates some awareness of the broader social context within which prisons operate and is not solely preoccupied with the internal dynamics of the institutions. It recognises the need to take account of the role played by prisons within the criminal justice system and the relationships which exist between individual establishments and the outside communities in which they are situated.

THE APPRECIATIVE RECEPTION

The broad remit which Woolf defined and the openness with which he conducted the Inquiry, undoubtedly raised expectations that a substantial and radical report would be produced. To a considerable extent he confounded the sceptics and produced a document which met with approval across the political spectrum and was acclaimed by penal pressure groups as the most important examination of the prison system this century. The Government too confirmed its acceptance of Woolf's central propositions in the White Paper *Custody, Care and Justice* (Home Office 1991a). In the midst of the acclaim which followed the publication of the Report one could be forgiven for believing that there had been nothing written on prisons since the Gladstone Committee published its report in 1895 (Departmental Committee 1895).

The extravagance of the praise, however, is somewhat curious when account is taken of the fact that much of what Woolf had to say was neither new nor surprising. It is not as if the lamentable defects of the prison system had hitherto been a closely guarded secret which was now being exposed for the first time. The mutinous behaviour of prisoners in April 1990 can hardly be described as being wholly without precedent, given the pattern of regular spring- and summer-time disturbances which had erupted in the 1980s. Neither can it be claimed that, when taken individually, Woolf's conclusions represent wholly novel and radical ideas. Most of the signposts which Woolf has erected had appeared in various guises in official reports and criminological literature over the past twenty-five years. Arguably what was new was their synthesis into a unique package of reforms which Woolf insisted 'need to be considered together and moved forward together' (para. 1.168). It is, therefore, not simply the content of the Woolf Report but its timing and delivery which provide the key to understanding its level of public acclaim.

The Woolf Report was published virtually twenty-five years after the Mountbatten Report (Home Office 1966). The intervening quarter-century had been a maelstrom for prisoners, prison staff and administrators. The demise of the rehabilitative ethos at the beginning of this period had left the Prison Service without a clearly defined mission. The May Committee (Home Office 1979) argued for 'positive custody' but the Service seemed to settle for 'humane containment' and often failed to achieve even that. In consequence, the task of prison staff came to be seen, at best, as an exercise in damage-limitation, so little confidence was there in the value of imprisonment. This ideological crisis coincided with a period of considerable organisational strain, brought about by the relentless growth in the numbers of prisoners, the deterioration of prison buildings and an operational preoccupation with issues of security and dangerousness. Against this backdrop industrial relations within the Prison Service deteriorated and industrial action by prison officers came to dominate the agenda for those responsible for running the Prison Service. The old dilemmas about what to do with prisoners were unceremoniously overtaken by a new and compelling urgency to do something about staff. Woolf acknowledged at the outset that: 'The Prison Service had already started to tackle some of the worst features of the prison system. . . . Long term problems were, for the first time being confronted' (para. 1.6). Fresh Start provided a new deal for prison officers and governors. Faith in a new managerialism took hold: governor grades were reincarnated as prison 'managers', who worked to achieve 'corporate objectives', within a re-designed public service. Such changes brought problems as well as dividends, as Woolf concluded the paragraph above: 'However, as often happens at times of change, the improvements that were being introduced brought with them periods of increased instability which made the prison system particularly vulnerable to disturbances. The riots interrupted that process of improvements' (para. 1.6).

A fundamental truth unearthed by Woolf during the course of his Inquiry was that many of those involved in prisons shared a common perspective on what was wrong with the system. Priorities differed, as did the detailed proposals for reform, but, by painting with a broad brush, Woolf succeeded in highlighting the common ground and skirting around the cracks of division. However, agreeing on the signposts and the general route to be followed is considerably less controversial than agreeing on the particular methods of transport and the timing of the journey. In addressing potentially controversial questions about the objectives which prisons should pursue, Woolf does not delve into an examination of the competing theoretical justifications and purposes of imprisonment, but adopts what might be described as a more pragmatic approach. He accepts, as given, the principles set out in the Prison Service's Statement of Purpose:

> The Statement of Purpose recognises that the Prison Service has three tasks: (a) to keep secure those whom the courts put in their custody; (b) to treat those who are in their custody with humanity; and (c) to look after those in its custody in such a way as to help them to 'lead law abiding and useful lives' (i) while they are in custody and (ii) after release.
>
> (para. 10.11)

Woolf stresses, however, that these tasks must be construed within the context of the criminal justice system as a whole and maintains that there are certain consequences which flow from this for their interpretation and realisation. The first of these is that prisons should operate less introspectively and demonstrate an awareness of a common purpose shared with other members of the criminal justice system. Thus, a primary objective of the Prison Service should be to ensure that prisoners are treated with justice. Woolf argues that the condensed language of the Statement of Purpose does not place sufficient emphasis upon this obligation. The Report notes that although there is a requirement to treat prisoners with 'humanity', this is not necessarily synonymous with 'justice' and that the Prison Rules should be amended accordingly (para. 10.23). Woolf's definition of justice extends beyond issues of procedure and due process to encompass prison conditions: 'If the Prison Service contains that prisoner in conditions which are inhumane or degrading . . . then a punishment of imprisonment which was justly imposed, will result in injustice' (para. 10.19). Since the Woolf Report, the Government has agreed to the publication of the Report of the European Committee for the Prevention of Torture and Inhuman or Degrading Treatment or Punishment (Council of Europe 1991). This condemned conditions in three large local prisons in England as both inhuman and degrading. The Government's response pointed to improvements being made and rejected the Committee's judgements.

Woolf also insists that, as an integral component of the criminal justice system, the Prison Service has an obligation to discourage crime and reduce the likelihood of reoffending, especially by co-operating with the Probation Service in delivering effective throughcare. The Report, however, draws a distinction between the old discredited model of rehabilitative *treatment*, whereby the offender was sentenced to imprisonment *for* reformative treatment, and the new rehabilitative approach. This can be accommodated within the sentencing framework of 'just deserts' and is based not upon a concept of treatment, but on *providing opportunities* for prisoners to minimise the negative effects of custody and to prepare themselves for release without recourse to further offending. Hence, it is the promotion of individual responsibility and the prevention of 'a creeping and all pervading dependency by prisoners on the prison authorities' (para. 14.13), that imbues and characterises Woolf's conception of the rehabilitative task.

Finally, Woolf acknowledges that, as part of the criminal justice system, prisons must be seen to uphold law and order, and that a central task for the Prison Service in this respect is the maintenance of security within establishments. He emphasises, however, that 'attention paid to security should not be at the expense of the other aspects of the role of the Prison Service' (para. 10.39).

Working from the existing Statement of Purpose Woolf reaches a synthesis, namely 'a proper balance between security and control on the one hand and humanity and justice on the other' (para. 10.44). This synthesis of ideas, painted with a broad brush and at this particular juncture in history, is at the heart of Woolf's successful reception. First the Report gives hope, reinforcement and direction to those who aspire to the re-establishment of a rehabilitative purpose in prisons. Doubtless this tradition was never totally abandoned, although the disillusionment surrounding its unfulfilled expectations arguably drove its expression underground. Second, despite appeasing this particular sector of consumer interest, Woolf skilfully avoids alienating the potentially competing faction of the 'law and order' lobby. The task of looking after prisoners with humanity and helping them to lead law-abiding and useful lives is presented in the Report not as a wishy-washy act of do-gooding, but as an obligation on the part of the Prison Service to protect society by helping to reduce reoffending. The Report's proposals on how this should be accomplished also help to allay anxieties that Woolf is soft on offenders. The emphasis he and Tumim place upon enabling prisoners to be held responsible and accountable for what happens to them in prison is wholly consistent with the neo-libertarian ideology current within the Conservative Party. Indeed the then Home Secretary, Kenneth Baker, speaking at the publication of *Custody, Care and Justice*, announced that the White Paper was entirely consistent with the principles and proposals set out in the Citizen's Charter.

Finally, the third constituency with which Woolf establishes a rapport may be described as the 'justice' lobby. By emphasising the need to redress the existing imbalance between security, control and justice, Woolf deliberately raises the profile of justice in prisons and enhances its status as a critical objective which the Prison Service must achieve in order to ameliorate the existing crisis. In so doing he advocates the other side of the libertarian coin which specifies the duties and obligations which the state owes to the citizen, or in this case, the prison authorities owe to the individual prisoner.

PRISONS AFTER WOOLF

The essays in this volume critically review the contribution which the Woolf Report makes to specific areas of prison policy. It has been divided into three parts. In Part I consideration is given to the practical and theoretical issues which have to be addressed if Woolf's vision of a 'proper balance' between security, control and justice is to be realised. In Chapter 1 Joe Sim provides a critical overview of the Woolf Report. He traces the history of prison disturbances in the UK since the mid-1960s and explicitly examines the extent to which there is a match, or correlation, between what he perceives to be the underlying crises in prisons and Woolf's proposals for change. He emphasises that the failure of Woolf to take adequate account of the unequal power relations between the prison and the confined and his disregard of the structural relationship between the prisons, the state and wider processes of discipline, regulation and control, lead to a myopic vision which diverts attention from a fundamental restructuring of prisons and the wider criminal justice process.

In Chapter 2 Roy King reviews the prospects of balancing the potentially competing demands of good order and humane regimes, by reflecting upon the similarities and differences in the recent history of the Scottish and English systems. He identifies the philosophical differences in the major reports that have followed crises in each country and how these have been translated into material variations in regimes. He emphasises that the success of policy initiatives will ultimately hinge upon whether prisoners, particularly the long-termers in high-security establishments, see, accept and trust the new order that arises from the present rhetoric.

The relationship between prisoner unrest and the prison environment is further developed in Chapter 3 by Silvia Casale who reflects upon the part which prison conditions can play in fomenting disorder. She emphasises that although poor conditions can degrade both prisoners and staff and erode co-operative relations, they are not the sole explanation of why inmates riot. They can, however, in collaboration with the deterioration of regimes, contribute to the breakdown of relations between inmates and the prison authorities. Lord Justice Woolf recognised that a high priority had to be given to improving prison conditions which, as Silvia Casale observes, are not simply comprised of the material state of the buildings but are 'the product of the physical environment . . . and the uses made of that environment'. Woolf's recommendations to provide access to sanitation, to restrict overcrowding and to develop national Accredited Standards are all broadly welcomed. However, Casale points out that certain impediments stand in the way of their realisation and she proposes specific mechanisms to overcome or limit these difficulties. She draws attention, for example, to 'the political resistance to legally enforceable standards' and the need for a system of independent enforcement, if 'compacts' between individual prisoners and their establishments are to have any real meaning.

The absence of a Bill of Rights and the reluctance of English judges to involve themselves in what they consider to be political and administrative decisions, have been seen as fundamental stumbling blocks to the improvement of prison conditions. Norval Morris, for example has observed:

> The problem of course, is that you don't have a Bill of Rights by which the law can find leverage. Under the European Human Rights Conventions you get very close to it and that's of course the reason why you are the most frequent failed defendant in that Court. Your standards aren't worse. The reason is of course that English judges are never answerable for prison conditions. They ought to be.
>
> (1990, p. 29)

Morris echoes the sentiments of the European Prison Rules (EPR) (which are persuasive rather than authoritative), especially EPR5:

> The protection of the individual rights of prisoners with special regard to the legality of the execution of detention measures shall be secured by means of a control carried out, according to national rules, by a judicial authority or other duly constituted body authorised to visit the prisoners and not belonging to the prison administration.

The appointment of a judge as Her Majesty's Chief Inspector of Prisons does not meet this requirement because he deals with no individual cases, but is confined to the inspection of entire establishments, inquiries and specific thematic reviews.

Access to justice, emphasised by Woolf as a critical element of a stable and safe prison environment, is directly explored in Chapters 4 and 5. Genevra Richardson addresses the question of what civil rights prisoners retain and what additional rights it is legitimate for them to claim because of their incarceration. She describes the existing legal position, examining decisions of the English courts in public and private law cases, together with the growing body of decisions from the European Court of Human Rights (ECHR), and concludes that although in some respects the legal status of prisoners has been strengthened over the last twenty years, enormous gaps remain. The absence of a Bill of Rights and the failure of primary legislation to provide prisoners with any enforceable rights have ensured the persistence of wide areas of administrative discretion and a continued lack of effective and readily accessible means for the expression and redress of grievances. The chapter considers whether the domestic courts, aided by the ECHR, can realistically be expected to intervene further or whether the preferred way forward lies with strengthened extra-judicial supervision. The importance Lord Justice Woolf attached to the involvement of prisoners in decision-making is welcomed, as is his endorsement of an effective, independent review mechanism which, Richardson believes, could greatly facilitate the provision of real accountability and even justice in prisons. Woolf's avoidance of the term 'rights' and his promotion of the concept of 'legitimate expectations' is, however, considered with some caution. Richardson concludes that 'the shift from rights to expectations can be seen as a valuable initiative building on recent developments in public law', but she points out that if 'legitimate expectations' are to have any real meaning, and are to offer any real protection to prisoners, then the notorious flexibility of the concept must be restricted and the nature of the expectations specified with some precision.

Access to justice in prisons is arguably most accentuated in the handling of prison disciplinary hearings. It is in relation to adjudications in prisons that the courts have intervened most readily. Stephen Livingstone in Chapter 5 chronicles the steps taken since the Hull Riot in 1976 to meet the requirements of natural justice. English and Irish cases have been taken to the House of Lords and the judgments of the European Court of Human Rights have been applied. Woolf's proposals and the White Paper's response are assessed in the light of this recent legal history. Already Boards of Visitors have relinquished their adjudicatory role and serious cases are to be referred to the Crown Prosecution Service with a view to criminal proceedings. The impact these changes will have upon the decision-making processes and the administration of justice in prisons raises important empirical questions for future research. Livingstone, however, introduces a note of caution by reminding the reader of the limitations of law in regulating the disciplinary power of prison authorities.

The Woolf Report emphasised how the process of judicial review would be the ultimate safeguard, not only in disciplinary proceedings but in all prison matters:

> We recommend that Prison Rules should make provision for establishments to offer a 'contract' to each prisoner in its care. The 'contract' would not be drawn up in a way which would give the prisoner private rights (that is a right to damages) but it would, in a case which was appropriate, be dealt with by the grievance procedure and it could provide a platform for an application for judicial review.
> (para. 12.123)

Woolf, however, recognised that access to the courts should not dominate the running of prisons, rather it should underpin working practices which promote an awareness of justice at all levels. The Inquiry elaborated the significance of inmate–staff relations as a causal factor in the riots. One prisoner from Strangeways recorded in an affidavit:

> The disturbance was intended as a protest not so much against prison conditions in terms of overcrowding, lack of privacy, 'slopping-out', lack of exercise and so on but more a protest against the oppressive regime conducted within the prison by prison officers. The oppression consisted of abuse by the officers of their powers and violence from the officers to inmates together with a complete failure by senior prison officers to fairly conduct the laid down grievance procedures.
>
> (para. 3.81)

The Report notes that another inmate,

> a former policeman, said that prison officers had their own system of control which was nothing to do with Home Office guidelines. There was no redress against prison officers and in his view the situation was so serious that those outside the prison had to be involved. He pointed out that, although only a very small minority of prison officers were bullies who verbally abused and degraded people, it was difficult to go to a prison officer to complain about another prison officer.
>
> (para. 3.79)

Although the management at Strangeways was praised by Woolf for its leadership and 'impetus in the right direction' it appears that not all staff shared the enthusiasm for an enhanced regime:

> I have little doubt that while the majority of officers' attitudes could not be described as other than correct and some officers were sympathetic in their attitude, a small minority of officers were still by their actions creating a divide between staff and prisoners and spoiling the good work of the majority. They created the impression among prisoners, whether justified or not, that staff could behave oppressively.
>
> (para. 3.89)

In Part II of the Woolf Report an entire chapter is devoted to issues directly concerning prison staff. It reviews the implementation of Fresh Start, the Prison Department's recent staffing policy, and notes the disappointment of many staff who claimed to have witnessed no enhancement of regimes and no increase in job satisfaction. Prior to the riot officers at Strangeways, like their colleagues elsewhere, would have been negotiating new working arrangements for a reduction of their average weekly hours from 45 to 43, to take effect from Sunday, 1 April 1990. Such negotiations were destined to raise anxieties since, at best, only half the reduction of hours was to be made up by extra staff. This could only exacerbate staff feelings about shortages and their ability to manage and control prisoners. It is possible that prisoners sensed such anxieties; some might have perceived this as a weakness and therefore an opportunity for a disturbance, whilst others might have had a diminished confidence in the staff's ability to contain disorder. 'A minority suggested that some prison officers wanted a riot and encouraged inmates to riot in order to justify their dispute with management on staffing levels' (para. 3.78).

In Chapter 6 J. E. Thomas explores the conception and evolution of Fresh Start and reflects upon the consequences this has had for the management of establishments. He considers the issues of recruitment, management and supervision of prison staff as important foundations for the implementation of Woolf.

Examples of arbitrary and oppressive behaviour by prison officers were predominant in complaints about the maltreatment of prisoners. Such complaints, however, were not restricted to uniformed staff or to prison governors. At Strangeways, for example, it was alleged that one prisoner in the punishment cells had been forcibly injected with drugs for control purposes, although the Inquiry was unable to establish the truth of this matter. However, the Report notes that when giving evidence one medical officer of the prison

> quite inappropriately suggested that drugs could be used for controlling prisoners when they were no more than a nuisance. It is possible therefore that the control of the administration of drugs was not as strict as it should have been.
>
> (para. 3.87)

Further evidence from Strangeways also indicated that 'there existed among prisoners a suspicion that largactyl was being used too frequently "down the block" for control reasons rather than medical reasons' (para. 12.132). Irregular use was categorically denied by the doctors responsible for medical treatment at Manchester. The Report does not imply or infer that dissatisfaction with health care was a critical factor in triggering the Prison disturbances in April 1990. However, it does recognise that medical treatment is a significant cause of prisoner anxiety and unrest and, whilst unable to make findings as to individual complaints, confirms the failure of the Prison Medical Service to uphold, as a matter of principle, National Health standards of treatment. Woolf recommends assiduous care in following regulations and in communicating professionally 'the medical reasons and the necessity for any treatment given' (para. 12.133).

In Chapter 7 Roger Ralli describes the evolution of prisoner health care, charting landmark developments in the Prison Medical Service over the last thirty years. It now appears that National Health Service standards in prisons are to be promoted by the Prison Health Service becoming a purchaser, rather than a provider, of health care. Roger Ralli explores the implications of this and the ethical dilemmas faced by doctors working in the prison environment. Writing from the perspective of someone working within the Prison Health Service, he specifically examines the provision of care for two categories of prisoner given special attention by Woolf – drug users and prisoners who are HIV positive – and describes what the Prison Health Service has achieved in respect of both since the Woolf Report was published.

In Part II of this book consideration is given to the likely impact of the Woolf Report upon five special groups of prisoners – the unconvicted, long-termers, the mentally disordered, vulnerable prisoners and women prisoners.

Rod Morgan writes after a long involvement with the problems of the unconvicted (King and Morgan 1976) and with the special knowledge of being one of Lord Justice Woolf's Assessors. He notes that official attention has been largely focused on sentenced prisoners because of the historical commitment to their 'treatment and training', from which the unconvicted are exempt, and because the unconvicted have seldom been involved in serious unrest. However, periods of remand, which were at one time very short, have been extended significantly as cases have taken longer to process through the courts. Morgan points to the increasing proportions of unconvicted men in the prison population as a whole and their concentration in local prisons where overcrowding and conditions are typically at their worst. He welcomes the reductionist position taken by the Woolf Report but identifies fundamental difficulties in achieving 'a minimum resort to custody for the untried' and in improving conditions for those who are refused bail. He illustrates how competing aims create awkward dilemmas for penal practice. For example, the aim of keeping untried prisoners apart from the sentenced population, under a specific set of rules which acknowledge their legal status, is difficult to reconcile with the concept of community prisons. Morgan also supports Woolf's proposals to reduce the security category of remand prisoners, from Category B to Category C, unless there is evidence that they pose a greater risk. This is an issue which was previously addressed by Ashmore, Creamer, Evans, MacLean and Readman (1988) who concluded that it was not a viable proposition because many prisoners are remanded on specimen charges and many others on higher tariff charges which are scaled down at trial. However, if prisoners are to be redistributed within community prisons the recategorisation of remand prisoners may be an inevitable consequence. Rod Morgan provides clear principles which should guide government policy in relation to the untried and which could be applied by the area criminal justice committees in their discussions about pre-trial arrangements.

In Chapter 9 Keith Bottomley focuses on long-term prisoners (including lifers). He points to the increasing proportion of long-termers within the prison population and anticipates their numbers growing following the implementation of the Criminal Justice Act 1991. Bottomley considers the 'causes for concern' since the Mountbatten Inquiry (Home Office 1966), in particular the predominance of security and control and the consequent effects on policy. Since the report of the Control Review Committee (Home Office 1984), for example, more attention has been given to the development of small units for disruptive prisoners, than to the more positive proposals to improve regimes for the generality of long-termers. The lodging in Strangeways (and other large local prisons) of long-term prisoners who were disruptive in training prisons is a direct consequence of control policies and has been identified as a major contributory factor to the riot of 1 April. Keith Bottomley examines specific problems experienced by prisoners serving long sentences and reviews Lord Justice Woolf's recommendations and proposals which affect the balance of security, control and justice for this important group. He comments especially upon the development of sentence plans, the creation of contracts between inmates and their establishments and the promotion of community prisons, all of which should reduce uncertainty for prisoners and so contribute to greater security. The chapter also considers the present strategies to cope with the 'hard core' minority of disruptive prisoners, most notably the Special Units, transfers to local prisons under Circular Instruction 37/1990 and segregation under Rule 43. How soon long-term prisoners will benefit from the improved regimes outlined by Woolf, and generally supported by the Government, is an open question. It is already eight years since the Control Review Committee put forward the proposals which are now endorsed by Woolf. The opening of 'New Generation' prisons could help to realise Woolf's ambitions for long-termers, by providing smaller units and better regimes. So far, however, only one has opened (Woodhill at Milton Keynes) and only one more is planned (at Doncaster); it remains to be seen, therefore, whether long-termers will benefit from them.

Adrian Grounds discusses the continuing presence of the mentally disordered within the prison population in the light of the Woolf Report, the recommendations made by the Reed Committee (Department of Health/Home Office 1991b, 1992c) and recently published research. He concludes, as does Reed, that the failure to divert mentally disordered offenders to NHS psychiatric services is not due to a lack of legal avenues for transfer, but to a lack of available resources, most notably the inadequate number of places in regional secure units (RSUs). The prospects for reducing the numbers of mentally disordered people in prison hinges critically upon the extent to which forensic psychiatry services 'survive and develop' within the reformed structure of the NHS. Adrian Grounds views the area criminal justice committees as having a significant role to play in influencing health authority purchasers and advocates that health and social services should be represented on the Area Committees. Effective liaison and planning are seen as vital, not only to facilitate and encourage diversion from prison, but to ensure that care in the community is able to contribute to the resettlement of those mentally disordered offenders who remain within the prison system. The degree of political commitment to these objectives is open to question. The White Paper *Custody, Care and Justice* supports a reduction in the use of imprisonment but does not respond to Woolf's proposal that the Prison Department should recognise a special responsibility for those mentally disordered offenders who remain in custody. Ministers' reactions to Reed's *Final Summary Report* (Department of Health/Home Office 1992c) give no timetable for implementation, although some funds have been committed for more RSU places.

The Prison Department's responsibility for vulnerable prisoners is discussed by Adam Sampson who considers the future for sex offenders in prison. He sets out clearly the current conflict which exists for prison managers between protecting sex offenders from attack and providing them with an active regime. He supports, as a first step, Woolf's proposal to establish a new Prison Rule which would distinguish those prisoners separated for their own protection from those segregated in the interests of good order and discipline. Sampson recognises, however, that there are numerous obstacles to be overcome in establishing normal regimes for sex offenders. The development of sex-offender treatment programmes in prisons, identified by Woolf as requiring 'more attention', is critically examined in this chapter. The Prison Department's initiative, and the optimistic predictions of success in reducing the rates of recidivism, are assessed in relation to a series of practical problems which define the context in which such programmes are to run. Sampson warns that unless fundamental weaknesses are addressed the benevolent efforts to provide treatment could leave sex offenders in a worse position than before the Woolf Report.

Similarly there are unresolved difficulties in respect of women prisoners, who were excluded from the Inquiry. Such disregard is entirely consistent with earlier reports and inquiries and has given rise to the claim that penal policy for women has largely evolved by adapting policy initiatives created for the male majority. In Chapter 12 Elaine Player considers how Woolf's proposed reforms, which were designed to resolve the underlying problems of disorder in male establishments, affect women's prisons. Differences in the size and composition of the male and female prison populations present fundamental dilemmas for the establishment of community prisons for women and for the promotion of distinct regimes for women on remand. Elaine Player argues that, if the principles underlying Woolf are to be realised in female establishments, fundamental questions about equal treatment and equal opportunities must be resolved. The resolution of these questions would, she suggests, prompt substantial changes in the women's system which would differ, both in nature and extent, from those envisaged in the male system. They should, she argues, be subject to a separate policy review.

The contributors to Part III shift the focus away from the internal problems of prisons to the relationships between prisons and the community. Woolf has stressed, however, that virtually all prisoners will eventually be released from custody and that their ability to resettle successfully without further offending will be significantly affected by the opportunities they have had to maintain family ties and develop relationships with agencies in their home communities. The National Prison Survey (see Walmsley, Howard and White 1992), conducted in 1991, revealed that the average distance travelled by a visitor was 62 miles (p. 44). Prisoners' suggestions for improvements confirmed the importance they attached to their visits: longer and more frequent visits; conjugal visits; and being in prisons near family and friends, were widely advocated (p. 35).

The Woolf Report is critical of the insularity of prisons, in relation to their detachment from other parts of the criminal justice system, their isolation from the wider community and their distance from most prisoners' homes. In Chapter 13 Jenny Roberts provides a valuable reminder that 'the community' is not a single entity and that 'the relationship between prisons and the communities they serve is at least ambivalent'. The isolationism of the Prison Service is often matched in the wishes of the general public who have no desire whatsoever to reduce the separation and stigmatisation of prisoners. Jenny Roberts reviews the major recommendations made by Lord Justice Woolf to improve the relationship between prisons and the community. She describes and endorses the advantages of community prisons but is sceptical about the prospects for their realisation. The changes proposed in the White Paper 'seem somewhat marginal' to a community-based approach and, in consequence, 'we must . . . assume only a limited commitment to community prisons and a continuing preference for managing the prison estate as a whole, giving consideration of security, discipline and economy precedence over community links'.

In remote prisons the immediate prison world, and its largely delinquent subculture, assume great importance. When prisoners are nearer home, however, their primary connection is more likely to be in the community since telephone contact is cheaper and visits can be afforded more often. Woolf recommended community prisons so that prisoners would normally be held close to home and this principle appears to have been endorsed in the White Paper.

> Location near home is likely to lead to greater stability and will enable programmes to be linked more closely to the opportunities available to the prisoner after release.
>
> (para. 5.13)

However, it is a principle which immediately yielded precedence to the emptying of police cells and the reduction of overcrowding. Jenny

Roberts's doubts thus seem to be well founded. If the more recent reduction in the prison population (following the implementation of the 1991 Criminal Justice Act) is to persist, the Prison Department could be encouraged to adopt proximity for the largest possible number of prisoners. It could also demonstrate its commitment to assisting prisoners to 'lead law-abiding and useful lives in custody and after release' by setting targets for a regular reduction in the distance travelled by visitors. More generally, it could take the opportunity to revise its thinking on allocation.

Woolf's insistence upon greater consultation between prisons and community agencies is also applauded by Jenny Roberts, although she points to an important distinction between the consultative structures, designed to facilitate shared responsibility for the resettlement of offenders, and the Criminal Justice Consultative Council and area committees, which are concerned with the criminal justice process and, in particular, the relationship between prisons and the courts. The setting up of the national and local groups is seen by Roberts as entirely consistent with Woolf's view that the ultimate aim of all the criminal justice agencies should be the reduction of crime. Thus, although there is a distinction between the criminal justice fora and the local consultative structures which promote resettlement, the various bodies may be seen as complementary if the former ensure that prisons contain only 'the irreducible minimum of offenders'. Again, however, the realisation of this symbiotic relationship appears to Roberts to be some distance away. Although the White Paper gives a commitment to establish the Criminal Justice Consultative Council and the area committees, Woolf's original proposals have been substantially altered and the coordination of services has been painfully slow.

In Chapter 14 Vivien Stern suggests a number of practical ways in which the voluntary sector, or non-governmental organisations (NGOs), could assist in both the consultative process and in the provision of services. Voluntary organisations tend to be pressure groups as well as providers of services and it is argued that their experience in these areas could help to forge the links which Jenny Roberts has identified as missing in the communication between prisons and criminal justice agencies, community bodies and government departments. According to Vivien Stern the campaigning experience of voluntary organisations could help to prevent the implementation of Woolf becoming 'buried in the press of day to day events in a traditionally crisis-prone service'. In addition, the standard methods of working adopted by the voluntary sector may be of value in helping to develop and reinforce widespread consultation and openness of communication within an organisation more used to closed systems of decision-making and policy development. Vivien Stern points to the track record of non-governmental organisations in helping to bring about major changes in dealing with juvenile offenders, in setting up successful employment and housing projects (which provide valuable links between the prisons and the community) and in the promotion and protection of human rights for prisoners and other vulnerable social groups. This wealth of experience and expertise is described as a critical resource which should be harnessed and used to secure the changes recommended by Lord Justice Woolf. Stern emphasises, however, that the task of NGOs must extend beyond this watchdog role in order to promote widespread change throughout the Criminal Justice System. From this perspective the Woolf Report should be seen as the beginning rather than the end of the reforming process.

COMMENT

The obvious and inescapable irony is that it took a major riot to generate the full and independent inquiry that academic commentators, pressure groups and politicians had been urging for many years. More than a decade ago several contributors to this volume wrote:

> There had been no searching appraisal of them [prisons] since the work of the Gladstone Committee of 1895. The Royal Commission of 1964–6 which might have illuminated 'the course ahead for a generation' had been disbanded in disarray and events had moved on dramatically since then. Rupert Cross had concluded his delightful Hamlyn Lectures as long ago as 1971 with the message that 'no matter what the source may be (Advisory Council, Departmental Committee, Inter-Departmental Committee or Royal Commission) we want another Gladstone Report'.
>
> (King and Morgan 1980, p. 8)

The authors sought debate, policy formation and action: 'But it had better be quick if the 1980s are not to be very much worse than the 1970s. Attica and Santa Fe could happen here.' (p. 8.)

> Ominously, particularly at Long Lartin and Hull, but also at other establishments, prisoners declared that real change only followed prisoner disorder as had occurred at Strangeways.
>
> (Home Office 1992c, para. 3.139)

It would be unfortunate if the Woolf Report and its implementation were to be viewed as a reward for disorder, yet this may be the cost of having failed to heed the earlier calls for another Gladstone Report. The next danger may be that the pursuit of justice is overtaken by the perceived prerequisite of greater security. In this respect the Prison Inspectorate's report on an unannounced visit to Strangeways is not encouraging:

> The overwhelming physical security arrangements appeared to the Inspectors as oppressive and inimical to a constructive regime. We

> believe that there are many points in the report which if acted on now can save trouble in the future.
>
> (Home Office 1992d, p. 1)

It seems that attention still has to be paid to the dilemma that 'the more control authority imposes, the more control it will need to maintain its grip; imposed control for its own exclusive purpose is self defeating' (Perrie 1981, p. 11).

It appears that during the process of refurbishment at Manchester an opportunity to create small units was passed up in favour of increased security at the end of each landing and in the roofs. Woolf has provided both the philosophy and the opportunity for necessary major change, yet it would seem that the 'biggest problem is actually influencing people, getting people to identify with the philosophy and actually to implement it on a day to day basis' (Rutherford, 1993). What Rutherford's quoted senior police officer was saying about his sergeants and constables can equally be applied to members of the Prison Service – at all levels.

When the Woolf Report and the White Paper *Custody, Care and Justice* were published, the then Home Secretary, Kenneth Baker, predicted a timescale of 25 years for total implementation. It seems to us, however, that there must be clear and immediate evidence for prisoners, staff and administrators that the ship has been turned. What signs are there that this has happened?

A year after the Woolf Report was published the Prison Reform Trust issued a questionnaire to all governors of prisons to discover whether a series of Woolf's proposals, which had no major resource implications, had been put into practice. They concluded that, 'the overall impression is one of strong commitment to the Woolf programme' (Prison Reform Trust 1992b, p. 21). However, running through the majority of responses, they detected a number of impediments to the process of reform. These 'darker undercurrents' related to serious limitations of resources, frustration on the part of governors over their lack of autonomy and an enduring lack of confidence by governors in their relationship with Prison Service Headquarters:

> Much more could (and should) be done, but not without increased resources – particularly staffing. When the final two hours of staff contract time under Fresh Start are lost in April 1992, we may have to consider (reluctantly) reducing our regime delivery.
>
> (p. 24)

> Most of the positive responses in the questionnaire refer to arrangements already in place prior to Woolf. Further resources must be made available before significant further improvements are possible.
>
> (p. 24)

> Food for prisoners remains a real issue . . . I believe the ration scale is

far too small and far too restrictive . . . Purchasing from prison farms guarantees mediocre quality. I do not blame the caterers entirely, but I would welcome contracting out food supply and preparation.

(p. 23)

I need more *disposable* finances at local level. I need more delegated personnel authority.

(p. 25)

No-one sees any response from Prison Service HQ and that is a source of alarm. There are words of approval about Woolf but no action. Dashed and frustrated expectations could lead to trouble.

(p. 23)

The managerial effectiveness of the Prison Service has been reviewed recently by Admiral Sir Raymond Lygo (Home Office 1991o), who recommended turning the Prison Service into an Executive Agency. This and a number of other recommendations have been accepted by the Home Secretary and have been included in the changes required by the move to Agency status on 1 April 1993. This has meant that although ministers remain ultimately accountable to Parliament for the Prison Service's operations, they are less involved in the day-to-day running of the Service. This falls to a newly appointed Chief Executive who is responsible for advising ministers on policy matters and who has a considerably larger degree of managerial freedom than his predecessor, the Director General. Governors, too, have greater authority and responsibility delegated to them to facilitate the efficient running of their establishments. A system of contracts effectively specifies operational objectives and responsibilities at every layer in the hierarchy and the performance of staff is to be judged in relation to the fulfilment of their contractual duties.

The significance of these structural changes for the development and implementation of the Woolf Report was not lost on the governors who responded to the Prison Reform Trust questionnaire:

Perhaps rather than looking to Woolf we should first look to the later report by Admiral Lygo. It seems to me to be an essential first step towards getting the Prison Service away from being a political pawn and may in the end prove more beneficial to the cause of humanity for prisoners than all the preceding reports together.

(Prison Reform Trust 1992b, p. 25)

The Government has emphasised that Agency status is not a step on the road to privatisation and has made clear that the Prison Service will remain a part of the Home Office and that its staff will continue to be civil servants. However, the Government is simultaneously encouraging increased involvement of the private sector in supplying specific services, such as education and catering, and in managing both new and existing prisons – a rumoured 50 per cent of the prison estate is destined to be 'market tested'. In effect an internal market has been created whereby competition will be encouraged within the Agency itself and between the Agency and privately run (contracted-out) establishments. Whether this will speed the delivery of Woolf or divert attention from its agenda is a critical question. One obvious danger is that, as ministers distance themselves from the operational concerns of the new Prison Agency debates about resources will be increasingly defined in terms of internal good husbandry and relegated from the political agenda.

In February 1993 the Prisons Board issued its paper *Vision and Values* (Prison Department 1993), which includes an unrevised Statement of Purpose and explicates a series of 'values' which should be adhered to by prison staff in achieving six 'principal goals'. This 'vision' of the future incorporates a clearly stated commitment to giving prisoners reasons for decisions and, 'where possible', involving inmates in discussions about matters which affect them. However, an important opportunity has been missed to re-emphasise the weight of *justice* in striking a proper balance with *security* and *control*. The word 'justice' appears only once in the entire document, under the heading of 'Values', where it is asserted that providing 'care' for prisoners requires staff to treat them with 'fairness, justice and respect as individuals'. The list of 'principal goals', however, whilst specifically identifying the maintenance of 'order, control and discipline', omits any explicit reference to 'justice'.

One consequence of imposing a market economy on the prison system is that prisoners are being formally acknowledged as 'customers', along with the general public. They figure as a special group in the Citizen's Charter, even though sentenced prisoners still forfeit the right to vote. This change of status will need to be carefully protected if it is to have real meaning. In line with the National Health Service the Prison Service is destined to engage in more formal contracts for service. It will be important for stability and justice to ensure not just the efficiency but also the quality of service – a variable conspicuously omitted in a recent survey of the gains to be expected as a result of shifts from the public sector to the private sector (Parker 1992).

Prisons have been likened to bombs; secure containers with an explosive mixture inside. That may be an extreme simplification but it embodies the starting point of the Woolf Inquiry. The ensuing Report advocates changes that will remove many of the precipitating factors of riots, damp some of the flashpoints and reduce opportunities for disorder through better procedures for control and security. The identification of 'justice' as a primary element of the new ethos and the stress upon prisons being an integral component of the criminal justice system are important steps forward. Woolf's recommendations and proposals were painted with a broad brush, establishing general principles and leaving much of the finer detail for future development. The Government's response in the White Paper *Custody, Care and Justice* has largely followed in this tradition and offers little fine tuning. In this context, however, such an approach creates vagueness and uncertainty. The contributors to this volume have examined carefully the content, potential and likely impact of the proposals and the Government's response. They have thus elaborated detailed policies for realising Woolf's potential and for establishing justice alongside control and security to the benefit of prisoners, prison staff and the general public.

Towards the end of Part I of his report Lord Justice Woolf wrote: 'A riot should be a rare and unusual event' (para. 9.58). We would add to that Judge Tumim's more recent comment: 'Hope lies in the development of balanced and integrated regimes with the sensible involvement of inmates in running their own lives, which includes addressing the reasons that brought them into prison' (Home Office 1992c, para. 5.21). The fact of imprisonment inevitably, and intentionally, serves to depress prisoners. Once their sentence has begun, however, their opportunities for change and recovery are compromised while hope and stimulus are absent. Equally there is much in prison to cause anger and such energy needs to be diverted into positive action, aimed at preparing prisoners for release. That is less likely where justice and stability are weak. The agenda before the Prison Service requires political commitment and an undertaking from the most senior managers of the Service through to the landings of individual establishments. It must also engage the rest of the criminal justice system as well as prisoners and their families. The Woolf Report has created a legitimate expectation of major change.

NOTES

1 Hansard, 2 April 1990, Col 893.

2 Lord Justice Woolf's statement is recorded in the transcript of the Inquiry at Manchester on Tuesday, 26 June 1990, pp. 1–3.

Part I

CONTROL AND PRISON CONDITIONS

1

REFORMING THE PENAL WASTELAND?

A critical review of the Woolf Report

Joe Sim

> . . . it is clearly of great value to the cause of 'stability', compliance and conservatism in general, that as powerful an institution as the judiciary, so solidly embedded in the structure of power constituted by the state, should be thought to be altogether removed from the struggles proceeding in society, and should be held to be free from the ideological commitments which beset mere 'politicians' and other people. It is this presumption which has made High Court judges such useful chairmen and members of royal commissions, departmental committees, and particularly committees of inquiry into 'delicate' matters concerning the conduct of agents of the state, in cases where police violence, the killing of civilians by soldiers, etc., have occurred. The record shows that the state can, at the least, expect that the reports which are produced will say all that can possibly be said in favour of its agents. There may be no deliberate intention to 'whitewash'; but wrong-doing by the agents of the state is made to assume a very blurred and uncertain character. The insistence on the political independence of the judiciary has a powerful legitimating resonance; and it is all the more powerful because judges, however traditionally-minded they may be, do not always act as allies of the government and the state, even in cases which involve 'security'; and because no defendant, however antipathetic to the court, need take it for granted that his cause is lost in advance because of judicial animus. This is no small matter either. All the same, the bias remains, and constitutes an important bulwark in the defence of the status quo.
>
> (Miliband 1982, p. 121)

Lord Justice Woolf's Report on the Strangeways disturbance received the same uncritical acclaim as Lord Scarman's inquiry into the disorder in Brixton published a decade earlier. Across the sociological and political spectrum, as well as in the media, Woolf's analysis and his policy prescriptions for the future based on the triumvirate of security, control and justice were endorsed by many as the political and philosophical panacea for alleviating the deep and destructive problems confronting the prison system in the UK. Mary Tuck, one of Woolf's assessors, described the Report as a 'massive, thoughtful and practical prescription for the reform of the prison system . . . [it was] received with acclaim and consensus . . . [it] was so penetrating, profound and went to the heart of the problems of the Criminal Justice System' (1991, pp. 1–5). Barry Sheerman, the Home Affairs spokesperson for the Labour Party argued that the Report 'provides a unique opportunity for reform of our penal system. There has been an unparalleled degree of support for the proposals amongst all those concerned with prisons . . . The Report must be implemented without delay' (*Guardian* 22 July 1991). The *Guardian* simply called it a 'masterly diagnosis' (*Guardian* 25 June 1991) while NACRO thought it was 'an historic opportunity to create a prison system structured to take us into the 21st century' (NACRO 1991b, p. 3).

In this chapter I shall deconstruct the hagiography surrounding the report and provide a critical analysis of a number of Woolf's key recommendations. Before considering these criticicisms however, I want to provide a brief but critical overview of the events leading up to the establishment of the Inquiry through analysing developments in penal policy since the mid-1960s, particularly those aimed at reasserting and resurrecting good order and discipline within a penal network that was assailed by a series of interlocking crises (Fitzgerald and Sim 1982). The history of conflict between the confined and their gaolers and the failure of the state to restore good order and discipline provides the sociological and political backdrop for the emergence of Woolf's proposed reforms.

WOOLF IN CONTEXT

While the Strangeways disturbance was the immediate precipitating factor in the genesis of the Woolf Report, it is important to remember that this disturbance came at the end of a series of often violent confrontations in British prisons over the previous twenty-five years. These confrontations have been recognised and well documented in a number of academic and official publications (Fitzgerald and Sim 1982; Home Office 1984; King 1985; Scraton, Sim and Skidmore 1991). As Michel Foucault noted, the disturbances which occurred on a worldwide basis from the 1960s were not simply a challenge to the physically brutalising conditions which confronted many of the confined each day and night, but were also a sustained reaction to the desperate alienation engendered by the philosophically barren 'machine for elimination' which the modern prison had become (Foucault cited in Simon 1974, p. 155). Within the UK the state's response to the disturbances that erupted in the male, maximum-security, dispersal prisons was built on the ideological assertion that the disorder was orchestrated by a small number of subversive recalcitrants who, once identified, could be removed from the main body of the prison population before the contamination of deviance could spread any further (King 1985). The less viable, but no less important disorder in women's prisons, was explained through identifiying the unique biological and psychological factors that drove criminal women to confront male and state authority (Carlen, *et al.* 1985). These ideological assertions in turn led to a series of coercive strategies designed to contain the disorder: transfer and solitary confinement, medicalisation, violence and militarisation (Sim 1991a). By the mid-1980s it was clear to many that these strategies had failed and that the state had not secured hegemony within the institution. There were a number of reasons for this failure.

First, the emergence of a newly radicalised prisoners' rights movement in the early 1970s meant that alternative definitions of, and explanations for, the prison crisis developed which challenged state and media representations of the 'truth' about life inside (Fitzgerald 1977). Second, the academic challenge mounted by those coming from the radical wing of British criminology again provided an alternative conceptualisation of the crisis. In particular, these accounts argued against the individualised explanations of prison conflict and called for a more complex analysis which included focusing on the meaning that the confined gave to their lives, in what Roy King and Kenneth Elliott called the 'electronic coffins' of the maximum-security dispersal prisons (King and Elliott 1977, p. 3). Third, the contradictions within the state itself and the sometimes bitter conflicts between different individuals and strata also contributed to the denial of hegemony. As Bob Jessop has pointed out,

> there is never a point when *the* state is finally built within a given territory and thereafter operates . . . on automatic pilot according to its own definite, fixed and inevitable laws. Nor . . . is there ever a moment when all state managers will simply follow universal rules to define their duties and interests as members of a distinct governing class.
>
> (Jessop 1990, p. 9, emphasis in the original)

The ongoing disputes between management and prison officers before and after the introduction of Fresh Start and the confusion and conflict between different state servants during the Strangeways demonstration provide clear illustrations of the fractured dislocation within the state concerning penal policy. Finally, the challenge to the state's hegemony came from below, from prisoners themselves (Sim 1991b). Not only was conflict endemic between 1966 and 1986 but it was often intensified by the very responses utilised to maintain order. As one prisoner noted after the arrival of the militaristic MUFTI squad to restore order at a particular prison:

> These Mufties batoned, kicked and elbowed every prisoner who happened to be in their way . . . it was decided to go on the offensive and that meant wrecking everything around them in revenge for the injuries inflicted on their innocent fellow prisoners by the Mufties.
> (MacLaughlin 1987, p. 82)

From the mid-1980s the spread of the disorder from long-term to the short-term and remand prisons and the ongoing and particular disorder in women's prisons provided a clear illustration of the still fragile nature of the modern prison's social order and the institution's lack of legitimacy in the hearts and minds of many of the confined.

It is within the political context of state failure to achieve hegemony that the Woolf Report emerged. As with a number of official publications emanating from the Scottish Office in the late 1980s, Woolf's analysis has been seen as a significant and historical moment on the road to fundamental penal reform. In the next part of this chapter I will critically assess this contention through focusing on a number of major themes and issues contained in the report: Woolf's methodology; the issue of the responsible prisoner and *his* relationship to prison contracts (Woolf did not discuss women, a point I shall return to below); the role of prison staff; and finally the politics of Woolf. Taken together, these critiques challenge the reformist rhetoric contained in the Woolf Report and other official publications, a rhetoric, which I have noted elsewhere:

> masks a series of fundamental problems . . . in the prescriptions for the way forward. From the prisoners' perspective the proposed reforms will do little to satisfy many of the demands they have made in the last twenty years and may simply be pouring petrol on prison fires that are still smouldering in the wake of the various disturbances in the late 1980s.
> (Sim 1991b, p. 9)

DECONSTRUCTING WOOLF'S METHODOLOGY

There has been much discussion concerning the methodology which underpins the Report and the difference between Woolf's Inquiry and previous inquiries into the prison system in the UK (Morgan 1991). This issue has been highlighted with particular reference to the fact that prisoners were allowed to present evidence, principally through writing letters and in interviews conducted by the assesssors to the inquiry. Altogether the Inquiry received 607 letters from those institutions in which disturbances had occurred – the 'target establishments' – and a further 603 from those in 'non-target establishments' – that is those prisons which did not experience disorder. Mary Tuck has argued that 'the letters gave vivid and personal reality to the experience and sufferings of prisoners' (Tuck 1991, p. 4). At one level this strategy of allowing prisoners to articulate their views and supporting this with open debate in public seminars was very different from the philosophy and methodology behind previous state inquiries where issues were quickly closed down and the Home Office view prevailed from the beginning. The inquiry chaired by Mr Justice May (Home Office 1979) was a classic example of this process (Fitzgerald and Sim 1980). However, as Rod Morgan has noted, Woolf's Inquiry was still confronted with a series of methodological problems. There was, for example, the issue of 'structured inequality' inherent in presenting evidence to a state inquiry. In this case, the Prison Department within the Home Office established a Woolf Support Unit which collated 236 pages of written evidence from the Department and also presented 'a huge portfolio containing no fewer than 80 annexes'. Morgan also points out that 'there were substantial misgivings' within the Home Office concerning the public seminars. However, he argues that these problems were overcome and that the Inquiry 'was based on the principles of openness and participation, of fairness to the greatest possible extent between parties' (Morgan 1991, pp. 13–30).

A close examination and rigorous deconstruction of the final Report raises some serious questions about this contention. Despite the apparent openness and fluidity in the Inquiry's methodology, it is clear that the accounts by prisoners were still treated with scepticism. In other words, whose account was to count in the last analysis was based on a hierarchical vision of penal truth in which the definition of reality articulated by the confined was secondary to the reality defined by state servants. There are a number of examples of this in the final draft of the Report which touch on some fundamental areas of prison life. For example, the scathing critique made by prisoners of the regime at Dartmoor – a critique which goes back to the nineteenth century (Atholl 1953) – is significantly qualified by Woolf's remark that 'it is important to remember these accounts by prisoners were not given on oath. They have not, unless they were given in oral evidence been subject to cross examination' (Woolf 1991, para. 5.27). Similarly, the Report cites a letter from one prisoner who argued that 'if prisoners are treated like animals, sworn at, degraded and psychologically toyed with week after week, they in turn lose their respect for society at large' (para. 14.3). Once again, the Report qualifies the prisoner's testimony: 'this letter reflects the prisoner's relationship with the Prison Service. We do not suggest that it accurately reflects the experience of all prisoners in prisons; or that it is an accurate and fair description of life in prison' (para. 14.4). Finally, prisoners' accounts of the Pucklechurch disturbance, in which they maintained that they were beaten and strip-searched, is again heavily qualified. At the same time, the Report points to the limitations of the inquiry in confronting these issues:

> It is possible that some of the screams and yells of pain which were allegedly heard by inmates could be attributed to the use of C and R [Control and Restraint] holds. It is accepted that C and R was used for

> bringing some prisoners into the cells. Others' screams and yells might have been deliberately misleading – 'put on' by inmates who wanted to make out that they were being hurt. For the reasons I explained at the public hearing and set out in Section 2 of this Report, it is not possible for me to make any findings about these allegations. I am conscious, however, that my inability to do so would be unfair to staff who were not in a position to rebut these and other allegations which were made in public. This is, I am afraid, a limitation of an inquiry of this sort – it is not practical to do more than record the fact of the allegations and the fact, which is equally important, that they are denied.
>
> (para. 8.142)

In contrast, no such qualifications are made with respect to the evidence given by state servants in general and prison officers in particular. Thus, the Report notes that 'the overwhelming impression created by [Prison Service staff] evidence is that the vast majority of the staff have a deep sense of loyalty to the Prison Service. They have a genuine desire to see conditions for prisoners improve' (para. 13.2). This uncritical acceptance of staff benevolence can be contrasted with the evidence contained both in the Report itself and more widely in prisoners' autobiographies as well as in the critical sociology literature on prisons. In the Report, Woolf notes that the largest number of comments in the prisoners' letters were about prison officers. The subject was 'mentioned in 294 letters, 245 of these letters (40 per cent of all respondents) were critical and 49 (8 per cent) favourable or neutral' (Annex 2E, ch. 2, para. II2). Even when a 'small minority' of prison officers are criticised for 'irresponsible behaviour' as after the Pucklechurch demonstration – the behaviour involved telling surrendering prisoners that their arms and legs would be broken – this is again done with some heavy qualifications:

> There is no doubt that at the time the inmates were very frightened (I use that word advisedly) and even if the remarks made to them when waiting on the lawn were made in jest, they could, and did, cause considerable fear to the inmates. When considering these criticisms the long hours that management and staff had been on duty should be taken into account. Each member of staff must have been extremely tired and . . . close to exhaustion.
>
> (para. 8.188 (30–1))

As noted above, the experience of confinement articulated in the Report and the role of prison staff in that experience can be contrasted with the repressive reality described in prisoners' autobiographies, accounts which go back to the second half of the nineteenth century (Sim 1990). More recent accounts have included the racism experienced by black prisoners

(Hercules 1989); the sexism experienced by confined women (Carlen, *et. al.* 1985; Padel and Stevenson 1988); the violence and the humiliation experienced by Irish prisoners (Conlon 1990; Hill 1990); and the particular patterns of brutalisation that are part of the everyday lives of the confined (Scraton, Sim and Skidmore 1991). This is not the place to explore the different and rich epistemological and ontological debates concerning definitions of reality that have developed within social sciences in recent years due primarily to the impact of feminist theory and methodology (Harding 1987; Smith 1987) and to Foucault's insistence that knowledge and power are linked to the production of truth (Kritzman 1988, pp. 255–67). It is important to note, however, that Woolf's analysis fails to convey in any strong sense alternative definitions of reality or different visions of penal truth. Rather, the Report, to use the words of Carol Smart, directs its gaze downwards towards prisoners thus reinforcing 'an overall impression that these are people who *need* to be researched, these are the ones who are out of step with "social norms" or who are causing the problems' (Smart 1984, pp. 150–1, emphasis in the original). Conversely the Report rarely gazes upwards to look at, in Smart's phrase, 'the locally powerful' who in the case of the confined would be the prison officers. The lack of any critical analysis of the role and daily practices of prison staff constitutes the second major weakness in Woolf's analysis.

WOOLF AND THE PRISON OFFICERS

Much of Woolf's discussion of prison staff is concerned with the perennial and debilitating issue of industrial relations, the impact of the Fresh Start reforms and the hostility of rank-and-file officers to the largely detrimental impact which they maintain these reforms have had on their everyday lives. Woolf, in this respect, has followed closely in the footsteps of the May Inquiry whose discussion of prison officers also revolved around the question of industrial relations and his attempt to construct a line-management solution to the crisis of authority in prisons in the late 1970s and early 1980s (Fitzgerald and Sim 1980). However, transforming the problems generated by prison officer power into a question of managerialism only reinforces the prevailing view that the conflict between the confined and prison staff is largely bureaucratic. Rather this conflict is more fundamental and revolves around the philosophical question of how the majority of officers see penal policy which in turn relates to the political questions raised by their often unfettered discretion and lack of accountability. Woolf fails to consider these questions in any depth nor does he analyse the role of staff in the deterioration in prison regimes, a situation that has developed 'not only because of the widespread industrial action taken by officers but also because of the strident culture of discipline, regulation and masculinity which underpins their everyday work' (Sim 1991b, p. 20). From the perspective of the confined, a significant element in the different protests that have occurred in the last twenty-five years in institutions such as Parkhurst, Hull, Gartree, Wormwood Scrubs, Dartmoor, Strangeways, Peterhead, Durham 'H' Wing and Holloway has been the role of officers in the formal and informal regulation of their behaviour (Fitzgerald 1977; PROP n.d.; Padel and Stevenson 1988; Scraton, Sim and Skidmore 1991). The recent interviews conducted by Elaine Genders and Elaine Player in which a mere six officers out of 101 did not refer to black prisoners in racist or pejorative terms only underlines the inbred conservatism of their occupational culture (Genders and Player 1989). As one remarked: 'they [black prisoners] remind me of a monkey colony, they keep together in a flock and are always scratching each other's back and hissing together when they're under any threat' (pp. 50–1). To argue, as Woolf does, that the role of prison staff 'should be a skilled professional [one] within a disciplined service' (para 13.9) fails to understand the dynamics of their occupational culture, the operationalisation of power in their everyday interaction and the discourses of authoritarianism and masculinity which underpin this interaction. As Mick Ryan has noted:

> no number of formal rules will secure justice unless the prison officers deliver it in their daily rounds, in their intimate relationships with those over whom they exercise great and sometimes regrettably, unyeilding power. About how to persuade officers to deliver justice in this sense, the Report has very little to offer . . . The culture of the prison and those who run it is far more resistant to in-service training than the Report imagines. A more convincing strategy would be to combine this training with a hefty infusion of more skills from the outside in order to confront the prison officer with other ways, and above all else, other expectations. But either way it's going to be an uphill struggle. Of course there are decent, progressive prison officers but the service is Janus-faced, and we hear of far too many potentially unruly officers, sporting menacing 'slashed peaks' and getting a basic wage of over £15,000 a year, who have not the slightest intention of 'going soft'.
>
> (Ryan 1992, pp. 10–11)

THE RESPONSIBLE PRISONER AND THE PRISON CONTRACT

The third dimension I wish to highlight is Woolf's argument concerning the responsible prisoner and prison contracts. Both are central to his vision for future penal arrangements.

The following extract provides a clear illustration of how the responsible prisoner is to be conceptualised:

> Prisoners must . . . be given the opportunity to make choices. They must be held accountable for those choices. Prisoners must come to recognize that it is for them to make positive use of their sentence. They should have a responsibility for how they serve their sentence and for how they will live after release. It is right that the Prison Service should provide every opportunity for prisoners to exercise that responsibility.
>
> (para. 14.14).

The concept of responsibility is underpinned by a second recommendation, the introduction of prison contracts. The report argues that a series of contracts should be established which would specify the obligations of the state to its servants and to the confined. Area managers, for example, would have a contract with prison governors which among other things 'would be a statement of what the establishment should be achieving during the year ahead and what it should be seeking to do in the longer-term' (para. 15.35). Prisoners would also receive contracts:

> In that 'contract', the establishment would state in as precise terms as possible, what it would provide for the prisoner. In return, the prisoner would agree to comply with the responsibilities which the 'contract' placed upon him . . . The prisoner would also receive progressively more under the contract as he progressed through his sentence. On the other hand, he could lose for a period of time some of the features of his 'contract' in consequence of a finding of ill discipline.
>
> (paras. 12.120–12.122)

Woolf's construction of the responsible prisoner and the social contract between the state and the confined has added another dimension to the current debate concerning the relationship between the free market and the process of punishment (Ryan and Ward 1989). The classical liberal notion of free-floating, responsible individuals contracted to the wider society through the neutral arbitration of state authority has thus worked its way into the discourse of twentieth-century penal reform. However, as a number of writers have pointed out, this classical conceptualisation of human behaviour, and the philosophy of utilitarianism which underpins it, is problematic. These writers have noted how classical liberalism failed to consider the material impact of wider structural relationships on individuals living in a grossly unequal society. Choice for many was (and is) severely restricted because of the divisions which flow from these structural relationships which are manifested along the fault lines of social class, gender, race, age and sexuality. Within this model, the state, despite its inherent contradictions and dislocations, reinforces these divisions. I do not intend to pursue this argument here as it has been well documented and analysed elsewhere (Held *et al.* 1983).

This wider critique of contract can, however, be related to three specific points concerning the conceptualisation of responsibility and contract within the Report and their applicability to the prison system. First, responsibility is defined and defended on the state's terrain. Conversely this means that definitions of irresponsible behaviour will also be defined by the state. The point made by Michael Adler and Brian Longhurst in relation to *Opportunity and Responsibility* (Scottish Office 1990) can be applied equally to Woolf. As they note, 'prisoners may find themselves in a very vulnerable position if and when they act "irresponsibly" and take decisions which land them in trouble' (Adler and Longhurst 1991 p. 7). In fact, Woolf is quite clear on this issue: those prisoners who do not exercise responsibility in a 'constructive and co-operative way' will be 'held responsible for this as well' (para. 14.14).

The prisoner's contract will also be tied to penal control. Thus a prisoner will receive 'progressively more' from the contract as he passes through the system. But 'he could lose for a period of time some of the features of his "contract" in consequence of a finding of ill discipline. The "contract" would therefore be a way of introducing greater incentives into the system' (para. 12.122). Responsibility and the contract are therefore directly linked to prisoner co-operation which is to be defined by the state or more precisely by its servants in the shape of prison officers. However, as noted above, it is precisely the highly discretionary, non-accountable pyramid of power within which prison officers work, and which allows their definitions of responsible and irresponsible behaviour to prevail, which has been a major factor in the conflict between the confined and the prison system in the last twenty-five years. The continuous enforcement of the many and diverse petty rules and regulations which govern prisoners' lives has allowed prison officers to define quite early and categorically what is acceptable behaviour (Scraton, Sim and Skidmore 1991, ch. 4). Woolf's conceptualisation of responsibility therefore does little to challenge this imbalance in power, it is simply reinforced in the Report.

The second weakness in the Report's support for prison contracts relates to the fact that the notion of the responsible prisoner is applied only to male prisoners. Woolf consciously excluded women from his investigation maintaining that it 'would not be right to investigate or make findings about' confined women, sentencing policy, prisoners from Northern Ireland and 'other important matters' (para. 2.18). Even if women had been included, there are still some fundamental questions to be asked about the general applicability of responsibility to a group within the prison population who are systematically denied responsibility and rationality at every stage of the criminal justice process (Carlen 1983; and see Chapter 12). A similar point can be made about the applicability of the social contract to women's prisons. As Carole Pateman has noted, within liberal democratic theory the contract is a particularly patriarchal phenomenon that has reinforced the control and regulation of women's lives. In Pateman's view it has 'helped to obscure coercion and violence in civil society . . . [and] gives the appearance of freedom to sexually ascriptive domination and subjection. Contract . . . hides the figure of the armed man in the shadows behind the civil individual' (Pateman 1988, p. 121). Simply applying the social contract to women's prisons will therefore do little to challenge the wider structures of patriarchal domination which shape and give meaning to women's lives within and without institutions (Walby 1990).

The third problem with applying the social contract to prisons is that it depoliticises the fact and nature of confinement by turning the prisoner into a consumer of prison 'services' – a customer. As Marx and Engels recognised long ago, to discuss social relationships in terms of contracts mystifies the wider, often hidden power relationships which underpin and shape observable reality. The contract does little to challenge these relationships, rather it asserts and confirms them (Lefebvre 1969, p. 113). Furthermore, as David Edgar has pointed out, conceptualising social relationships simply in terms of customers and consumers of services is also problematic: it limits the power of the consumer; it subtly alters the feasible grounds of complaint 'from collective concerns to the shortcomings of an individual transaction'; it is concerned with 'differentials rather than with the quality of treatment'; and lastly it 'homogenises the relationships we have with the outside world, denying their specific (and essential) character' (Edgar 1991, p. 28). Russell Keat has developed this theme in arguing that the notion of the consumer 'is based on an entirely voluntaristic view of human agency which denies altogether the relevance of social conditions in determining human action' (Keat 1991, p. 11). The metamorphosis of the prisoner into a consumer is therefore likely to fracture and atomise the prison population still further, marginalising the social and political context of the prison experience and transforming the discourses of discipline and punishment which underpin penality into politically neutral and individually safe questions of satisfaction or dissatisfaction with the commodity or service on offer within an individual establishment.

DISCIPLINE, THE STATE AND THE POLITICS OF WOOLF

In the final part of this chapter I want briefly to explore the dynamics of the Woolf Report from another angle, and to position it within the broader context of the direction of penal policy and the state in the 1990s. There are two problems in particular that I wish to highlight. The first is concerned with the relationship between the Report's recommendations and the ongoing issues of discipline and coercion which lie at the heart of contemporary penality (Garland 1990; Sim 1990). The second problem relates to the place of the prison in the wider context of developments within the state in the last decade, particularly the consolidation of what has been termed the 'strong' or 'authoritarian' state and the concomitant subversion of the brittle structures of democratic accountability and civil liberties within the institutions of state and civil society (Hall 1988). As I shall illustrate, the model of accountablity, which is mainly implied rather than clearly explicated in Woolf, will do little to confront this broader issue and may ultimately reinforce the drive towards the centralisation of social authority and power through the ideological dressage of limited penal reform.

I noted at the beginning of this chapter how the Woolf Report had transcended the divisions between politicians, penal reformers and media personnel and how it united the different interests of these groups on the ideological terrain of penal reform. However, in concentrating on what they understood to be the positive aspects of the Inquiry these commentators missed an obvious and crucial sociological point, namely that many politicians and state servants – despite the contradictions and conflicts between them – are still committed to maintaining the prison's social order through repression. The coercive strategies discussed above, which have been utilised in the last twenty-five years and which have often brought further dislocation, none the less remain central in the repertoire of responses available when the 'exhaustion of consent' leads to the breakdown of institutional authority and control (Hall *et al.* 1978, p. 218). The solutions offered by Woolf to deal with the crisis are unlikely to marginalise the ideological and material support for these strategies. Indeed in his speech in the House of Commons on the day that Woolf reported, Kenneth Baker, the then Home Secretary, was quite explicit about the message that prisoners and those in the wider society should receive. After condemning 'utterly the small minority of the prisoners who joined in [the] orgy of destruction' at Strangeways and other prisons, he then outlined the reforms which had been introduced following the disturbances. These included: establishing a new incident control centre; overhauling contingency plans; clarifying lines of responsibility; training more staff in the new and improved techniques of riot control; increasing the stock of riot-control equipment; and reviewing the physical security of prisons. He went on to point out:

> The country will not tolerate the kind of disgraceful behaviour witnessed last April. We must make clear our utter condemnation of it by introducing a new deterrent. We shall therefore, as we have already made clear, bring before the House proposals to create a new offence of prison mutiny, which will carry a maximum penalty of 10 extra years in prison.
>
> (Hansard 25 February 1991, col. 659)

Finally, he referred to the prison building programme, the jewel in the government's penal crown, and indicated that another 12 new prisons were to be opened by 1993. It was only after listing these changes that Baker turned to the issues which many prisoners had identified as important in the genesis of the disturbances: overcrowding, slopping out, the lack of rehabilitation and the fracturing of family ties (Hansard 25 February 1991, col. 660).

In September 1991 the Home Secretary reiterated his coercive intentions in his speech to the annual conference of the Boards of Visitors. He announced that the offence of prison mutiny would be included in the Queen's speech to Parliament and the nation the following November. Furthermore, he made it clear that

> prisoners must understand that they will have to pay the price for rioting – by spending longer in prison and by waiting longer for improvements in prison conditions . . . The repairs required will . . . have to be made at the expense of other improvements the prisoners themselves would like to see.
>
> (*Guardian*, 7 September 1991)

He repeated this argument at the Conservative Party Conference in October and added some further dimensions to his vision of the prison's future: ten years for aiding and abetting escapes, a privately run prison, 'plus the promise that prisoners will quickly learn that rioting was not "a cost-free option"' (*Guardian*, 10 October 1991).

Baker's emphasis on maintaining order through coercion has been supported most notably by the Prison Officers' Association. At its annual conference in May 1990 the Association called for the establishment of an emergency task force of 1,000 officers to deal with prison disturbances. This force would be 'trained in riot strategy and tactics and armed with CS gas, rubber bullets and stun grenades. The Army including the Special Air Service would be summoned to help if prison staff and police failed to terminate the riot' (Power 1990, p. 654).

The emphasis on paramilitarism can be seen in the Woolf Report itself. Woolf points to the advantages of the 'new' Control and Restraint (C and R) techniques which have been developed to replace the infamous MUFTI techniques secretly introduced in the late 1970s (Fitzgerald and Sim 1982, p. 22). By April 1990, 2,234 members of staff had completed basic C and R training. The target was 4,200 staff who would then have refresher courses. Woolf hoped that 'as standards within the prison system improve . . . a reduction in the C and R training programme will be possible' (para. 9.92). At the same time, he conceded that the use of C and R techniques was 'closely related to a military operation' (para. 12.152).

The marginalisation of coercion and discipline in recent debates about the future of the prisons and their subordination within Woolf's reformist rhetoric can be linked to a set of wider issues which are also marginalised in the Report but which are likely to have a crucial influence on the nature and form of imprisonment in the 1990s. In particular, there is the question of the democratic accountability of state institutions. Although the term tended to be used often uncritically in the late 1980s, it was none the less part of a key political debate which emerged during the decade in the UK and Europe where it was linked to the issues of citizenship and human rights (Andrews 1991). Within the UK this debate has had a particular resonance in the context of more general sociological and political discussions about the emergence of the authoritarian or strong state (Hall 1988). The consolidation of this state form can be seen not only in the criminal justice sytem through the centralisation of power, the militarisation of different institutions and the fracturing of already heavily circumscribed civil and political liberties but also within state welfare provision where the erosion of welfare rights has been legitimated through the ideological construction of the 'genuine claimant' (Hillyard and Percy-Smith 1988; Squires 1990).

The drive towards the centralisation of power and the concomitant marginalisation of democratic accountability in the 1980s, provides a sharp contrast to the evolutionary and highly conventional view of accountability implicit in the Woolf Report. The few references which mention accountability only underline the Report's conventional stance. Thus Woolf notes that 'the Home Secretary, assisted by one of his junior Ministers, is directly responsible for all aspects of Prison Service work' (para. 12.35). This pluralistic, organisational model of the prison hierarchy can be contrasted with the critiques which have been made in relation to the problems associated specifically with prison accountability and the nature of power within the institution (Maguire *et al.* 1985). More generally, it can also be contrasted with the failure of the parliamentary model of politics, which in its present form, has failed to deliver a sustainable model of accountability built on the regulation and control of state institutions and their servants. Recognising this process means moving beyond the highly restricted model of accountability proposed by Woolf, for as Bob Jessop has noted:

> In practice democratic rights are often eroded by a number of very serious obstacles resulting from deliberate political action and/or the unintended effects of particular institutional arrangements . . . Moreover, even where such deliberate barriers to formal democracy are minimized in the electoral process, similar barriers may be erected to prevent elected representatives controlling the exercise of state power. This is most evident in the insulation of key parts of the governmental system from effective control through legislative assemblies and/or popular consultative bodies with real teeth. Here we could mention the forces concerned with law and order (police, secret services, military). . .
>
> (Jessop 1990, p. 177)

Jessop's point can be equally applied to the issue of prisons as a 'force concerned with law and order'. Indeed, it could be argued that it has been the failure of the parliamentary model of democracy to deliver a supportive, rights-based regime based on the accountability of those who manage the system that also contributed to the crisis behind the walls. Woolf's model of accountability will do little to challenge the perception held by the confined that there is little control, regulation or fairness within the system notwithstanding the principles of justice and independence which Woolf argues should be introduced into future penal arrangements. As Mick Ryan has pointed out, even here there are problems in that the principles set out for allowing an independent voice to be heard in grievance procedures 'are far too restrictive'; while in the case of disciplinary hearings, Woolf's proposals to allow a sentence of 28 days loss of remission to be 'awarded' by prison governors 'is a heavy one . . . [which] should be reduced' (Ryan 1992, pp. 9–10). These issues are pursued in Chapters 4 and 5 respectively.

CONCLUSION

Taken together, the issues discussed in this chapter raise some serious questions about the viability of the Woolf Report to provide a programme that will tackle the prison crisis and deliver far-reaching and fundamental change. Already the portents for the future are not good. The sharp rise in the prison population in the first nine months of 1991, the continuing debate over the treatment of remand prisoners and the ongoing issues concerning deaths in custody have all been highlighted in one form or another since Woolf reported. In addition there have been further disturbances in Leicester, Moorland, Durham, Lindholme, Frankland, Everthorpe, Shotts and the Crumlin Road. These disturbances indicate that the troubling issues confronting the confined remain unresolved. At the same time their expectations that reforms – however limited – may be introduced in the wake of Woolf (and *Opportunity and Responsibility* (Scottish Office 1990) in Scotland) have been heightened. If the authorities fail to strike an ideological chord with the imprisoned by providing a vision for the future which deals humanely and seriously with these heightened expectations then they might find that the fire next time will burn even more severely in British prisons with catastrophic consequences for all concerned.

ACKNOWLEDGEMENTS

This chapter is dedicated to the memory of Jim Hewitt.
Thanks to Jenny Burke for her support with this chapter.

2

ORDER, DISORDER AND REGIMES IN THE PRISON SERVICES OF SCOTLAND, AND ENGLAND AND WALES

Roy D. King

In May 1990, just after the prisoners came down from the roof at Strangeways, the Scottish Prison Service published *Opportunity and Responsibility* (Scottish Office 1990), the third in a series of policy and discussion documents intended to take the Service 'along the road of change'. Given that the subtitle of the document was *Developing New Approaches to the Management of the Long Term Prison System in Scotland*, the obvious comparator for the prison system of England and Wales is the Report of the Control Review Committee, *Managing the Long Term Prison System* published six years earlier (Home Office 1984). But while the timing of the two reports *is* important, it is not *just* an accident of timing that it may be more appropriate to compare the Scottish document with the White Paper *Custody, Care and Justice* (Home Office 1991a); and with the Report of Lord Justice Woolf (1991) on *Prison Disturbances April 1990*, to whose recommendations the White Paper seeks to give effect.

In this chapter, therefore, I propose to review the prospects of having good order and good regimes in our prisons by reflecting upon some of the similarities and differences in the Scottish and English experience and the way in which the two systems now approach their common task. If the focus of the discussion leans rather heavily towards higher security and longer-term prisoners that is deliberate. Prison systems should have few difficulties in running decent regimes for medium-term prisoners in medium or low-security. The test cases for prison systems lie in providing regimes for the high-turnover, remand and short-term prisoners – where it is essentially a test of management and logistics; and for long-term, high-security, difficult and dangerous prisoners – where it is a test of philosophy and will. In a vitally important sense the stance a prison service adopts towards its most difficult prisoners sets the tone for the rest of the prison system.

ORDER AND CONTROL

In his foreword to *Opportunity and Responsibility*, Malcolm Rifkind, the (then) Secretary of State for Scotland, wrote as follows:

> It is clear that the old objectives of 'treatment and training' are outmoded. A new approach is required, which will recognise the mutual responsibilities of the prisoner and the prison authorities and ensure that the long term prisoner is encouraged to address his offending behaviour and offered an appropriate range of opportunities to use his time in prison responsibly for personal development.
>
> (Scottish Office 1990, p. 4)

There was little mention of 'treatment and training' in the Report of the Control Review Committee (CRC) either – for the phrase had been officially buried by the Report of the May Committee five years earlier (Home Office 1979). But the new approach adopted by the CRC, unpicking much official thinking on security and control of the recent past, did not attract the same level of ministerial blessings that Rifkind bestowed upon *Opportunity and Responsibility*. In part this was because of the political climate in which the CRC was conceived and its report given birth. The CRC was established in the wake of further disturbances in the dispersal system – at Albany and Wormwood Scrubs in May and June 1983 – and the Committee had scarcely met before the Home Secretary announced changes to the parole system which at once increased the numbers of long-term prisoners and decreased the most powerful incentive towards good behaviour – the prospect of early release.

In the circumstances the Committee did well to seek a way out of the tangled history of the concentration/dispersal dilemma in the possibilities offered by unit management and 'new generation' prison design. In the short term the CRC successfully headed off demands for a return to something akin to the punitive control units of a decade earlier, through a strategy of developing small long-term units operating a variety of essentially positive regimes for difficult prisoners (see Chapter 9). Adventurous though some of these ideas were, and notwithstanding the references to sentence planning and the provision of individual programmes for prisoners, the report stopped short of locating the control problem clearly within the very structures of imprisonment and the organisation of prison life itself. Although it argued for more research on these matters the report never quite broke free – in spite of its rejection of a control classification – from the idea that control problems in prisons are essentially the product of an identifiable minority of disruptive prisoners (Home Office 1984, paras. 86–8).

But the lack of a positive Foreword from the Home Secretary to the Report of the Control Review Committee also reflected the fact that Home

Office officials were themselves divided over some of its recommendations and the costs of implementing them. Nevertheless, ministers were persuaded to appoint three outside academics[1] to a Research and Advisory Group (RAG) – amongst other things, 'to advise on the planning, coordination and evaluation of the proposed long-term prisoner units' (Home Office 1987b, p. 1). The deliberations of RAG were largely devoted to the attempted identification of the 'intransigent troublemakers' because they dominated official thinking about control problems in prisons (see King and McDermott 1990a).

It is intriguing, moreover, that all of the proposed small units so far established continue to reflect this view of control problems and offer alternative specialist ways of controlling such individuals – a 'highly structured' (restricted) regime, but with some degree of psychological assistance at Lincoln, a moderately structured regime with psychiatric oversight at Parkhurst, and a more loosely structured regime with a high degree of psychological assistance at Hull. None involves 'inmate participation in the running of the unit' (Home Office 1987b, pp. 41–3). Considerable discussion took place over the possible establishment of a fourth unit (and even a fifth) which might be more sociologically informed and concerned with the *mutual responsibilities* of staff and prisoners (cf. Rifkind, in Scottish Office 1990, p. 4, quoted above) in maintaining 'order' rather than with imposing 'control'. Such a unit would have wider implications for the prison system as a whole, but it has yet to be established.

It should not be forgotten that the CRC Report led directly to the examination of new generation architecture (Home Office 1985a), and this in turn has profoundly influenced design briefs for new prisons – if not yet for the custody of high-security prisoners. Valuable work on regime activities was also carried forward through Dunbar's brief secondment to the Prisons Inspectorate (Home Office 1985b). Nevertheless, as changes occurred in the composition of the Prisons Board, the implementation of the report was more narrowly confined to the technicalities of control than it might have been and certainly narrower than might be expected of *Opportunity and Responsibilitiy* (Scottish Office 1990).

Opportunity and Responsibility had its own unpicking of earlier themes to accomplish. The Scottish system had not been without its history of troubles, particularly at Peterhead, which had been traditionally used not just for prisoners of peculiarly high-security risk but also, and perhaps more so, as a 'sin bin' for prisoners whose control had proved problematic in what the Scots refer to as the 'mainstream' prisons. As a result Peterhead acquired a unique reputation as a prison which took a no-nonsense approach to matters of discipline and control.

There were well-publicised, though shortlived, rooftop incidents at Peterhead in 1972, 1979 and 1984. But in 1985, members of staff were taken hostage in two incidents and it seemed as though the seriousness of incidents had moved to a new level. During 1986 serious damage was also done to the fabric of a number of Scottish prisons, and a member of staff was held hostage for four days in Edinburgh Prison in October, to be followed in November by a similar incident in Peterhead. The following year saw a further wave of hostage-taking incidents: in Barlinnie in January, Shotts in September, and both Shotts and Peterhead in October. By then, however, some pretty draconian restrictions had been introduced into the regimes in the long term prisons, especially at Peterhead.

These incidents were every bit as serious as those that had occurred earlier south of the border. But surprisingly the first of the Scottish Prison System's consultation documents on policy, *Custody and Care* (Scottish Office 1988a), which was published just a few months after the latest hostage taking in Peterhead, was singularly low key on the question of control. Instead it sought to set out a 'coherent corporate philosophy' for the system within a framework 'intended to make possible a better quality of life for inmates and encourage better, professional standards for staff at all levels' (paras. 1.1, 1.4).

Later that year, however, a new discussion paper, *Assessment and Control* (Scottish Office 1988b) took a somewhat different tone. The future of Peterhead was under review and a new maximum-security unit for 60 prisoners in four groups of 15 was planned for Shotts (para. 8.10) – though it was not made clear whether this was simply for 'security risks' or 'control problems' or both. It also called for new arrangements for the 'identification of potential troublemakers in advance' (para. 1.8) and the development of a new system of 'profiling for individuals assessed as potential control risks' (para. 1.9). In this it went much further than had the CRC Report (see Cooke 1991, p. 98), although its proposals to extend the range of facilities for difficult prisoners were broadly in line with the emerging policy in England and Wales. There were plans to supplement the short-stay Segregation Unit at Inverness with a similar unit at Perth, and the long-stay Special Unit at Barlinnie with a new special unit at Shotts where 12 prisoners might spend up to a year out of the mainstream and receive intensive specialist advice from both psychiatrists and psychologists (paras. 9.7–9.12).

A small-unit strategy was not new to either system. The Control Review Committee built upon the experience of C Wing at Parkhurst and indeed a remodelled C Wing was the first of the new units to be established. In Scotland the Barlinnie Special Unit, which dated back to 1973, had attempted to find a different way of handling 'difficult and dangerous' prisoners after the problems of the 'cages' at Inverness. But neither system had yet grasped a satisfactory way of integrating special units into the structure of the system as a whole or of engineering the environment of the 'mainstream' (in Scotland) or 'normal location' (in England and Wales) so that special procedures, of whatever kind, would be less necessary. In essence, the problem was one of the extent to which prisoners might be given some sense of say and participation in what goes on; and if they had more say, whether they would come to have a different kind of stake in the maintenance of good *order* instead of being required to conform to a predetermined regime, and when failing to do so, have to be brought under *control.*

The position of Barlinnie Special Unit is crucial. Any outsider who has visited both the Barlinnie Special Unit and B Hall at Peterhead under lockdown conditions will have seen both ends of the spectrum of possible regimes for difficult and dangerous prisoners. They might be forgiven for thinking that a system that could contain both at the same time must border on the schizophrenic – although no doubt many experienced prison staff might wish to argue that both are necessary in the real world of imprisonment. However that might be, the two situations – Peterhead and Barlinnie – offer extreme examples of what is possible and models, or perhaps tendencies would be a better word, towards which the rest of the system might wish to go (or find itself pushed or pulled).

The official Scottish attitude towards the Barlinnie Special Unit has always been, and to some extent continues to be, ambivalent. From the outset it was distanced from the rest of the system by its 'experimental' status, although it was not set up as a serious experiment in any scientific sense and it had been in existence for fifteen years before any worthwhile research evaluation was carried out (Cooke 1989a, 1989b). The divisions within the Scottish system about Barlinnie have been well publicised through the autobiographical accounts of Jimmy Boyle (1977, 1984) and there is little doubt that the Scots have been on the horns of a dilemma: having set it up, it went much further than they had intended, particularly in terms of its visits policy, but they have been unable and increasingly unwilling to close it down because of the publicity that would attract. For much of its history Barlinnie has been something of an embarrassment to the Scots – famous but marginalised (Coyle 1989).

The significant difference between the two prison systems in this regard, however, is simply this: *in Scotland the Barlinnie Special Unit has somehow survived, whereas in England and Wales no such unit has yet come into being.* In England and Wales the question of setting up a Barlinnie-style special unit in the wake of the CRC report was the subject of fascinatingly oblique discussions at the Research and Advisory Group. Eventually, after allowance had been made for what the Prisons Board would consider to be unacceptable excesses, a model was established incorporating the essential element – 'a high degree of prisoner participation in decisions about the way in which the unit operates' – into the RAG proposals, if only as the second option for a potential fourth or fifth unit (Home Office 1987b, para. 145). The first option was for a regime organised 'according to psychological principles': although RAG specifically excluded a 'token economy', the discussions centred on a social learning environment with some clear behaviourist leanings (paras 129–30).

Since RAG published its report, however, events have moved on. Further changes in the Prison Department representation on RAG were accompanied by a marked shift away from option two in favour of option one – thereby reinforcing the offical discourse on control that locates the problem in individuals. In spite of that the difficulties in actually identifying prisoners suitable to fill the units – predicted by King and McDermott (1990a) – was confirmed by Bottoms who reported (to a special conference at York on special units for difficult prisoners which took place on the day following the outbreak of the riot at Strangeways) that there had in fact been a dearth of candidates, and that this had led the Department to decide to restrict 'the eventual size of the special unit system to four units' (Bottoms 1991, p. 10). The space identified at Frankland had already been put to another use; and the plans even for the preferred psychologically based unit at Milton Keynes had been undermined by renewed suggestions that the 'special task of the fourth unit explicitly be to tackle those who cannot be contained elsewhere' (Bottoms 1991, pp. 10–11) even in the existing special units. If such a policy were adopted, noted Bottoms, it would drive a coach and horses through CRC's and RAG's principle that none of the long term units should be regarded as places of last resort.

A year later RAG itself was dissolved (Home Office 1991d, para. 34). By then the Woolf Report had also noted the current Prison Service thinking about the need for a 'more *structured* regime' at Milton Keynes (Woolf 1991, paras. 12.289–12.290) but without further comment. In part, no doubt, this was because Woolf hoped that special units would become less necessary once it was recognised that the key to the problem of difficult prisoners lies 'in the management of the prison system as a whole and in the provision made for the generality of prisoners' (para.12.295). In any event a Barlinnie-style unit had thus been effectively first postponed and then simply removed from the agenda. What eventually is established in Milton Keynes, now re-christened Woodhill, can be expected to send a critically important message for the future of policy in England and Wales.

In terms of the strain between what might be termed the Peterhead and the Barlinnie tendencies *Opportunity and Responsibility* (Scottish Office 1990) is remarkable for the candour with which it distances itself from its predecessor *Assessment and Control* (Scottish Office 1988b). The later report makes clear that the proposal for the new maximum-security unit at Shotts – which *would have been* to accommodate some 60 of the 120 or so potentially very difficult prisoners identifed in *Assessment and Control* – was to be dropped (Scottish Office 1990, p. 47, para. 2, p. 53, para. 19). The Report makes no bones that the change of heart is because the proposal had been seen as 'promoting an ethos which relegated prisoners to be little more than the objects of a management process' (p. 47, para. 3) and that this was 'contrary to the main message of the earlier consultation paper *Custody and Care* [Scottish Office 1988a]'. The Report reiterates a flexible small-units strategy and concludes by spelling out the two key assumptions underlying its policy for small units:

> Firstly, small units must be seen as complementary to the mainstream. Secondly, we no longer believe that it is appropriate to think in terms of identifying a specific number of prisoners who present such difficult management problems that they will require to be accommodated in small units (as was implied in *Assessment and Control*). What is clear is that, at any one time, the number of prisoners who can be accommodated in small units will be a minority. *The value of such units lies as much in the ability to pioneer innovative approaches, the lessons of which can be applied to the mainstream generally, as in the capacity to provide for a limited number of prisoners who are having difficulty settling to their sentence.*
>
> (Scottish Office 1990, p. 59, para. 16, emphasis added)

This is a quite remarkable statement. It constitutes a threshold over which neither the CRC nor RAG was quite prepared to step. It reflects, perhaps, what might be called the marginalisation of the Peterhead tendency in favour of the Barlinnie tendency. Indeed in the rest of the document the Scottish Prison Service returns unmistakably to the themes expressed in *Custody and Care* (Scottish Office 1988a) and spells them out in a series of briefly expressed policy objectives. Although the document is less than comprehensive, and there are a number of important matters on which *Opportunity and Responsibility* is silent, in others the statements rank alongside those contained in the White Paper *Custody, Care and Justice* (Home Office 1991a). But what is most remarkable about *Opportunity and Responsibility* is that it was the product of offical thinking and consultations, as part of a self-correcting process, that took place over a period of approximately three years. There was undoubtedly a major process of review continuing within the Home Office in the seven-year interval between the Report of the Control Review Committee and the publication of *Custody, Care and Justice*. But it is most unlikely that the White Paper would have appeared at all, or taken the form it did, without Strangeways and the massive, and very public, intervention of the Woolf Inquiry.

Words, of course, are cheap: even when, perhaps especially when, published on glossy paper. Getting the right words is no doubt an essential prerequisite for getting the right action. But no one who has observed prison matters over the last quarter of a century, or who has any feel for the history of imprisonment, can be optimistic about the capacity of prison systems to be changed – or to stay changed. In the concluding part of this chapter I seek to review the extent to which the two systems have got the right words, and the prospects for turning those words into action as far as regimes are concerned. But first it is necessary to say something of what needs to be done.

PRISON REGIMES

The sharp impoverishment of prison regimes in England and Wales – at least from the late 1960s to the mid-1980s – was well documented (King and McDermott 1989) before the establishment of the Woolf Inquiry. So too was the fact that the deterioration in prison regimes had occurred alongside, and apparently in spite of, a major growth in both capital and current expenditure (see Home Office 1979, para. 6.95). These expenditures provided a huge increase in the prison estate and major improvements in the staff: prisoner ratios (Morgan 1983; King and McDermott 1989), but contributed very little to improvements in prison regimes. Recognition of these unpalatable facts provided the rhetorical justification for Fresh Start (McDermott and King 1989). There is much less published information about the situation in Scotland. The May Committee reported that, at least in regard to current expenditure, the Scottish Prison Service had benefitted in much the same way as had England and Wales (Home Office 1979, para. 6.95). The increases in staffing between 1965 and 1978, for example, were only marginally less for Scotland (82 per cent) than for England and Wales (88 per cent), although Scotland had a sharper growth in the prison population – 50 per cent compared with 38 per cent. Whether this staff increase was accompanied by a decline in prison regimes cannot very clearly be ascertained: the Annual Reports *Prisons in Scotland*, give remarkably little information and there appears to be no published research for Scotland on the subject. However, it is clear from *Custody and Care* (Scottish Office 1988a) that the Scottish Service considered there to be scope for improvement.

Although there are no historical data available on which to compare the two systems, some research on Scottish regimes was commissioned in the wake of *Custody and Care*. The work was carried out by Jon Vagg but has unfortunately not been published. However, it is clear from the draft interim report (Vagg n.d.), that the data offer few, if any, points of direct comparison with similar work conducted in England and Wales. The National Prison Survey (NPS) (Office of Population Censuses and Surveys 1992; see Walmsley, *et al.* 1992) now provides some interesting additional data for England and Wales, but comparison of the data from different sources is not straightforward.[2]

It is clear that the Scottish prison system suffers less from overcrowding than its counterpart in England and Wales. In 1987 the official overcrowding in England and Wales stood at 113.2 per cent (population over 'certified normal accommodation' – CNA) although this concealed wide discrepancies between the grossly crowded local prisons and remand centres on the one hand and the under-used open prisons and institutions for young offenders on the other: all told, 30 per cent of the total prison population were 'three'd up' and a further 10 per cent doubled up in cells designed for one. By the time of the National Prison Survey, conducted in January and February 1991, 1,812 prisoners were three'd up and 11,286 were two to a cell. Unconvicted inmates were most overcrowded – only 18 per cent had a cell to themselves (Walmsley, *et al.* 1992, p. 22). In 1988 – after the Scots had ironed out the worst mismatches between the designations of institutions and the categorisation of prisoners in a process engagingly referred to by all concerned as 'Grand Design' – Vagg reports that the total population was only 5,215 as against a design capacity of 5,759 places. Even after allowing for some remaining mismatches in various institutions only just over a hundred prisoners (less than 2.5 per cent of the population) were 'three'd up' (Vagg n.d., ch. 2, p. 5).

With regard to sanitation it is hard to make comparisons using available data. Vagg found very wide variations amongst the 129 separate 'regime units' he identified in the availability of sluices (he did not count WCs), wash basins and showers. Some rather uncertain comparisons *could* be made with King and McDermott's (1989) study of five representative prisons in the Midland Region of England and Wales, but so much depends on the peculiarities of the penal estate in the two systems that generalisation would be hazardous. Perhaps all that can be said here is that the less crowded state of the Scottish system, other things being equal, is likely to put less of a strain on sanitary facilities. The NPS found that 54 per cent of prisoners wanted a WC in their cell but better food, access to telephones, canteen, information on reception, TV in cell and visits were seen as more important improvements (Walmsley, *et al.* 1992, p. 33).

One major difference between the prison systems in Scotland, and England and Wales is that the former has relied much more on 'progressive systems' to reward good behaviour through variations in regimes, both between different prisons and between different units within the same institution. As a result it would seem likely that more prisoners in Scotland eat their meals in association than in England and Wales where associated dining had been largely phased out except in the lowest security establishments. The NPS records that 31 per cent of prisoners ate in association (Walmsley, *et al.* 1992, p. 27). Ironically CRC looked towards better progression through the prison system in terms of privileges and so on, whereas *Opportunity and Responsibility* sets its face against it in favour of raising the threshold of basic amenities and services.

Vagg collected no data on work that could be related back to the identified regime units. However, it is possible to make some comparisons about the employment of prisoners in the two systems from figures published in the Annual Reports and which are reproduced in Table 2.1.

Table 2.1 Employment of prisoners in Scotland, and England and Wales

	Scotland (1990–1)		*England and Wales (1988)*	
	No.	*%*	*No.*	*%*
Industry, farms, etc.	1,974	40.2	9,960	21.1
Works, kitchen, cleaners	1,538	31.3	13,820	29.3
Training and vocational	268	5.5	2,660	5.6
TFF/pre-release	42	0.9	560	1.2
Full-time education	0	0.0	5,480	11.6
Unoccupied	1,093	22.2	14,730	31.2
Average Daily Population	4,915	100.0	47,210	100.0

Source: For Scottish data, Scottish Office (1991, p. 31); for England and Wales, Home Office (1989f, Table 10.1, p. 146). Figures for England and Wales either not published, or published in different form for subsequent years.
Note: Data include all prisoners, male and female, convicted and unconvicted. Figures for unoccupied include those not available for occupation as well as those who are available but effectively unemployed.

It can be seen from Table 2.1 that the Scots rely much more heavily on industrial workshops, farms and gardens with 40.2 per cent of their population so occupied as against 21.1 per cent in England and Wales. The proportions employed in works, domestic activities and kitchens are similar, as are those for prisoners engaged on training courses and pre-release or training for freedom schemes. There are, however, major reported differences in the numbers of unoccupied (31.3 per cent for England and Wales against 22.2 per cent for Scotland) and for those in full-time education (11.6 per cent for England and Wales against no reported figure for Scotland). There are clearly many Scottish prisoners engaged in educational activities – the most recent Annual Report, for example, cites 882 prisoners who were entered for external examinations – but it is not clear where these are included in the statistical returns. It seems evident that the accelerating decline in workshop-based and similar employments, which has been such a feature of the system in England and Wales (from 47.8 per cent in 1968 to 43.7 per cent in 1978 and 21.1 per cent in 1988), and a partly compensating growth in daytime education (from zero in 1968 to 2.4 per cent in 1978 and 11.6 per cent in 1988), has not occurred, or has been less marked, in Scotland. The available data do not indicate whether the Scottish system contains the same 'padding' – where hugely under-employed prisoners are nominally assigned to workshops or cleaners – which was once so blatant, and to some extent is still apparent, in England and Wales. The NPS records that 59 per cent of prisoners said that they did some work: 23 per cent were employed as cleaners; 20 per cent were in workshops; and 14 per cent were involved in preparing and serving meals.

Unfortunately Vagg offers no data on either hours out of cell, or hours in employment which between them would probably give a better shorthand indication of the nature of prison regimes than any other variables. Instead he gives details of time spent in associated recreational activity. On average, in the 83 'normal' regime units (the other 46 regime units were in one way or another 'special') prisoners had 17 hours of associated recreation per week. For units with convicted adult offenders this rose to 22 hours per week and for units with untried adults or with young offenders it fell to 14 hours a week. Presumably, where prisoners had no employment, this associated recreation was the only time they had out of cells, and if that assumption is correct it matches the bleakest situation to be found in England and Wales. But these average figures masked wide variations from as much as 50 hours in some units with enhanced regimes to virtually zero in some (post-rioting) restricted regimes and segregation units.

Once again it is extremely hard to make comparisons with the findings from King and McDermott's (1989) study, partly because Vagg appears to have included only formally timetabled associated recreation whereas King and McDermott regarded all time out of cells, which was not spent at work or in education, as association. More importantly Vagg provides only weekly figures (including, but not differentiating, weekends) whereas King and McDermott give daily figures (excluding weekends). Perhaps the safest assumption, given the problems with the data, might be that as far as convicted prisoners are concerned, prisoners in the enhanced regime units of the Scottish system probably get more associated activity than their counterparts in England and Wales, whereas those in the ordinary or restricted regime units probably get less. Perth prisoners, for example, could progress from 18.75 hours a week in C and D halls through to 39.25 hours per week in E hall: most prisoners in Nottingham (the nearest comparator from King and McDermott's study) would get around 35 hours a week of non-work association. The NPS found that the prison population as a whole spent an average of 14 hours locked up on the day before the interview took place, 2 hours longer than Prison Service policy and 5 hours longer than specified in the contract for the Wolds, Britain's first prison contracted out to private management (Walmsley, *et al.* 1992, p. 24).

Further comparisons are possible by drawing on the results of a survey carried out for the Central Research Unit of the Scottish Office by Wozniak and McAllister (1991) and some hitherto unpublished findings from the King and McDermott study (together with some reference to the NPS). However, important methodological differences between the studies of Wozniak and McAllister, and King and McDermott mean that the comparisons have to be treated with some caution. The work of King and McDermott was carried out between 1985 and 1987 in just five prisons, although they were chosen to be representative of the adult prison system for males in England and Wales. The Wozniak and McAllister study involved an attempted census coverage of all staff and prisoners in the Scottish system carried out in 1990 and 1991. King and McDermott's work was conducted on the basis of long periods of participant observation in each of the prisons and the researchers were at pains to identify themselves as independent of the Prison Service. They also made extensive use of tape-recorded interviews, although the data reported here were drawn from self-completion questionnaires which were targeted at all the staff on duty and all the prisoners in custody on a given day at the end of the fieldwork in each establishment. The Wozniak and McAllister study relied exclusively on self-completion questionnaires administered by research personnel who were presumably identifiable, if not necessarily identified, as part of the system.[3]

The overall response rates for the studies by King and McDermott and Wozniak and McAllister were broadly similar but there were differences in response rates from prison to prison. King and McDermott's published data make prison by prison comparisons and show distinctively different patterns of regime and ratings of regime variables in different prisons (King and McDermott 1989, 1990b, 1992; McDermott and King 1989). In contrast the Wozniak and McAllister data so far only relate to the total sample (Wozniak and McAllister 1991). Therefore when one compares these English and Scottish studies, it is only possible to compare aggregated data for the two systems, ignoring any differences between prisons. A further warning is required. Although there is considerable overlap between the studies in the variables addressed there may be important variations in the wording of questions and in the range of possible answers. Thus many questions invited the respondent to rate services and facilities on a scale of 'goodness' and 'badness': however Wozniak and McAllister used a five-point scale with a middle category that allowed respondents to indicate the service was 'OK', whereas King and McDermott restricted their respondents to choices of 'very little' or 'quite good' and 'rather bad' or 'very bad'. Nevertheless one has to make the best of what is available and in the comparisons which follow attention is focused largely upon staff and prisoners in the two systems who were prepared to rate their experience as 'rather bad' or 'very bad'. On this basis, and for all the variables on which it is possible to make comparisons, Scottish prisoners rated their experience more highly or at least no worse than did prisoners in England and Wales. There are several areas where it seems likely that these responses (with all their limitations) reflect real differences in regime (or at least real differences in expectations of what the regime should be). Thus only 35 per cent of Scottish prisoners compared to 63 per cent of English prisoners considered the state of their clothing to be 'poor' or 'very poor'. And whereas 47 per cent of Scottish prisoners thought that facilities for recreation, indoor and outdoor exercise were 'fairly bad' or 'very bad', some 59 per cent of the English prisoners rated indoor exercise and recreation as 'bad' or 'very bad', and 63 per cent regarded outdoor exercise and recreation in these ways. A little more than a third of the prisoners in the Scottish system (37 per cent) gave negative responses on the conditions of their toilets and showers compared with 45 per cent of the English prisoners who thought their showers to be poor, and 49 per cent who thought the same about the toilets. It is possible that prisoners in the two studies were responding to somewhat different modalities of these variables, but the differences appear to be sufficiently large to indicate real differences. On the other hand there was very little difference in the proportions rating food negatively (Scotland 64 per cent, England 65 per cent) or the canteen (Scotland 51 per cent, England 55 per cent). Unfortunately the reported data relating to visits and relationships with the outside world were collected in ways that do not permit direct or meaningful comparisons.

The NPS asked prisoners to rate aspects of their regime as 'good', 'bad' or 'no opinion'. Only 13 per cent rated the food as good; 51 per cent said it was 'bad'; and 36 per cent had 'no opinion'. More than a third (38 per cent) had a 'bad' opinion of the provision of underclothing, while 45 per cent expressed 'no opinion'. No ratings were given on the other variables.

With regard to the various services on offer the differences in ratings between the Scottish and English prisoners were apparently quite small – except in relation to the chaplaincy. Although the vast majority of prisoners in both systems appeared to rate the chaplaincy favourably, nearly twice as many English prisoners (24 per cent) as Scottish prisoners (13 per cent) rated it negatively. Again most prisoners were relatively positive in their views of education with only a fifth of the Scots and a quarter of the English prisoners rating it as bad or very bad. In both cases about a third of prisoners expressed negative views of social work and welfare services, but in both systems it was the medical service about which most prisoners expressed dissatisfaction – 57 per cent in Scotland and 62 per cent in England and Wales (the NPS confirmed prisoners' positive views of education).

One of the most striking differences, however, between the two earlier surveys was that relatively speaking, many fewer prisoners in Scotland expressed negative views about their relationships with hall officers – 16 per cent in Scotland thought these relationships were tense or very tense, compared to 35 per cent in England and Wales describing their relationships as poor or very poor. In both services the relationships between prisoners and governor grades were seen as being worse than with hall officers, but again the situation was less bad in Scotland where 27 per cent thought relationships with hall governors were tense or very tense, and 28 per cent thought the same with regard to other governor grades. In the research by King and McDermott no distinction between different governor grades was drawn for this purpose, but 48 per cent thought the relationship was bad or very bad. The NPS asked similar questions but received significantly different responses: 41 per cent said that their relationships with officers were 'good' and only 9 per cent described them as 'bad'. Sixty-one per cent said they never saw the governor but relations with governors were described as 'good' by 19 per cent and 'bad' by 9 per cent.

Fewer comparisons are possible on the basis of published data in relation to staff responses. Intriguingly Scottish prison officers were more critical of their mess facilities, with 69 per cent describing them as poor or very poor compared with 32 per cent south of the border; and 70 per cent of the Scots felt the same about facilities for relaxation compared with 58 per cent of their English counterparts (King and McDermott 1991). In spite of this Scottish prison officers were much more positive towards Fresh Start, with 54 per cent claiming that it had improved their job compared with only 38 per cent who took this view in England and Wales. Relationships between officers and governor grades seemed to be better in Scotland – with only 25 per cent compared with 44 per cent in England and Wales complaining of poor relationships. It is not possible to make a point for point comparison on relationships with the various specialist grades, but overall there does not appear to be much difference between the two systems. Very few staff were prepared to rate their relationships with fellow officers as being poor, though once again more did so in England and Wales (12 per cent) than in Scotland (4 per cent).

These data do not, of course, provide objective measures of the actual state of regime activities and facilities in the two systems. They do suggest, however, that if these qualitative ratings in Scotland have the same kind of relationship to regime factors as has been found in England and Wales (King and McDermott 1989) then the situation in Scotland might not have deteriorated to quite the same extent as had been the case in England and Wales. Nevertheless, it is clear that both systems now recognise there is a need for dramatic change. How, then, do they respectively address the problem of improving regimes? And with what prospects of success? It is to these matters that I now turn.

OPPORTUNITY AND RESPONSIBILITY: CUSTODY CARE AND JUSTICE – THE WAY AHEAD?

In reviewing the prospects for the future, space precludes a fully worked out analysis. In what follows I can do no more than try to catch a few of the straws in the wind.

Although it could be argued that at various points there is a significant glossing of the Woolf proposals in *Custody, Care and Justice* (Home Office 1991a), the White Paper was probably more faithful to the spirit of Woolf than commentators expected (King 1991). Subject to the more systematic analysis throughout this volume, the initial concerns were centrally with the failure to take on Woolf's seventh recommendation – for a new rule limiting the numbers of prisoners in each prison to the level of certified accommodation – and the failure, except in regard to sanitation, to provide a timetable for implementation. The main questions were thus whether the resources would actually be provided to accomplish change and, if so, when.

Two issues continue fundamentally to cloud the horizon with respect to implementing the White Paper: the first concerns the law and order context within which Woolf has been received, and the second involves the legacy of industrial relations disputes. From the outset of events at Strangeways the tenor of the public pronouncements by ministers was, to say the least, shrill. Perhaps that was not surprising when the issues were shown live each night on television. But when the Woolf Report was published Kenneth Baker spoke first and at length to the House of Commons about the minority of destructive prisoners and the need for a 'new deterrent' – the irrelevant and unnecessary offence of 'prison mutiny' – as well as the many and various improvements to security and equipment to be put in place before addressing the central matters raised in Woolf's diagnosis and recommendations. No doubt this could be dismissed as necessary political window-dressing – a diverting sideshow for the backwoodsmen before the administration could set its hand to the main event of penal reform. If so, it has been an act meticulously sustained. Thus at the PRT Conference in London in July 1991, at the height of speculation as to what the White Paper could contain, Kenneth Baker first trumpeted the vast prison-building programme since the May Report as a major government accomplishment before going on to indicate, rather residually, seemingly reluctantly and somewhat bleakly – or so it seemed to the audience – that Woolf had set an agenda that would occupy us for the next quarter of a century (Baker 1991).

Moreover, there is no mistaking the conditional nature of the reform package embodied in *Custody, Care and Justice.* In the Introduction it is made clear that the provision of new resources 'will depend on the effectiveness with which the Prison Service makes use of its existing resources and on what the country can afford' (Home Office 1991a, p. 4). Woolf, of course, had catalogued the appalling state of relationships at just about every level to do with prisons as being at the heart of the problems of the service. Indeed, at a conference held at All Souls College, Oxford, he indicated that he had considered organising his whole report around the theme of relationships – those between ministers and the Service were too close, between headquarters and establishments and governors and prison officers too bad, between prison officers and prisoners too unfortunate, and between prisoners and their families, and prisons and the rest of the Criminal Justice System they were too lacking. Most of these areas, of course, get attention in various parts of the White Paper. But in case there should be any mistaken belief that through Fresh Start the Prison Service was to be allowed to put the troubled history of industrial relations behind it, the identity of the 'real' culprit is spelled out in the fourth chapter. Although the chapter begins with the statement that the staff of the Prison Service are its 'most valuable asset' it ends with the assertion that without a sea change in industrial relations 'there can be no assurance that the resources devoted to the Prison Service will be used effectively and efficiently in a way which fulfils the obligations of the Prison Service' (Home Office 1991a, paras. 4.1, 4.25). In the immediately preceding paragraphs the 'pit bulls' of the Prison Service unions are called upon to make a commitment to match that of the Government. The Government is simply construed as standing 'ready to play its part' – without any reference to its own Rottweiler pedigree in these matters.

Nevertheless, the Woolf package and the way it is embraced by the White Paper is comprehensive and impressively detailed. One has to suppose that its substantive programme for reform will outlast the ephemeral political and industrial relations context in which it was born.

From these points of view the situation in Scotland looks much better. Both *Opportunity and Responsibility* and the commentary accompanying its introduction were remarkably free of either the invective against prisoners or the undercurrent against staff which has been seen south of the border. Instead the focus was squarely upon how to balance the various forces that impinge upon the Scottish prison system in such a way that the 'mutual responsibilities of the prisoner and the prison authorities' are fully recognised (Scottish Office 1990, p. 4). As a document and a programme for reform, however, it is neither comprehensive nor detailed, contenting itself more with principles than with practice. It must be repeated that some licence is involved in making direct comparisons between *Opportunity and Responsibility* and *Custody, Care and Justice* – the former was limited to long-term imprisonment even though it was hoped that its underlying principles would be applied across the system as a whole in due course (Scottish Office 1990, p. 64). And it did not have the authoritative weight of a report such as Woolf's behind it. It is not surprising, therefore, that there are important omissions.

One such omission concerns staffing. The welcome absence of raking over the embers of industrial disputes in Scotland is unfortunately part of a general absence of *any* discussion about staffing. It would appear from the evidence adduced earlier that Scottish prison officers are more positive towards Fresh Start than those in England and Wales and seem to enjoy better relationships with each other, with governor grades and with prisoners. Nevertheless it has to be axiomatic that the provision of a decent quality of life for prisoners will require the fullest support of prison staff at all levels. At a recent series of workshops with senior managers in the Scottish Prison Service, the point was forcefully made that any attempt to deliver a high quality package for prisoners without attention also being given to raising the quality of life for staff would be fraught with difficulties. That such a point was made in the course of a training programme which will extend across all grades of the service, however, suggests that at least this will be kept at the top of the Scottish agenda.

When the dust settles there will be no mistaking that *Opportunity and Responsibility*, the Woolf Report, and *Custody, Care and Justice* are all essentially about redrawing the balance of potentially conflicting forces within prison systems. What was essential for Woolf was the need to temper the traditional concerns about 'security' and 'control' with an equal concern for 'justice' – indeed to insist that the maintenance of security and control were actually predicated upon the prior existence of a proper sense of 'justice' (Woolf 1991, paras. 1.148–1.151). It is clear that for Woolf 'justice' embraces a number of things: treating prisoners with fairness, humanity and respect (including the provision of decent facilities and programmes) as well as the notion of due process. In the White Paper, Woolf's concerns with security and control were more loosely subsumed under the generalised notion of 'custody' whilst some of the matters which Woolf had included under the umbrella of 'justice' were (helpfully it has to be said) separated out under the heading of 'care'. In Scotland, a central chapter of *Opportunity and Responsibility* addresses the need to hold in balance the respective drives towards greater 'security', the maintenance of 'order' and the provision of better 'regimes'. There is hardly a mention of 'justice' in *Opportunity and Responsibility* though it should be noted that with the adoption of Woolf's recommendation that Boards of Visitors should no longer adjudicate, the disciplinary system in England and Wales becomes 'more closely akin' to that already in place in Scotland (Home Office 1991a, para. 8.9).

Whilst there are important and subtle differences of inflection in the way the ideas are expressed, all three reports are identifiably products of their age. All look to the world outside prison as a comparative base for normalising life inside; all stress the need to provide greater opportunities for prisoners with staff playing a facilitative role; all look towards the assumption of greater responsibility by prisoners – although it is only in Scotland that the concept of the 'responsible prisoner' is worked out and placed centre stage. All of them use as reference points, albeit for different parts of their respective analyses, aspects of market situations – Woolf and the White Paper in their taking up of the concepts of 'contracts' and 'compacts' for the delivery of services, whilst the Scottish Prison Service eschews contracts but effectively goes still further in its subsequent development of the concept of responsible prisoners as customers and consumers of services for which the authorities are providers.

The assumption that the product of this analysis is somehow in everyone's best interests is enshrined in the White Paper's assertion not only that it reflects 'the relevant principles for better public service identified in the Government's recent White Paper "The Citizen's Charter"' but also that prisoners too 'remain citizens even though they have been charged with or convicted of committing an offence' (Home Office 1991a, p. 5). Taken with a suitable pinch of salt there is, in fact, good reason to welcome a return to the Beccarian diet of responsibility and justice in prison, if only as a corrective to the ways in which what goes on in prison has too often been conceptualised with scant regard for either. But it would be as wrong now to pretend that prisoners, or for that matter much of the citizenry outside prison, were equal partners to a social contract as it was when the philosophers of the Enlightenment first suggested it. One only has to imagine the reaction to a Scottish prison governor, for example, who might be foolhardy enough to take this market analogy to its logical conclusion – by suggesting that the 'customer is always right' – to recognise that we are in a Kiplingesque world of the 'just so' story. It remains easy to see how prisoners will be taken to task for not keeping their part of the express or implied bargains – but how effective their remedies will be for failures to deliver on the part of the authorities remains very much to be seen.

Leaving aside the fact that the recognition of prisoners' citizenship rights has been the outcome of a struggle, the suggestion that prisoners will best acquire a sense of responsibility when they have meaningful opportunities to exercise it, can and should become a powerful lever for change. But it is intriguing that there is a major difference as to how the ideals of *Opportunity and Responsibility* and *Custody, Care and Justice* are to be achieved, a difference which seems to characterise the current styles of the two prison systems. In Scotland the approach now emphasises strategic planning, but allows, so far as is possible, prisoners, staff and managers to set their objectives within that broad framework. In England and Wales the approach is much more legalistic and bureaucratically managed. The White Paper accepted Woolf's recommendation that the already evolving system of contracts between area managers and governors be extended both upwards to regulate relations between the Director General and the Minister (Home Office 1991a, para. 3.6), and downwards to define the legitimate expectations of prisoners (para. 7.20), with the whole process subject to routine monitoring to measure performance against the contracts (para. 7.11). In time a codified set of standards, against which institutions may become accredited, may eventually be enshrined in revised Prison Rules (paras. 6.14–6.22).

One example will have to suffice to illustrate the difference of style. In Scotland one of the main instruments for breathing life into the concept of the responsible prisoner is the sentence planning initiative. Sentence planning, it will be recalled, also figured in the CRC Report and is a significant element in the White Paper dealing with programmes for prisoners. But while the White Paper, following Woolf, points to the importance of prisoners being given reasons for decisions, and being consulted more than they are on issues which affect their daily lives (Home Office 1991a, para.

7.20) it is apparent that sentence plans will be bureaucratically managed: they have already been *provided for* some categories of prisoner and will be *provided for* others (paras. 7.16, 7.19, emphasis added). It would be a pity if in England and Wales sentence planning simply provided prison officers with another opportunity to exercise control. There is certainly nothing in the documentation for England and Wales, as there assuredly is in Scotland, to suggest that each prisoner will 'share in a decision-making process relating to how he spends his sentence' (Scottish Office 1990, p. 30). There is no doubt that the Scots do intend to implement their participative style of sentence planning, one element of which – a self-completion personal-development file – is already being piloted. To the extent that this involves a shift towards the empowerment of prisoners and gives them some control over some aspects of their lives, it constitutes another modest victory for Barlinnie over the Peterhead tendency.

But it will not be easy for the Scots to deliver important and meaningful choices and it is by no means clear what will be the mechanism for ratcheting up the threshold quality of life and making relevant opportunity choices available. The Scots, it seems, have taken a very laid-back view of regime monitoring. Unlike the situation in England and Wales – where prison officers (especially principal officers) now feel that they spend more and more of their time providing performance indicators of what others think should be happening – in Scotland it may be possible for officers to spend more time actually doing what they should be doing. But whilst the outcome of regime monitoring in England and Wales needs to be treated with some caution as superiors are told what they want to hear, we should not forget that in Scotland at present it is very hard to come by any data at all about the quality of regimes.

It is just conceivable that both systems have now adopted a style of approach that is appropriate for their situation. The reduced weight of the routine monitoring process in Scotland, coupled with a greater level of participation in the strategic planning process, may be possible in a system which is small and where relationships – relatively speaking at least – are reasonably good. It may work, and if it does it could make for a greater sense of satisfaction for both staff and prisoners who will have each exercised some real responsibility. But expectations have undoubtedly been raised and the danger is that the prisoners now completing their own personal-development files will find the prison system's ability to meet their needs even more wanting than they might otherwise have done.

Whether or not that works for Scotland, there would be little prospect of it succeeding in England and Wales – the heavier emphasis on defining standards, establishing contracts and monitoring performance has been made necessary not just by the greater size and complexity of the system, but by the very absence of goodwill that has left it floundering for so long. There has to be a better chance now of improving standards than at any time in the recent past – but it may be at the cost of a more beleagured staff and a more litigious prison population.

NOTES

1 The three academics were Professor Tony Bottoms, Professor John Gunn and Professor Roy King. The present author left RAG shortly before the first RAG report was published because his involvement in field research produced a conflict of responsibilities. He was not replaced.

2 The National Prison Survey was conducted by the Office of Population Censuses and Surveys (OPCS) and was based upon a 10 per cent sample of the male population and a 20 per cent sample of women prisoners.

3 NPS interviews were conducted by OPCS researchers.

3

CONDITIONS AND STANDARDS

Silvia Casale

INTRODUCTION

The Woolf Report presents a broad vision of what prisons ought to be like for those who live and work in them. The approach rests on twelve central recommendations, reproduced in the Introduction to this volume, which encompass a number of interrelated issues that define the quality of life in prisons (Woolf 1991, para. 1.167).

The following critical analysis of the Woolf recommendations as they relate to prison conditions is in no way intended to detract from the achievement of the Woolf Report which marks a milestone in prison history. It is the result of the first really open inquiry into the underlying causes of unrest in the prison system. This chapter is concerned with prison conditions. It uses the term to mean more than the physical environment of prison establishments. Prison conditions are not made up merely of the bricks and mortar of prison buildings. They are the product of the physical environment of a prison and the uses made of that environment.

A cell thirteen feet long by seven feet wide by eight feet high, with no running water and small high barred windows (as in many cells at Strangeways at the time of the riot) is a poor physical environment for living. If prisoners have to share that environment 'locked up for excessive periods of time' without access to integral sanitation, it is true to say, as the Woolf Report did of Strangeways, that 'conditions within the prison were still of a wholly unacceptable standard' (para. 3.55). When the European 'inspectors' visited Brixton, Leeds and Wandsworth in 1990 they concluded that:

> the cumulative effect of overcrowding, lack of integral sanitation and inadequate regimes amounts to inhuman and degrading treatment.
> (Council of Europe 1991, para. 57)

The Woolf Report recognises that poor prison conditions degrade both prisoners and staff. They erode professionalism, tolerance and human relations. While conditions are not the sole explanations of unrest, when conditions and regimes both deteriorate, relations within prisons break down. Unrest may be seen as a symptom of that breakdown. Relatively small changes for the worse can trigger a seemingly disproportionate reaction. The impact of poor conditions depends on the degree to which prisoners are subjected to them without alleviation. Mobility, activity, time out of cell, access to showers and changes of kit are aspects of regime which may alleviate the effects of poor environment.

Over the years the debate has tended to focus on certain aspects of prison conditions – notably slopping out and overcrowding. The latter has become a watchword for all that is wrong with the prison system. This oversimplification ignores both prisoners' willingness to tolerate degrees of overcrowding in preference to dislocation (allocation to a prison far from home) and examples of establishments with a positive ethos despite overcrowding. The following discussion examines the Woolf recommendations with respect to these and other aspects of prison conditions. Some of the central recommendations of the Woolf Report deal specifically with conditions, while others have indirect implications for the prison environment. This chapter will consider in detail the three recommendations in the Woolf Report most directly concerned with prison conditions:

— the timetable for providing access to sanitation;
— the new Prison Rule to limit overcrowding;
— the national Accredited Standards.

ACCESS TO SANITATION

The Chief Inspector of Prisons has focused public attention on the question of prison sanitation and hastened the long overdue end of slopping out (Home Office 1989g). This most conspicuous 'symptom of an archaic prison system' (Woolf 1991, para. 1.192) has for years been the subject of severe criticism from inside and outside the prison system with limited effect.

The Government has undertaken to provide access to sanitation at all times for all prisoners by 1994 (Home Secretary's announcement of February 1991). The White Paper *Custody, Care and Justice* confirmed this commitment and the deadline of the end of December 1994 (Home Office 1991a, para. 6.8). The fact that this should have happened years ago does not mean that it is not still a major achievement. It marks a great step forward in eliminating the squalor of prison life for prisoners and prison officers. The refurbishment programme is 'the clearest signal possible that the Prison Service is to be committed to bringing the prison system up to acceptable and just standards' (Woolf 1991, para. 1.193).

The Prison Service has been committed to an extensive programme of refurbishment but this has been somewhat changed by the promise given by Kenneth Baker, then Home Secretary, to end slopping out by 1994. A good example of prison refurbishment can be found at Stafford, a Victorian prison where integral sanitation is provided by elaborate reorganisation of the accommodation space. In the rows of cells on the landings, the middle cell of every three neighbouring cells has been taken out of use as living accommodation, divided in two and converted into two toilet/washrooms, with access from the adjoining cell. The result is an 'en suite' room with a sink and lavatory for each remaining cell providing living accommodation. This model provides a higher standard of physical environment than other options currently used in the refurbishment programme.

However, the installation of integral sanitation cannot await full refurbishment. While the programme of refurbishment is an opportunity to bring the physical environment in prisons up to an acceptable standard and so establish a firm basis for decent prison conditions, sanitation focuses on one condition only. The model predominantly chosen for the refurbishment programme eliminates slopping out by providing a lavatory and sink in the already small existing prison cell. Even when there is a screen of sorts, the prison cell becomes in effect a toilet. This model compares unfavourably with the Stafford model: there are obvious problems of hygiene and odour.

It is not an ideal environment when one prisoner is living in the toilet, but when prisoners share the cell, the living conditions are inadequate. The short-term effect of refurbishing and installing sanitation is to increase cell sharing, as cells are temporarily removed from use. When the work is accomplished the living area of the cell is diminished by the space taken out for the toilet area. Many of the cells were below the space standard required for double cells in new prison buildings even before the refurbishment work. Where a lavatory is simply installed in an existing cell it is clearly unacceptable for that cell to be certified for more than one inmate.

One of the risks associated with all models of refurbishment is short-term overcrowding, as cells are taken out of use for modernisation. The more serious problem of continued reliance on cell sharing as the norm is exacerbated in the Stafford model by the fact that the conversion of three cells into two with integral sanitation reduces the total number of cells available as living accommodation by one third (Casale and Plotnikoff 1989). There is also the danger that once the physical amenities are provided, prisoners will be assumed automatically to have a better quality of life. If prisoners lose even the minimal activity and contact with other people necessitated by slopping out, life in prison may become more sterile, in more senses than one.

The installation of lavatories in cells is only one route, and a capital intensive one, towards providing all prisoners with modern sanitary conditions. Another is to allow prisoners out of their cells when they need access to sanitation. This has cost implications of a different kind. Clearly it involves some capital outlay to improve communal sanitary facilities: this would entail modernising and extending the existing recesses which are frequently inadequate for the size of the prisoner populations they serve. However, the biggest potential costs lie in the staffing levels needed to ensure access at all times. At night, the problem is hard to solve except by increases in staff, use of mechanical unlocking systems or a change in policy and practice concerning locking cells at night for some categories of prisoner.

It is important to consider the implications of constant access to sanitation in relation to regime provision generally. Where prisoners are afforded the opportunity to participate in a full daytime schedule of activities, access to sanitation during the day is provided almost automatically during activity time, without additional staffing to unlock and escort. This happens in most training prisons but only to a limited extent in local prisons. Prisoners taking part in classes may have access to sanitation in the education department. Moreover, physical education usually provides an opportunity not only for use of the toilet but also of showers; sometimes this is even linked in to kit change. The relatively low staff to prisoner ratio generally accepted for physical education makes it a particularly useful means of enhancing conditions as well as activity.

Regime developments have important implications for conditions. The current focus on regimes is an opportunity to manage both activity and conditions in imaginative new ways to the improvement of both.

REGULATION OF OVERCROWDING

It is important to view the recommendations of the Woolf Report together. The recommendation for provision of access to sanitation must be read in conjunction with the proposal for a new Prison Rule to limit overcrowding. The vision behind these two recommendations is the creation of a decent environment to be used by a reasonable number of people – the foundation of good conditions.

The proposed Prison Rule limiting use of accommodation seems at first glance a radical innovation today, when CNA (the certified normal accommodation level for a particular establishment, which indicates how many prisoners it is designated to hold without overcrowding) has ceased to have much bearing on reality. However, the Woolf Report is in effect restating an existing principle: a prison should normally be occupied under its CNA.

The new terminology of 'normal occupancy' has supplanted CNA as a working guide to levels of accommodation. This is not because the accommodation has changed. Time has only caused the often ancient plant of the prison system to deteriorate and previous programmes of refurbishment have not kept pace with that decline. The building programme has not kept pace with growing numbers. 'Normal occupancy' has come into use because the Prison Service has lived so long with overcrowding that CNA has become irrelevant to day-to-day operations. Expectations have shifted. Normal occupancy is a euphemism: it stands for a prison establishment's customary level of overcrowding.

The Woolf recommendation marks a return to the concept of CNA. To ensure that the principle is applied, Woolf urged a new Prison Rule to be in force by the end of 1992 requiring every establishment to keep within its CNA, except for temporary fluctuation to the extent of 3 per cent over CNA for not more than one week in any quarter (Woolf 1991, para. 1.190). Parliament would have to be apprised of any departure from this rule. This places a limit on the capacity of individual establishments but does not deal with what happens to excess population.

Taken together with other measures, this is intended to provide a way out of the perennial problem of overcrowding. However, as a mechanism focused on prisons, it ignores the importance of sentencing practice in determining the size of the prison population. The Woolf Report does discuss the need to 'reduce the prison population to an unavoidable minimum' (para. 10.70) and specifies groups of people who might be diverted from custody, including remand prisoners, fine defaulters and mentally disordered offenders. However, it does not include in its brief the sentencing process.

What happens if the courts consistently commit more people to prison than the total of CNA of all prison establishments combined? Are the extra prisoners to be held in police or court cells? On 31 March 1991 such facilities held 767 prisoners (NACRO 1991d) in accommodation designed for short-term stay and offering wholly inadequate conditions for long-term imprisonment. Alternatively, is there to be an endless prison-building programme to meet the demand created by the courts? Several organisations giving evidence to the Woolf Inquiry stressed the dangers of continual expansion and the tendency of the courts to fill whatever prison places are available. The consensus seems to be that prison building is an ineffective means of reducing overcrowding; it merely results in moving the goal posts.

> We share forcefully the wish . . . to see a reduction in the prison population, but we cannot accept the implication that this should be achieved at the expense of proper conditions for prisoners and staff.
>
> (Woolf 1991, para. 11.4)

The Woolf Report's endorsement of the prison-building programme must be taken together with the recommendation for a new Prison Rule to limit overcrowding. The new buildings are viewed as replacements for dilapidated plant and as a means of eliminating existing overcrowding.

Whether or not the proposed new Prison Rule could represent a workable mechanism to eliminate overcrowding appears, in the wake of the White Paper, *Custody, Care and Justice*, unlikely to be tested in practice. The

White Paper affirmed that one of the Prison Service's priorities should be to end overcrowding (Home Office 1991a, para. 1.34). It also devoted considerable attention (Home Office 1991a, ch. 5) to the question of reducing overcrowding by flexible use of the prison estate and to the problems of balancing this approach with the need to hold different types of prisoners separately and to locate prisoners near home.

The White Paper does not, however, accept the recommendation in the Woolf Report concerning CNA. Although the White Paper refers to the Criminal Justice Act 1991 as taking forward government policy to promote community penalties and stresses that 'a custodial sentence should be used only to punish the most serious offences' (Home Office 1991a, para. 1.6), it also reiterates the Prison Service's obligation to implement the court's decision by keeping the prisoner in custody (para. 1.21). This appears to allow little scope for dealing with overcrowding. It would seem to rule out mechanisms for adjusting the prisoner population to a reasonable ceiling corresponding to the number of places available. One such mechanism is a periodic balancing of release and intake of prisoners, based on a determination of which individuals might return to the community with least risk to the public, but this would require legislation.

The English system already incorporates discretion to adjust the prison population. Parole is an obvious example. It may be that it is not for the Prison Service to decide whom it will receive and release. However, it is time to recognise that overcrowding will not disappear for good unless processes are introduced with the specific aim of readjusting the level of the prison population created by remand and sentence decisions.

The White Paper's considered opinion 'that the prison system is in sight of providing sufficient places to match the average size of the prison population' is predicated upon two large conditions: 'Subject to the sentencing decisions of the courts and, in particular, to the effects of the Criminal Justice Act 1991' (Home Office 1991a, para. 6.12). During 1992 there was a sharp fall in the prison population: down from 47,055 on 1 October 1991 to 45,918 on 1 October 1992. Moreover, since the Criminal Justice Act came into force in October 1992, the first few months of its operation witnessed a substantial drop in the prison population: from 46,120 on 27 September 1992 to 42,255 on 18 December 1992. A change in Home Secretary, and complaints about parts of the Criminal Justice Act by a small but vocal group of sentencers has led the Government to review implementation of the Act. By the spring of 1993 the prison population has begun to rise again.

As the Woolf Report implies in its discussion of reducing the prison population, there are already more people in prison than belong there. It has been argued many times that the prison system cannot improve if it continues to be used without restraint as a dumping ground for the social, health and criminal justice systems. The fact that this area was not part of the Woolf brief was a serious limitation. The Prison Rule on restriction to CNA cannot stand alone, even if it were politically acceptable. Its efficacy is linked to assumptions about changes in sentencing, as are the White Paper's statement about the priority to end overcrowding. It is, however, questionable whether the 1991 Criminal Justice Act will be able to sustain its apparent reductivist influence over sentencers' decision-making in the medium and long term.

ACCREDITED STANDARDS

Apart from the focus on sanitation and overcrowding, the Woolf Report recommends other changes which have major implications for prison conditions. Chief among these is the recommendation for a system of standards. The Woolf Report proposes a national system of Accredited Standards with which, in time, each establishment would be required to comply and which would eventually be incorporated in the Prison Rules and so 'would be legally enforceable by judicial review' (para. 1.187). Ultimately, this process would establish nationally acceptable levels of conditions across the system which would be enforceable. The eventual goal is clear but the time frame is vague: 'For the time being, the national standards would have to be aspirational' (para. 1.187). This statement rests on a recognition of how far the system as a whole is from achieving acceptable standards. It is realistic but it compromises the potential for change.

The White Paper accepts the recommendation for standards and devotes an entire chapter to this subject. It gives a clear commitment to a code of standards concerning prison conditions and regimes 'focused directly on the service to be provided for prisoners' (Home Office 1991a, para. 6.15). This is at once a recognition of the need for standards and an acknowledgement that, for real improvement, standards must cover all elements of provision contributing to the quality of life in prison. The White Paper also gives a clear indication about the level at which standards should be set. It establishes the following general criteria: 'prisons should aim to provide decent but not lavish conditions. Conditions should be of a standard which fulfils the Prison Service's duty to provide humanely for prisoners and to preserve human dignity' (para. 6.1).

The White Paper's position on accreditation is more equivocal. It appears that the best way of signifying when standards have been met is still an open question and that whether accreditation represents the best option will be given further consideration. 'The government will consider whether a system of certificates of accreditation is the best way of signifying when the standards have been met, as the Woolf Report recommended' (Home Office 1991a, para. 6.20).

The argument for voluntary accreditation seems to be that enforceable standards cannot be established until the system is up to standard. This ignores the dynamic potential of standards as a force for change rather than as a reflection of the status quo. A system which is not in breach of standards needs them only to prevent backsliding. Although the ability of the prison system to go backwards as well as forwards should not be underestimated, this relegation of standards to the role of guarding the back door to progress is a concession to the lack of political will to speed up change in the prison system.

The White Paper agreed with the Woolf Report that enforceability 'should be considered when the standards can be met consistently in all establishments' (Home Office 1991a, para. 6.21). Logically, enforcement mechanisms would then operate to ensure no slippage of levels of achievement. The political resistance to legally enforceable standards in this country stems from hypocrisy. There is great reluctance to establish enforceable standards which parts of the system might breach. This is ironic in a prison system which daily flouts its written rules. For example, Prison Rule 3 requiring separation of unconvicted from convicted and sentenced prisoners is frequently honoured in the breach. The routine integration of unconvicted and convicted prisoners in many local prisons in this country runs counter to European Prison Rule 11 (3) and flies in the face of international law (International Covenant on Civil and Political Rights, Article 10, 2a, ratified by the United Kingdom in 1976). It seems that it is acceptable to breach written rules, and even binding international legal instruments, provided that there is no mechanism to enforce compliance. If the prison system can withstand the moral and legal pressure to comply with domestic and European prison rules and international treaty, it is doubtful whether a code of accredited standards will exert more effective pressure. The absence of an enforcement mechanism for the national standards, at least in the first instance, is a serious limitation. Accreditation is a tame process, relying on professional pride or embarrassment as a motivation for compliance.

The US federal model of accreditation, developed by the Commission for Accreditation for Corrections, involves voluntary submission by individual establishments to assessment according to a three-tier system of standards. All mandatory standards must be met before the establishment may receive accreditation; 90 per cent of essential standards must also be met and 80 per cent of important standards (American Correctional Association 1981). The accreditation process operates across the different jurisdictional divisions in the United States, where there are codes of standards at the federal, state and local levels. It serves the function of drawing together establishments in different jurisdictions on the basis of a national code, a function which does not fit in the English context where the model would require modification.

The Steering Group on Standards (of which the author is a member) was set up by the Prison Service in the autumn of 1991 to take forward the proposals in the White Paper by developing a framework for standards for the prison system through a process of discussion with all levels of the Prison Service and with outside organisations. In the course of its work, it is consulting about many of the issues raised above, as well as considering the relevance for the English context of various models of standards and accreditation.

One model is the tiered code of standards, as used in the US accreditation system. Its main advantage lies in its adaptability for establishments whose starting points on the road to standards are very different. The enormous variation in conditions and regimes across our prison system means that a single tier of standards might be pitched too low for some of the more advanced establishments or so high for others as to seem unattainable in the foreseeable future. The drawbacks of tiered standards lie in their relative complexity and in the very real danger that the bottom tier is set to reflect the status quo and is used to justify this as an acceptable level of provision, obviating the need for further progress. In our current system there is a tendency to blame failures in performance on lack of resources. That is an oversimplification which serves in some cases to mask poor management or poor staff attitudes. However, there are times when, with the best will in the world, it is impossible to achieve targets because of budgetary and other considerations beyond the governor's control. A prison establishment may receive a draft of extra prisoners because of occurrences in the system at large. There is unlikely to be a concomitant adjustment of resources. The resulting adverse effect on conditions might mean that an establishment failed to achieve standards. The process of accreditation under such circumstances would be conspicuously flawed, like a relay race in which some teams had no baton.

Whatever lessons may be learned from other jurisdictions, it would be wrong to expect too much from the analogy with the American experience of accreditation. The context is materially different. The accreditation process which has been in place in the United States for over a decade operates against a background of minimum standards at the federal, state and local level and of active judicial intervention to enforce standards. Accreditation has its place as a vehicle for professional recognition and development of good practice but it is no substitute for a system which obliges compliance.

The local, state and federal prison systems in the United States have been struggling to make minimum standards operational. The specificity of some of the American codes of standards has a direct bearing on the question of compliance. There is less room for varying interpretations, a problem besetting the European Prison Rules, whose vague wording and qualified statements of principle create loopholes and allow circumvention.

Various mechanisms to enforce compliance have emerged in the American context. In some cases the courts have actually ordered closure of substandard facilities, as in the case of the 'Tombs' detention facility in

New York City. In Texas the Federal District Court in *Ruiz* v. *Estelle* (1980) set out standards for many aspects of prison conditions and appointed monitors to investigate and report to the court on compliance. The process lasted for nine years (Deitch 1990). In some jurisdictions cases were settled by 'consent decrees', negotiated agreements for precise timetables of change in conditions at particular establishments.

There are a variety of options available for facilitating the enforcement of standards. Codes of standards may incorporate their own timetables and mechanisms for compliance. The arguments for a code of standards specifying incremental levels of prison conditions and regimes have been made before (Casale and Plotnikoff 1989).

Any system of standards, whether for voluntary accreditation or for enforceable compliance, must address the diversity in current conditions. It must be applied through a process of establishing targets and deadlines in establishments individually, and of monitoring. Such a process would force the prison system step by step and establishment by establishment to acceptable conditions.

The English system has the advantage of a Prison Inspectorate which could be adapted to the role of monitoring and commenting upon compliance. It is a role which would necessitate some changes. The current recruitment of the staff of the Inspectorate from the senior governor grades of the Prison Service and from civil servants, should be balanced by a complement of people from outside. It may not be reasonable to expect a dynamic approach to standards from a group of experts drawn solely from within the system. The process should be independent and should be seen to be so.

A disadvantage of the English system lies in the status of prisons as premises of the Crown. This confers Crown Immunity against prosecution for violations of standards applicable outside the prison system. The Woolf Report did not go so far as to advocate the abolition of Crown Immunity for prisons, but welcomed the references to equality with standards in the community made in the Prison Service bulletin 'Prison Board Priority 1991/1992 – Hygiene in Prisons' (Home Office 1991p).

The Woolf Report also describes in detail the partial lifting of Crown Immunity with respect to food hygiene. This change, which came into effect in April 1992, is a significant, though limited, step forward. In other jurisdictions, such as the United States, codes of standards for prisons stipulate that prisons should be inspected by the relevant outside authority in the area outside the prison (Casale 1984). This approach has many advantages. It uses the skills of experts in substantive areas relating to living or working conditions; it brings people from outside the prison system into the system, breaking down the barriers between the establishment and the rest of the community; and it opens up the system to external scrutiny.

In 1985, the Chief Inspector of Prisons recognised the obstacle that Crown Immunity presented to improving standards in prisons:

> If public confidence in the standards of hygiene applied to public institutions, such as prisons, is to be maintained, it may well be that the ending of Crown Immunity is the price that will have to be paid.
> (Home Office 1985c, para. 3.06)

The Steering Group on Standards has been considering *inter alia* the link between standards, governors' annual contracts and prisoners' compacts. The annual contracts between the governor of an establishment and the area manager might form the natural vehicle for planned progress towards achievement of standards. Successive contracts would address the incremental timetable for compliance through the short-term and longer-term use of the establishment's resources.

In turn the prisoner's compact might reflect the commitments in the annual contract to specified regime provision. A workable system of compacts for individual prisoners rests on the assumption of agreed levels of provision. A governor's contract would establish these within a particular establishment, whereas national standards would establish levels applicable to all prisons. Without an assumed basis of standards, compacts would become unwieldy: they would have to specify aspects of prison conditions as well as of regime and sentence planning. If compacts are predicated on the notion of an agreed level of core conditions established by a system of standards, then local compacts with individual prisoners would be confined to the fine detail of regime, i.e. the individual's access to particular facilities and to activities tailored to sentence planning.

Without the foundation of standards, emphasis on individual compacts carries the danger of fragmenting prisoners' already fragile power as a group to complain or exert pressure to improve their conditions. Monitoring or inspection of provision to prisoners based on individual compacts in the absence of standards is a less manageable mechanism for checking upon progress. There is also a risk of the excessive administrative burden of a system of contracts for each prisoner. However, the greatest risk lies in the perpetuation of inequities in the system if compacts and annual contracts operate without the framework of a national code of standards.

There are a number of other ideas put forward in the Woolf Report which have less direct, but possibly significant implications for prison conditions. The short-term options for implementing the idea of the community prison, with a variety of prisoner populations held close to home, could have a profound effect on the conditions experienced by prisoners formerly held in the training prisons. In the past, some of the worst conditions have fallen to the lot of remand prisoners and others held in local prisons. If the existing prison estate is redesignated to provide community prisons, then some of the former inmates of training prisons will find themselves in the former locals or in other prisons with a part-local function (such as Lewes or Bristol).

The principle acknowledging the importance of the separate status of remand prisoners refers specifically to separate conditions for remand prisoners (see Chapter 8). This might entail a new kind of remand centre, with entirely separate facilities and conditions governed by standards analogous to those contained in the terms for the tenders for running Wolds, the new remand establishment at Everthorpe. Alternatively, part of the community prison could be devoted to remand prisoners, with 'ring fencing' of resources.

The Woolf Report points to serious underlying difficulties in the prison system. These difficulties necessitate systematic rather than piecemeal change. The Woolf Report provides a broad vision of what the prison system and prison conditions should be like. What is missing now is the network of mechanisms to realise that vision. This chapter has tried to indicate ways in which the principles of the Woolf Report might be translated into practical mechanisms for systematic change.

4

FROM RIGHTS TO EXPECTATIONS

Genevra Richardson

PUNISHMENT AND RIGHTS

In the debate surrounding the present state of British prisons much has been made of the notion of prisoners' rights: the claim to a right can be a powerful political device. However, if the debate is to penetrate beyond rhetoric it is essential to examine more closely the nature of and justification for any claim to the existence of prisoners' rights. An individual asserts a right when she makes a claim to performance, either action or forbearance, on the part of another (Corbin 1919; Hohfeld 1919). The right is legal when the correlative duty is owed at law and moral when the duty is morally enforceable. This chapter will be based on the assumption that a core of basic or moral rights exists and that it should be reflected in law (Gerwith 1984; Pennock and Chapman, 1981).

Commentators who accept the existence of such rights, however, differ significantly as to their contents (Nozick 1974; Dworkin 1977; Campbell 1983). This uncertainty is only exacerbated when the relationship between punishment and rights is considered. While most who accept the existence of basic rights are prepared also to accept their partial loss through punishment, the extent of that loss is rarely specified. Thus the problems associated with the identification and specification of basic rights are greatly compounded when the individual possessor of those rights is the subject of punishment by the state.

In England and Wales imprisonment is the most severe form of state punishment. Individuals who are convicted of serious breaches of the criminal law are removed from the rest of society, deprived of their liberty and subjected to numerous other restraints frequently amounting to an alteration in their legal, and possibly basic, rights and obligations. If it is accepted that punishment may properly entail a loss of basic rights, then the precise extent of that loss must be dependent on the justification underlying the imposition of the punishment. Thus in principle, when the punishment is imprisonment, any alteration in a prisoner's rights, whether legal, basic, or both, can only be justified by reference to the recognised aims of imprisonment. Unfortunately the force of this statement is significantly reduced by the absence of any clear agreement as to the proper purposes of imprisonment. Nevertheless, despite this lack of agreement, it is possible to argue that no acceptable prison regime can justify the denial of all basic rights in the imprisoned: the prisoner must always retain some residue, whether the purpose of imprisonment is expressed in terms of retribution, rehabilitation, social protection or deterrence (see Richardson 1985b). Rather than favour a particular justification for imprisonment, this chapter will adopt a minimalist approach. It will argue that whatever the underlying purpose of imprisonment, that purpose can be met by the mere segregation of the prisoner from society.

Imprisonment will, thus, be regarded as justifying only the removal of those rights necessarily affected by the need to segregate, or more specifically by the need to maintain security and control. All other rights, whether legal or basic, should be retained. This approach accords well with the views of those who advocate adherence to the principles of minimum interference and normalisation within prison regimes (King and Morgan 1980). Arguably, however, the claim to rights in prisoners should not end with the recognition of a significant residue. Society, for whatever reason, has deprived prisoners of their liberty and in doing so has increased their dependence. Society thus has a duty to protect prisoners and to provide them with certain essential facilities. Whatever the merits of the debate concerning society's duty to provide such facilities to non-prisoners, it can be argued that prisoners, by virtue of their exceptional and involuntary dependence, are in a special position and are therefore entitled to additional rights against the authorities: rights for example to adequate medical, educational and recreational facilities. Finally, one further distinction needs to be made. Rights can be to substantive goods, a bed or warm clothes, for example, or they can be to a particular procedural protection, a fair hearing or the provision of reasons, for example. As will be seen, both the case law and the Woolf Report (Woolf 1991) tend to differentiate between substantive and procedural rights.

The discussion so far has centred on the notion of 'basic' rather than legal rights. In relation to prisoners there is a particularly strong case to argue that such basic rights should be reflected in the law. Legal recognition is essential to enable prisoners realistically to assert their rights. There is also an argument that the retention by prisoners of the legal rights ordinarily possessed by non-prisoners is itself a basic or moral right, encapsulated in notions of equal treatment before the law, and should be recognised as such by the law. Recognition by the law of the existence of a right does not, however, imply that the formal legal structure should be the primary mechanism for the enforcement of that right, and in the discussion that follows thought will be given to alternative enforcement mechanisms and their proper relationship with the courts.

This chapter will consider briefly the extent to which, in England and Wales, prisoners' rights are recognised by the current law, both statute and case law, and will draw some tentative conclusions concerning the attitudes of the courts to prisoners' claims. It will then consider the recommendations designed to promote justice in prisons contained in the Woolf Report, and will examine the alternative, extra-judicial mechanisms available for the protection of prisoners' legitimate interests.

THE PRESENT EXTENT OF PRISONERS' RIGHTS IN ENGLAND AND WALES

The statutory framework

Imprisonment in England and Wales is primarily governed by the Prison Act 1952. The Act, however, provides only the barest framework and certainly contains no comprehensive statement of the rights and duties of either the prison authorities or the inmates. It vests the Home Secretary with constitutional responsibility for the administration of the prison system in England and Wales and authorises him to issue rules for 'the regulation and management of prisons . . . and for the classification, treatment, employment, discipline, and control of persons required to be detained therein' (s.1 and s. 2.47). This he has done in the form of a statutory instrument, the Prison Rules 1964 and subsequent amendments.[1]

The Prison Rules are considerably more detailed than the Act, specifying, for example, the duties of Boards of Visitors and prison chaplains, listing the various offences against discipline, and laying down basic rules concerning letters and visits. They do not, however, as will be explained below, create rights in prisoners directly enforceable at private law. Indeed, although some are relatively specific, others vest considerable discretion in the governor or the Secretary of State. The Rules have therefore been supplemented by Standing Orders and Circular Instructions. The former are now published and are designed as formal statements of a prisoner's privileges and obligations, while Circular Instructions provide internal administrative guidance on specific issues and procedures.

The formal rules governing the management of prisons, whatever their constitutional status, however, do not, either singly or in combination, purport to provide a code of directly legally enforceable rights in prisoners. Indeed it is not profitable at present to search for such a code. In conformity with its traditional residual approach to such matters, the law in England and Wales chooses merely to regard the prisoner as retaining the rights possessed by non-prisoners, provided those rights are not removed by imprisonment.

In *Raymond* v. *Honey* in a speech now widely quoted to illustrate the legal status of prisoners, Lord Wilberforce stated that a prisoner 'retains all civil rights which are not taken away expressly or by necessary implication' (p. 10). At first sight this statement seems encouraging to those seeking to enhance the rights of prisoners, particularly since many of the express legal disabilities which used to attach to the prisoner have been removed. Of the few that remain section 4 of the Representation of the People Act, which effectively disenfranchises convicted prisoners, is perhaps the most significant.

Nevertheless, even on its face Lord Wilberforce's statement reveals some fundamental dificulties. In the first place, there is the incorrigible problem of identifying exactly what 'civil rights' are possessed by non-prisoners. That problem must be faced before it is possible even to start speculating on the impact of imprisonment on those rights. Second, the notion of 'necessary implication' allows extensive scope for judicial discretion in a sensitive area of public policy. Further, when set against the model for prisoners' rights discussed above, it is clear that Lord Wilberforce's statement is concerned exclusively with the retention of existing rights: no reference is made to the possibility of additional rights attaching to prisoners by virtue of their exceptional dependence.

With Lord Wilberforce's statement and the statutory background in mind, it is necessary to consider briefly the decided cases in order to obtain a clearer picture of how the assertion of rights by prisoners is in practice dealt with by the courts. It is convenient to start with the position in private law.

Private law

Duty of care

It is now well established that the prison authorities owe a duty of care to the prisoners in their custody and that prisoners are therefore entitled to compensation for injury incurred through any breach of that duty.[2] A prisoner like any other citizen has a right not to be injured through the negligence of another. In some respects the common law, in recognition of the exceptional vulnerability and dependence of prisoners, has gone further and has refined this general right in the prisoner's favour. It is now established that the authority's duty of care extends to providing one prisoner with reasonable protection against the assaults of other prisoners. Thus prisoners have a right to reasonable protection by the authorities against the intentional violence of other prisoners. Reported cases suggest, however, that the enforcement of this right by prisoners is not easy: courts appear reluctant to find a breach of duty on the part of the authorities.[3]

By contrast to the case of inter-prisoner violence, the fact of imprisonment has been used, presumably 'by necessary implication', to reduce the duty imposed on the prison authorities with regard to the provision of medical care. The prisoner's right to medical care, it seems, is inferior to that of non-prisoners. In *Knight and Others* v. *The Home Office*, a case involving the suicide of a prisoner awaiting transfer to a psychiatric unit, the High Court was unable to accept that a prison hospital was to be judged according to the standards appropriate to an ordinary psychiatric unit, despite the fact that the prison regularly contained a number of potential suicides.

Outside prison those injured at work receive special protection under the law. The law recognises that the relationship between employer and employee gives rise to special rights and duties. Within prison convicted prisoners can be required to work in prison workshops. A prisoner who is injured in the course of such work is not, however, offered the same protection as is available to other victims of 'industrial injury'. The courts have denied that the Factories Act applies to prison workshops[4] and have further denied the existence of the common-law relationship of master and servant.[5] The prisoner injured in the prison workshops has, therefore, to rely on the general principles of negligence. On the face of it the law deprives the prisoner of rights which apply to non-prisoners and does so with little justification, since there is no apparent conflict between the purposes of imprisonment and the objectives of either the Factories Act or the common-law rules. The willingness of the Home Office to provide *ex gratia* payments fails to alter that fact.

Prison conditions

The appalling physical conditions which prevail in a number of British prisons and which are discussed by Silvia Casale in Chapter 3, are well known. According to the notion of rights suggested above, a prisoner, who by definition is entirely dependent on the prison authorities for the conditions in which he or she lives, should be entitled to special rights guaranteeing an agreed minimum standard. Prisoners who have attempted to assert such rights in private law have, however, met with little success. The Prison Act 1952 does not define imprisonment nor does it specify the conditions which should prevail within a prison. Section 14 merely specifies that no cell may be used as sleeping accommodation unless it has been certified as adequate, and requires the certificate to specify the maximum number of prisoners who should be housed in each cell. Rule 23 of the Prison Rules, however, allows the maximum number to be exceeded with leave of the Secretary of State. The legal force of section 14 is thus effectively neutralised.

The failure of the primary legislation to provide any enforceable rights to minimum physical conditions is compounded by the court's attitude to the Prison Rules, which provide the most comprehensive legislative statement of the obligations of the prison authorities. While many of the Rules, such as Rule 23(2) itself, provide the authorities with considerable discretion, some are phrased in mandatory and relatively unambiguous terms, referring, for example, to a separate bed (Rule 24), or the provision of toilet articles (Rule 26). None the less the courts have denied that the Prison Rules vest prisoners with any special rights. An action for breach of statutory duty will not lie with respect to injury flowing from non-compliance with the Rules.[6] In any context the court's decision whether or not to allow an action for breach of statutory duty will be a matter of statutory interpretation and is likely to involve an assessment of the relevant policy implications. In relation to the Prison Rules those policy implications have been assessed overwhelmingly in favour of the authorities.[7] Thus, even if the conditions of a prisoner's confinement are in clear breach of the Prison Rules no action for breach of statutory duty can arise.

Thwarted by the court's attitude to the Prison Rules, prisoners have sought to use false imprisonment to challenge the lawfulness of the conditions within which they are being held. However, in *Williams* v. *The Home Office (No. 2)* Tudor Evans J held that imprisonment is justified in law by the order of the court and by section 12 of the Prison Act, and that it cannot become unlawful merely by reason of the conditions in which it is served. Until recently it might have been thought that subsequent case law concerning both prisoners and detained mental patients had slightly softened the impact of this ruling. However, the House of Lords in *R.* v. *Deputy Governor Parkhurst Prison, ex. p. Hague* has now put a stop to all such speculation. An action in false imprisonment is not available to a prisoner to challenge the conditions of his or her imprisonment.[8] None the less, their Lordships were at pains to stress that a prisoner retains the right to claim damages in negligence against the authorities in relation to any injury caused by a breach of the authority's ordinary duty of care. It remains to be seen how willing the courts will be in practice to find that duty breached.

It must be concluded from the above that the private law has generally been reluctant to uphold rights in prisoners. Residual rights have typically been restricted by a generous interpretation of the 'necessary implication[s]' of imprisonment, and additional special rights have been denied.

Public law

The dearth of support offered to prisoners by the private law has led to an increased reliance on public law. Through an application for judicial review a prisoner may claim that his or her interests have been adversely affected by the unlawful actions of the prison authorities. If such an application succeeds the unlawful, or *ultra vires*, decision or action can be quashed. Very briefly stated, a decision may be unlawful in this context if it is contrary to the express provisions of the empowering legislation, or if it involves the unreasonable exercise of discretion, or if it is taken in breach of certain procedural safeguards, namely natural justice or the duty to act fairly.[9] In certain areas of prison life the courts have been willing to use these public-law principles of legality to protect the interests of prisoners, and they have declared decisions taken in breach of the principles to be unlawful. The imposition of the public-law principles of natural justice on the prison disciplinary system, which is discussed in Chapter 5, is perhaps the best-known example of public-law intervention in prison affairs. Indeed the recognition in *R.* v. *Hull Prison Board of Vistitors, ex p. St. Germain (No. 1)* of a prisoner's right to a fair hearing can be said to have heralded the modern era of prisoner litigation. However, the assertion of public law rights by prisoners has not been limited to the disciplinary context.

Prisoners' correspondence and access to lawyers

For a person confined to prison the ability to maintain contact with the outside world is of considerable importance. Further, the ability to obtain independent legal advice is essential to the full protection of the prisoner's rights and interests. However, the relatively liberal practice which now prevails with regard to both access to lawyers and the exchange of ordinary correspondence only developed initially as a result of pressure from the courts. Two rulings by the European Court of Human Rights (ECHR), upholding a prisoner's right of access to the courts and the right to respect for correspondence,[10] supplemented by one decision of the House of Lords itself, *Raymond* v. *Honey*, and one of the Divisional Court,[11] were required before the Government finally amended the Prison Rules and Standing Orders sufficiently to bring them into compliance with the United Kingdom's obligations under the European Convention on Human Rights.

In more recent years this court-inspired liberalisation has been pursued as a matter of considered management policy. In the years following the publication of the Control Review Committee Report (Home Office 1984), the routine reading of correspondence was withdrawn, first in open prisons, then in Category C establishments and in 1991, following the recommendations of the Woolf Report, the Government finally abolished the routine reading of letters in all establishments, except dispersal prisons (Home Office, 1991a). Thus over the last twenty years the prisoner's rights of correspondence with the outside world have been greatly extended. Certainly the initial pressure for reform came in the form of a clear recognition of 'rights' by the ECHR, which was eventually echoed by the domestic courts. More recently, however, the liberalising steps taken by the Prison Service seem to have been inspired by the desire to rationalise the system and to facilitate the smooth management of inmates. The Woolf Report, while adopting this management focus by avoiding the rhetoric of rights and concentrating on the value to management of the maintenance of justice within prisons, none the less recognised the fundamental significance of the issues involved (see para. 14.274). It is heartening to see that the government has responded positively.

Segregation and transfer

As was suggested above, the prisoner's public-law right to a fair hearing has been taken very seriously by the courts in the context of prison discipline. In relation to segregation and transfer decisions, however, the judicial approach has been more restrained. In *R.* v. *Deputy Govenor Parkhurst Prison and Others, ex p. Hague,* a case involving the transfer and segregation of a prisoner under the 'ghosting' procedure contained in CI 10/1974,[12] the Court of Appeal refused to recognise a right to be heard either before the initial segregation under Rule 43 or before its renewal. The context was distinguished from that of a formal disciplinary charge where the Prison Rules specifically require a hearing, and it is evident that the Court of Appeal felt there were sound policy reasons against extending such procedural rigour to the decision to segregate. The Court further refused to recognise a legal right in the prisoner to be given the reasons for his or her segregation, although Taylor LJ states that '[no] doubt in many cases the governor will be able, as here, to give reasons at the time of the decision or shortly after'.[13]

Following the lead of the Court of Appeal, the revised Circular Instruction concerning segregation under Rule 43, remarks that 'inmates have no entitlement to be given reasons for their segregation under R.43', and states merely that 'the giving of reasons is encouraged as a sensible practice'.[14] However, irrespective of the procedural issues, the Court of Appeal in *Ex p. Hague* had declared the original 'ghosting' Circular to be unlawful because it was *ultra vires* the powers granted by the Prison Rules. The Circular was thus revised to ensure that any decision to segregate a transferred prisoner is taken by the governor of the receiving prison.[15] It is encouraging to note that this new Circular on 'ghosting', despite the lack of enthusiasm for the procedural rights of segregated prisoners displayed by the Court of Appeal, is significantly more demanding in procedural terms (Richardson 1993). It requires reasons to be given to the prisoner for both his transfer and his segregation, preferably before the event, and was accordingly welcomed by the Woolf Report. In formal legal terms, however, the prisoner still possesses no directly enforceable right to reasons.

The enforcement of the prison rules and conditions generally

Having failed in their attempts to claim special rights in private law, some prisoners have sought remedies in public law in relation to the Prison Rules and prison conditions generally. In the first place although the House of

Lords in *Ex p. Hague* has now confirmed that a deterioration in prison conditions cannot amount to a tort of false imprisonment, the House did reaffirm that a decision to hold a prisoner in intolerable conditions could be subject to judicial review.[16] Presumably the decision to hold a prisoner in intolerable conditions would be regarded as unreasonable and thus unlawful. What might amount to intolerable conditions is not, however, clear. Indeed the attitude of the judiciary to such issues in the past does not suggest that the threshold of tolerability will be set very high.[17]

Second, although it is now clear that the private law will provide no means of direct enforcement of the Prison Rules by way of an action for breach of statutory duty, the courts have accepted that section 4 (2) of the Prison Act imposes a public law duty on the Secretary of State to ensure compliance with the obligations contained in both the Rules and the Act.[18] It is thus theoretically possible for a prisoner to challenge the Secretary of State's failure to ensure compliance. However, many of the Prison Rules are expressed in such a way as to leave considerable discretion in the authorities, thus making it extremely hard to establish any unreasonable refusal to ensure compliance. In *R.* v. *Secretary of State for the Home Department ex p. McAvoy*, a case involving the transfer of a remand prisoner from London to Winchester, the court showed little enthusiasm for challenging the exercise of discretion by the Secretary of State.[19] Although the court accepted in principle that the Secretary of State must take into account the obligations relating to visits imposed by the Prison Rules when exercising his discretion under section 12 of the Prison Act, it was loath to police the degree of consideration given to those obligations. Once the Secretary of State affirmed that he had operational and security reasons for ordering the transfer, the court inquired no further. Thus the public law, by merely recognising a right in prisoners to the reasonable exercise of discretion by the authorities, provides no adequate mechanism for enforcing special substantive rights in prisoners.

Release

The selective early release of fixed-term prisoners at the discretion of the executive was introduced in England and Wales by the Criminal Justice Act 1967. The Act created a dual key system whereby the Secretary of State was empowered to release if recommended to do so by the Parole Board.[20] The Act and accompanying regulations imposed few procedural requirements: there was no obligation to provide a hearing, the prisoner had no access to the dossier on which decisions were reached and there was no obligation to give reasons, save after recall. The procedure for the release on licence of life-sentence prisoners was identical in many relevant respects but life-sentenced prisoners had no right of reference to the Parole Board. Their first review date would be set by the executive in consultation with the judiciary and was related to the period deemed necessary to reflect the gravity of the offence, the tariff period.[21]

As in the context of transfer and segregation, prisoners have sought to persuade the courts to recognise their procedural rights with regard to release. Again, until recently, they met with little success. The Court of Appeal in *Payne* v. *Lord Harris*, a case involving a mandatory life sentence, took an unsympathetic line which dominated the case law for a decade. Led by Lord Denning, the court held that parole was a privilege not a right, and there was no obligation on the Parole Board to give reasons for its refusal to recommend release. Indeed, according to the court, any such obligation would hamper the Board's work, provide ammunition for litigious prisoners and inhibit the production of candid reports. A similar judicial attitude was evident in *R.* v. *Secretary of State for the Home Department, ex p. Gunnell* when a recalled life-sentence prisoner sought to challenge the process of his recall. He argued that he was entitled to a written statement of reasons and a hearing before the Parole Board, involving at the very least the disclosure of police and medical reports. He was unsuccessful before both the Divisional Court and the Court of Appeal. The disclosure point was taken up again in *R.* v. *Secretary of State for the Home Department, ex p. Benson* where the Divisional Court reasserted that there was no general right to disclosure where parole was refused.

The disinclination of the courts to recognise rights in prisoners in the context of release decisions was not limited to strictly procedural matters. In *Re Findlay* two of the appellants were lifers who had been transferred to open prisons in the expectation of fairly imminent release. On the day that the then Home Secretary announced the introduction of a new restrictive policy on the release of certain categories of prisoner, they were transferred back to closed conditions and, in light of the new policy, could not then anticipate release before 1989 and 1993 respectively. The two men argued that, whatever the legality of the overall policy, their cases were exceptional and should be recognised as such. The Home Office never alleged that the return to closed conditions was related to the appellants' behaviour and, indeed, the court seemed to accept that it resulted exclusively from the change in policy. However, neither the Court of Appeal nor the House of Lords would accept that the transfer to open conditions, with all its implications, constituted exceptional circumstances. Further Lord Scarman, in the only speech provided by the House of Lords, dismissed any suggestion that the appellants had a legitimate expectation of early release.[22]

In the context of release, therefore, the domestic courts were reluctant to recognise any 'rights', whether procedural or substantive, in prisoners beyond those specifically included in the relevant legislation, although they have recently displayed a greater willingness to challenge the discretion of the Secretary of State.[23] In October 1992, however, a new system for early release was introduced by the Criminal Justice Act, which, in the case of fixed-term prisoners, allows greater openness and participation. Although oral hearings are not required, prisoners are now to have access to their parole dossiers and will be given reasons for the final decision.[24]

Unlike those serving fixed-term sentences, prisoners serving sentences of life imprisonment have been able successfully to claim rights guaranteed under the European Convention on Human Rights. In 1981 the ECHR held in *X* v. *The United Kingdom* that articles 5(1) and 5(4) of the Convention guaranteed a mentally disordered offender, compulsorily detained under a restricted hospital order, regular access to a 'court' to determine the lawfulness of his detention.[25] In 1987 in *Weeks* v. *The United Kingdom* these principles were applied to a prisoner serving a discretionary life sentence. The ECHR felt that the indeterminate sentence had been imposed for the purposes of social protection because of the prisoner's mental instability and potential dangerousness. Both of these conditions were susceptible to change over time and, as in the case of *X*, article 5(4) guaranteed the prisoner regular access to a 'court' in order to test the continued lawfulness of his detention. As neither the Parole Board nor the Secretary of State could constitute such a 'court', the United Kingdom was in breach of the Convention. Given a generous interpretation, this judgment carried broad implications for the release structure provided for all discretionary life sentences. The government, however, chose to take no action, presumably hoping that the case was special to its facts.

In 1990 the ECHR published its decision in *Thynne, Wilson and Gunnell* v. *The United Kingdom.* This judgment makes it clear that the principles expressed in *Weeks* cannot be restricted to the facts of that case alone. According to *Thynne, Wilson and Gunnell* the requirements of article 5(4) apply to all discretionary life-sentence prisoners who are detained, on the basis of their mental instability and dangerousness, after the expiry of the punitive, or tariff, period of their sentence. While the Court accepted that it might be hard to distinguish the punitive from the protective elements in a discretionary life sentence, it felt that at some point, however heinous the offence, the punitive element must expire, leaving the continued detention to be justifed solely on the grounds of the prisoner's potential dangerousness. A person's capacity to be dangerous may change over time and thus, on the principles of *Weeks* (1988), anyone detained solely on the grounds of their dangerousness, must be entitled regularly to challenge the lawfulness of that detention before a 'court'. When the Criminal Justice Bill was first published in November 1990, no concessions were made to the European ruling. Following widespread revolt in the House of Lords over the retention of the mandatory life sentence for murder, however, the Government finally introduced provisions, contained within the Criminal Justice Act 1991, to enable the Parole Board to order the release of discretionary life-sentence prisoners. Section 34 empowers the Board to direct the release of a discretionary life-sentence prisoner if it is satisfied 'that it is no longer necessary for the protection of the public that the prisoner should be confined'. The new scheme provides for the specification of the relevant (or tariff) period by the trial judge in open court, and empowers the Board to release the prisoner after the expiry of that period. It came into operation in October 1992, and in August rules were made specifying the procedures to be followed by the Board when hearing individual cases. Under the transitional arrangements provided by the Act the scheme has also been extended to apply to discretionary life-sentence prisoners sentenced before October 1992 who have reached their tariff date. Since October 1992, therefore, the release procedures for discretionary lifers have been radically changed. The tariff date will be declared in open court, the release decision itself is taken by an independent tribunal following an oral hearing and the executive veto has been removed. These are major improvements which could scarcely have been achieved without the intervention of the ECHR. Inevitably, however, some problems remain. It is particularly unfortunate that the government has followed the pattern adopted by the Mental Health Act 1983, and has required the Board to be 'satisfied that it is no longer necessary for the protection of the public that the prisoner should be confined'. Such statutory wording effectively creates a presumption against release, despite the expiry of the tariff period, which must be rebutted if the prisoner is to obtain release.[26] It is also important to realise that the new procedures apply only to discretionary life sentences certified under section 34. Thus it is possible that some offenders sentenced to life for offences for which that sentence is not mandatory will not receive the benefits of section 34. More significantly the new procedures do not apply to murderers, all of whom receive a mandatory life sentence. The decision whether or not to release a mandatory lifer still rests with the Secretary of State, but a review of the structure has been promised.

Finally, since the intervention of the ECHR in *Thynne, Wilson and Gunnell* the domestic courts have at last begun to shake off the deadening influence of *Payne*. In 1992, emboldened by the judgment in *Thynne, Wilson and Gunnell* and the impending reforms contained in the Criminal Justice Act, the Court of Appeal agreed to depart from *Payne* and to order the disclosure of the parole dossier in the case of a discretionary life-sentence prisoner whose case was considered prior to the implementation of section 34.[27] While it is still too early to predict how far this enthusiasm for the procedural rights of prisoners will extend, it is evident that the judiciary were prepared directly to depart from *Payne* in the case of mandatory life sentences as well.[28] In the event such intervention was rendered unnecessary by the Secretary of State's decision to allow mandatory lifers access to their dossiers and reasons for their release decisions.

THE ROLE OF THE COURTS IN THE PROTECTION OF RIGHTS

It should be evident from the above that the record of the domestic courts as a protector of the 'rights' of prisoners has been variable. The ability of the private law to provide any real protection is greatly inhibited by the court's attitude to the Prison Rules. There are no effective private law rights to sensible minimum standards. In relation to negligence the court's assessment of the implications of imprisonment has varied. With regard to inter-prisoner violence courts have been prepared to recognise special duties of protection on the part of the authorities, although they appear reluctant to find those duties breached. In the context of medical care, by contrast, the fact of imprisonment has led the courts to accept a lower standard of care from the authorities.

The inadequacies of the private law have led to greater reliance on public law, and in certain circumstances prisoners have met with considerable success. Most notably as far as domestic courts are concerned, the judiciary has intervened in the disciplinary system and has imposed fairly stringent procedural requirements on both Boards of Visitors and governors. Other areas of judicial activity have owed much to the involvement of the ECHR. In relation to prisoners' correspondence the domestic courts did eventually follow the European lead and recognise a right of access to the court, and in the context of early release the domestic judiciary displayed reluctance to recognise rights beyond those few expressly stated in the legislation until inspired to do so by the European Court.

It has been suggested elsewhere that the approach of the domestic courts to prisoners' claims in both public and private law displays considerable sympathy for the arguments of administrative convenience, typically offered by the authorities in response to any attempts to enforce rights in prisoners (Richardson 1985a). The judicial interpretation of the 'necessary implication' referred to by Lord Wilberforce tends in practice, therefore, to favour the authorities. The areas where the courts have been prepared to intervene in order to resolve uncertainties in favour of prisoners have typically been either those, such as prison discipline, where the context is 'quasi-judicial' and the courts feel confident and appropriately equipped with the armoury of natural justice, or those where rights which they might hold particularly dear, such as access to justice, are concerned. In the more 'administrative' areas of transfer and the conditions of imprisonment, the courts of England and Wales have shown little enthusiasm for acting as a mechanism for the enforcement of prisoners' interests. With reference to Lord Wilberforce's statement, therefore, the case law suggests that the interpretation of 'necessary implication' typically adopted by the domestic judiciary will tend to lead to the recognition of only a restricted residue of rights in prisoners. Further it is clear that the courts are reluctant to step beyond Wilberforce and to recognise additional special rights in prisoners.

THE WOOLF REPORT AND JUSTICE IN PRISONS

In the light of the above, it is encouraging to note the emphasis placed by the Woolf Report on the importance of justice within prisons (see section 9). By stressing the need to treat prisoners with justice and humanity the Woolf Report recognises both the substantive and the procedural aspects of a prisoner's 'rights'. The requirements of justice, according to Woolf, seem to encompass notions of procedural fairness, particularly the obligation to provide prisoners with reasons and with a satisfactory means of redress (para. 10.20). Thus the Report recommends that a prisoner be given reasons 'for any decision which materially and adversely affects him', not just the major decisions relating to transfer and release (para 14.300). This is a most important recommendation. The obligation to give reasons can both encourage better decision-making and, by providing an explanation, can render the decision more acceptable to those affected. Indeed the giving of reasons can be regarded as essential to any acceptable system of decision-making (Richardson 1986). It is, therefore, encouraging to see that the Government has accepted this recommendation in principle (Home Office 1991a, para. 7.20). However, the participation of interested parties before the decision is actually made is arguably of even greater importance to the acceptability of the ultimate decision, and here the Woolf Report is slightly more tentative in its recommendations. The Report urges the provision of extensive and regular information to prisoners and encourages the development of more frequent consultation with prisoners by governors before decisions are taken. In response to such calls for greater participation the authorities typically stress the need for governors to govern and for staff rather than prisoners to exercise the necessary discretion. Fears are also expressed concerning the ease with which powerful groups can dominate any representative structure (Woolf 1991, paras. 14.275–14.288). These may be significant reasons for caution, but the case for greater participation is strong. According to the approach adopted here, just as prisoners possess rights despite their imprisonment, so they remain responsible for their lives and should be entitled to participate in the decisions which affect them to the extent that that participation is compatible with the demands of segregation, or more specifically, of security and control. It is to be hoped therefore that the Woolf Report's preliminary suggestions will be taken up in earnest.

With regard to the more substantive aspects of imprisonment, which appear to be incorporated within the obligation to treat prisoners with humanity, the Woolf Report makes a number of recommendations. While the Report does not talk in terms of rights and, indeed, rejects any moves to encourage strict legalisation of prison life, it does, as described by Silvia Casale in Chapter 3, support the eventual introduction of a code of minimum standards. It also urges the Prison Service to drop the term 'privilege' and to refer instead to a prisoner's normal expectations (para. 14.32). Finally it recommends the introduction of a contract or compact between each prisoner and his or her prison (paras. 12.120–12.129). These contracts, which might eventually reflect the minimum standards expected of the particular prison, would not create private-law rights in prisoners, but would reflect the prisoner's 'legitimate expectations'. Thus the Woolf Report is not recommending the creation of substantive rights in prisoners, directly enforceable in private law. Rather, by recommending the eventual introduction of a statement of expectations with regard to both 'privileges' and minimum standards, it is placing the focus on public law. The notion of a legitimate expectation as an interest attracting the protection of the public law has been developing rapidly in recent years, and is seen by some as a welcome vehicle for the extension of judicial control over government action. Unfortunately from the prisoner's point of view it is a notoriously flexible notion.[29] In the first place the court must decide that an expectation is legitimate, before it will offer any protection. Second, once the existence of an expectation is recognised the court must determine its legal implications. With regard to the first issue, that of recognition, the publication by the Prison Service of a statement of expectations is likely to be sufficient. The second issue, however, may present greater difficulties. The extent of the protection offered to a legitimate expectation by the public law is unclear. A legitimate expectation to evening association, for example, is not a right to such association. Having recognised the existence of the expectation the court may decide that it must be met unless there are overwhelming difficulties in meeting it, or it may decide merely that the expectation should be met unless the prisoner is given a reason for the failure to meet it. A number of points should be made.

In the first place, it is unlikely that any government would agree to introduce a detailed code of substantive rights directly enforceable in court by prisoners, even if such a scheme were justified in penal and legal theory. In the absence of such a code, the conclusions drawn from the case law described above would suggest that the courts are unlikely to encourage prisoners' claims to directly enforceable substantive rights. A system which provides for the ultimate enforcement of a prisoner's specific entitlements through an application for judicial review, therefore, has much to recommend it. However, the history of prisoner litigation suggests that, save in certain well-defined circumstances, the courts incline to interpretations which favour the administration. This does not, of course, mean that courts will never adequately protect the interests of prisoners. Rather, it suggests that, if they are to do so, the framework against which they are required to act must be as specific as possible Thus if the notion of a legitimate expectation is to be relied upon to trigger legal protection, the nature of the expectation must be precisely expressed. Specifically the circumstances which might justify the failure to meet any particular expectation should be listed in detail.

Finally, it has been accepted throughout this discussion that the court's role in the protection of prisoners' 'rights' should be one of last-resort enforcement only. It is clear that at present the courts play a marginal role in most areas of prison life, but this lack of routine involvement is not necessarily to be decried. Even if suitably empowered the ordinary courts are unlikely to provide an effective mechanism for the routine oversight of prisoners' interests (Morgan and Bronstein 1985). As presently constituted they are not the most appropriate body to provide regular oversight. A specialised, but truly independent, lay body could be more accessible, could possess more relevant expertise and could be in a better position to achieve improved standards through conciliation. The court's role could then be limited to the provision of an ultimate means of enforcement. At present, however, the extra-judicial safeguards available to prisoners are sadly inadequate.

EXTRA-JUDICIAL ENFORCEMENT

Most aspects of a prisoner's existence are governed by administrative rules and guidelines. Indeed as Ditchfield has described, the 'bureaucratic-lawful' approach has become the dominant model of prison management within the United Kingdom (Ditchfield 1990). A prisoner who wishes to challenge a decision made in relation to such rules or guidelines, or any other decision relating to his or her treatment in prison, has a number of avenues of redress available. In the first place she may raise the matter internally within her own establishment and then, via the area manager, with headquarters. In 1990 a new internal system for dealing with prisoners' complaints was introduced. Evidence gathered by Austin and Ditchfield (1985) and Her Majesty's Chief Inspector of Prisons (Home Office 1987c) concerning the previous system had suggested that, while inmates were broadly satisfied with the management of 'applications' at wing and governor level, dissatisfaction was widespread among prisoners with regard to the old system of petitioning the Secretary of State, and such dissatisfaction was frequently echoed by staff. In September 1990 the procedures were amended to encourage greater confidentiality, speedier resolution and the provision of reasoned decisions but, while it is to be hoped that these new procedures will meet most of the criticisms, it remains an exclusively internal procedure.

In addition to the internal system of applications, a prisoner may raise a grievance with the Board of Visitors and this currently provides the most accessible mechanism for external review. Much has been written concerning the procedural vagaries of some Boards, their lack of conspicuous independence, their strong tendency to identify with management and the difficulties inherent in their dual role as complaints mechanism and disciplinary tribunal (Maguire 1985). In the light of these criticisms, Woolf recommended a strengthening of the Boards' complaints role and an end to their involvement in the disciplinary system. Even after the acceptance of this latter recommendation however, the question remains whether local Boards of Visitors can ever possess sufficient status and independence to provide, on their own, an adequate external safeguard of the rights and interests of prisoners.

If it be accepted, as suggested above, that the court's involvement in the oversight of prisoners' interests should be limited to the provision of last-resort enforcement, then there is a strong case for the introduction of a truly independent and appropriately empowered national body to whom prisoners would have access for the resolution of grievances. The internal departmental working party which was set up to consider the complaints' procedures prior to the recent reforms, however, concluded that, in view of the costs involved in establishing an independent complaints' investigator, the new internal arrangements should be introduced and established first before any further thought be given to the creation of an investigator. In contrast the Woolf Report took a refreshingly uncompromising position on the need for an independent element:

> the presence of an independent element within the grievance procedure is more than just an 'optional extra'. The case for some form of independent person or body to consider grievances is incontrovertible . . . A system without an independent element is not a system which accords with proper standards of justice.
>
> (para. 14.345)

The Woolf Report recommended the introduction of a Complaints Adjudicator to 'recommend, advise and conciliate at the final stage of the [grievance] procedure' (para. 14.349). While the precise details of the Woolf recommendations can be criticised for not going far enough (Richardson 1993), they have placed a welcome emphasis on independence and have succeeded in eliciting a positive response. The government is in the process of appointing a Prisons Ombudsman to provide both a central independent element within the greivance procedure and an independent 'appellate' tier for the disciplinary system. Whether this new figure, who for the present will enjoy no statutory status, will possess sufficient standing, resources or powers to be truly affective in either capacity remains to be seen.

CONCLUSION

This chapter has sought to argue that the claim to rights in prisoners is justified and should encompass both the retention of those general rights possessed by non-prisoners, in so far as they are not necessarily removed by the fact of imprisonment, and the acquisition of additional rights beyond those possessed by non-prisoners. At present the law in England and Wales inadequately reflects this claim. The statutory framework is essentially enabling and non-specific and the courts have been reluctant to recognise rights in prisoners enforceable in private law. In the assertion of public-law rights prisoners have achieved greater success, particularly in certain areas, but even here the courts have displayed considerable sympathy for the difficulties faced by prison management. The emphasis placed by the Woolf Report on the need to promote both substantive and procedural justice in prisons is therefore warmly welcomed. With regard to substantive rights, the shift in emphasis from rights to expectations can be seen as a potentially valuable initiative building on recent developments in public law, provided the nature of the expectations is specified with sufficient precision. In relation to procedural justice, the importance attached by the Report to provision of reasons and the need to encourage greater participation on the part of prisoners is of considerable significance, and could, if fully implemented, greatly improve the standard of internal decision-making within prisons. Finally, given the inevitable limits on the court's role, the introduction of an effective and accessible mechanism for the review of prisoners' grievances is essential, and it is therefore of the utmost importance that the new Prison Ombudsman be appropriately resourced and empowered.

ACKNOWLEDGEMENTS

Sections of this chapter have appeared in McCrudden and Chambers (eds) *Rights and Freedoms* (Oxford: Oxford University Press).

NOTES

1 SI 1964 No. 388.
2 *Ellis* v. *The Home Office* (1953) and *Christofi* v. *The Home Office* (1975).
3 *Ellis* (1953) and *Egerton* v. *The Home Office* (1978). But see *H.* v. *The Home Office* (1992).
4 *Pullen* v. *The Prison Commissioners* (1957).
5 *Davis* v. *The Prison Commissioners* (1963). The Home Office does have a duty to train prisoners adequately in the use of machinery, a duty that derives from the 'neighbour principle', *Ferguson* v. *The Home Office* (1977).
6 *R.* v. *Deputy Governor of Parkhurst Prison, ex p. Hague* (1991) confirming *Arbon* v. *Anderson* (1943).
7 See, for example, Lord Goddard, *Arbon* (1943) p. 255.

8 *R.* v. *Deputy Governor Parkhurst Prison, ex p. Hague* (1992).

9 See particularly *Council for Civil Service Unions* v. *Minister for the Civil Service* (1985).

10 *Golder* v. *The United Kingdom* (1983) and *Silver* v. *The United Kingdom* (1983).

11 *R.* v. *Secretary of State for the Home Department, ex p. Anderson* (1984). More recently the Court of Appeal has decided that the Prison Rules rule 33 is *ultra vires* the Prison Act in so far as it purports to allow letters to lawyers to be stopped or read in order to ensure compliance with the general restrictions on correspondence, *R.* v. *Secretary of State for the Home Department, ex p. Leech* (No. 2) (1993).

12 Circular Instruction 10/1974 *Dispersal Policy – Provision of Cells in Local Prisons.*

13 *R.* v. *Deputy Governor of Parkhurst Prison and Others, ex p. Hague* (1990) p. 698.

14 Circular Instruction 26/1990 *Removal From Association Under Prison Rule 43 and Youth Offender Institutions Rule 46 and Arrangements for the Management of Vulnerable Prisoners.*

15 Circular Instruction 37/1990 *Transfer of Inmates in the Interests of Good Order and Discipline.*

16 *Ex p. Hague* (1992).

17 *Middleweek* v. *Chief Constable of the Merseyside Police and Another* (1990).

18 *R.* v. *Deputy Governor of Camp Hill Prison, ex p. King* (1985).

19 See also *R.* v. *Secretary of State for the Home Department, ex p. McComb* (1991).

20 The Carlisle Report gives an account of the history of parole under the Criminal Justice Act 1967, see Home Office (1988e).

21 A clear account of the relevant procedures can be found in House of Lords (1989).

22 Lord Scarman, *Re Findlay* (1985) at p. 338.

23 See *R.* v. *Secretary of State for the Home Department, ex p. Handscomb* (1987), but arguably the courts were there motivated primarily by the desire to protect their own standing rather than the interests of the prisoners. See also *R.* v. *Secretary of State for the Home Department, ex p. Cox* (1991).

24 The early release structure is found in Criminal Justice Act 1991 Part II. The procedural requirements are non-statutory and are found in C.I. 26/1992.

25 *X.* v. *The United Kingdom* (1982).

26 For an account of the interpretation of the release provisions of the Mental Health Act 1983 see Peay (1989); and for further discussion in the context of life sentences and mentally disordered offenders see, Richardson (1991).

27 *R.* v. *Parole Board, ex p. Wilson* (1992). See Richardson (1993) for further discussion.

28 *R.* v. *Secretary of State for the Home Department, ex p. Creamer* (1992).

29 See particulary, *Re Findlay* (1985); *R.* v. *Secretary of State for The Home Department, ex p. Khan* (1985) and *R.* v. *Secretary of State for The Home Department, ex p. Ruddock* (1987). For further discussion see Forsyth (1988).

5

THE CHANGING FACE OF PRISON DISCIPLINE

Stephen Livingstone

INTRODUCTION

Prison discipline was a significant battleground of prison policy and practice in the 1970s and 1980s. Prisoners and their advocates stressed the link between perceptions of unfairness in the disciplinary system and unrest in prisons. Reformers criticised the division of discipline hearings into those by governors and those by Boards of Visitors, arguing that involvement in discipline confused Boards' roles in theory and their conduct of them undermined their effectiveness in practice. The courts became involved in reviewing and significantly reshaping the content of disciplinary procedures. Now that Woolf has recommended, and the Government has accepted, some of the main recommendations of the reformers, prison discipline may become less of an issue or may be entering a period of new questions in a new context.

PRISON DISCIPLINE: THE MILITARY MODEL

Prison discipline and the relevant Prison Rules changed little in the century after the Prison Act 1877. The composite Prison Rules 1964 followed the new Prison Act, 1952, but broke no new ground. Some offences in Rule 47 were akin to criminal offences, for example, '(4) commits an assault' and '(11) wilfully damages . . . property not his own'. Others were more clearly tailored to the internal concerns of the prison, for example, '(12) makes any false and malicious allegation against an officer' and '(18) disobeys any lawful order'. Most charges (usually about 95 per cent) were heard by prison governors but they could refer serious or repeated offences to the Board of Visitors and 'graver offences' and 'especially grave offences' were almost invariably referred. Accordingly, the penalties the Boards could order were significantly more severe. Governors' powers were limited by Rule 50 to a maximum of three days' cellular confinement and 28 days' forfeiture of remission, whereas the Board of Visitors could order up to 56 days' cellular confinement and up to 180 days' forfeiture of remission for 'graver offences'. For 'especially grave offences' there was no limit on the forfeiture of remission and, up until 1968, they could order corporal punishment for sentenced male adult prisoners.[1]

As a result of the Courts Act 1971, all prisons had 'Boards of Visitors' consisting of a mixture of magistrates and lay people. Previously local prisons had 'Visiting Committees', groups of magistrates appointed by Quarter Sessions much as they had been before the Prison Act, 1877, when they had borne authority superior to the governor for the control of the prison (see Martin 1975). Despite these useful modifications the quality of prison justice was, by all accounts, less than ideal. Official inquiries acknowledged a need for reform (Home Office 1975). More radical critics were scathing about what they saw as a 'kangaroo court' where prisoners rarely had an opportunity to present their side of the case fully and were routinely disbelieved by the governor or tribunal members. They could not even sit down during the hearing but instead had to stand facing two prison officers ('eyeballing' in prison terminology) (Fitzgerald and Sim 1979). Such summary procedures were not, however, deviations from the norm but very much represented the model to which the prison disciplinary system worked. As Edward Fitzgerald has described it, the model was that of the military, with prison analogised to an army, the prison authorities to military officers and prisoners to ordinary soldiers on parade (Fitzgerald 1985). In this model, discipline was something to be administered regularly in order to keep prisoners on their toes and reinforce their respect for authority. In this model, fairness of procedure was of little importance, the expressive function of punishment was uppermost with a premium on punishment being visibly and swiftly administered once disorder was discovered. That punishments were regular and swift was more important than establishing that an offence worthy of punishment had been committed, or ensuring that the person responsible for it was actually the one punished. However disturbing this model may have been generally, it was particularly disturbing when it came to the punishments handed out by Boards of Visitors. Their greater distance from day-to-day management than governors and the severity of their punishments, amounting to the equivalent of extra months or even years in prison, could hardly be analogised to confining soldiers to barracks or giving them extra drill for a few days. Yet no appreciably different procedural safeguards prevailed in Board hearings than those over which governors presided.

The way that many such hearings were conducted appeared to be a clear breach of the right to a fair hearing. Yet the courts had indicated in the case of *Arbon* v. *Anderson* (1943) that they would not regard a breach of the prison rules as giving rise to a remedy for the prisoner. This did not resolve the question of whether public-law principles of natural justice would afford remedies to prisoners as to all other citizens. The early indications however were not favourable. In *Fraser* v. *Mudge* Lord Denning made it clear that the military model held good and that judicial intervention would interfere with the swiftness and decisiveness that was essential to the role of disciplinary proceedings in prison. The route to the European courts also seemed barred. Despite the encouraging decision of the European Court of Human Rights in *Golder* v. *The United Kingdom*, where the Court ruled that the European Convention of Human Rights was applicable to prisoners, the Commission in *Kiss* v. *The United Kingdom* ruled that prison disciplinary proceedings did not amount to 'criminal charges' within the meaning of Article 6(1) of the Convention. As a result the procedural guarantees under Article 6, including the right to legal representation, were inapplicable in this context. In 1976, therefore, the prospects for change in the prison disciplinary system through the courts looked poor.

However, both the Weiler Report (Home Office 1975) and the Jellicoe Report (Martin 1975) indicated pressure for change both within the Prison Department and among lawyers. The courts also seemed readier to review the actions of public authorities (see Aldous and Alder 1985) and the introduction of 'judicial review' in 1978 opened a new avenue for prisoners. Then, not for the last time, a case arising out of a major disturbance in a prison was to produce a significant alteration in judicial thinking.

PRISON DISCIPLINE AND THE COURTS 1978–91

The watershed case was *R.* v. *Hull Prison Board of Visitors , ex p. St. Germain (No. 1)* and it arose out of the riot at Hull prison in 1976. The facts were extraordinary. In response to three days of riots, which left the prison largely uninhabitable, the authorities decided not to prefer criminal charges but instead to proceed against the prisoners through hearings before the Board of Visitors. As the prisoners had been dispersed to prisons throughout the country the panel of the Board (specially convened to adjudicate on the charges) had to travel all over England. In all they heard over 500 charges against 185 inmates. Nearly all were found guilty and severe punishments, up to 720 days' loss of remission, were imposed. The dispersal alone had a severe effect on the prisoners' ability to conduct their defence, as it made it difficult to consult with prospective witnesses before the hearing. However, these difficulties were compounded by the Board's refusal to allow them to call any witnesses or to cross examine even hearsay evidence given against them.

In 1978 the prisoners sought review of these proceedings, and of their 'convictions' and punishments, by the Divisional Court but were initially refused: the Court cited the military analogy and decided that it had no jurisdiction. That view was reversed, however, by the Court of Appeal which indicated that, whatever the value of the military analogy when it came to disciplinary proceedings by governors (only Shaw LJ being prepared to say explicitly that it was not helpful there too), it was inappropriate to disciplinary hearings before Boards. These often occurred a significant time after the alleged offences and were clearly judicial rather than administrative proceedings. Where serious punishments were involved, arguments of the need for speed and finality did not justify the exclusion of judicial oversight. Board hearings, therefore, were subject to a duty to ensure that prisoners received a fair hearing.

Ex p. St. Germain (No. 1) was clearly a landmark case, and it opened the way for judicial scrutiny of the content of procedures of prison disciplinary hearings that began with *R.* v. *Hull Prison Board of Visitors, ex p. St. Germain (No. 2)*. In time the division between the Court's jurisdiction over Board hearings but not those of governors would fall away with the House of Lords decision in *Leech* v. *Parkhurst Prison Deputy Governor. Leech* resolved a dispute between the Court of Appeal in England, which held in *R.* v. *Deputy Governor Camp Hill Prison ex p. King* that governors' hearings could not be the subject of judicial review, and its equivalent in Northern Ireland, which held the opposite in *R.* v. *Governor of the Maze Prison, ex p. McKiernan.* After *Leech* the view taken in Belfast prevailed and the rule of law, in form at least, was applicable to all prison disciplinary hearings.

Whether the rule of law applies in substance depends very much on the content of natural justice in prison disciplinary hearings. As the courts have often observed, most recently in *Lloyd* v. *McMahon*, the requirements of fairness vary, depending upon 'the character of the decision making body, the kind of decision it has to make and the statutory or other framework in which it operates'.[2] Prisoners' advocates have often argued that, as regards Boards especially, the kind of punishments involved suggest that the appropriate procedural model is the criminal law. However, the Divisional Court accepted in *ex p. St. Germain (No. 2)*, that hearsay evidence was admissible in prison hearings (subject to a right of cross examination) and so indicated that they would not go so far as to apply all the procedural protections of the criminal trial to adjudications in prison. Nevertheless they did move considerably away from the military model.

Through a series of decisions a number of safeguards have now been established, namely:

- prisoners should normally be allowed to call witnesses;[3]
- if the authorities are aware of a relevant witness that is unknown to a prisoner they should inform him/her;[4]
- prisoners should also be entitled to cross-examine witnesses for the prosecution;[5]
- they may apply for legal representation at the hearing;[6]

— where there is ambiguity in disciplinary charges this should be construed in favour of the defendant (especially as regards the mental element of the offence);[7]
— tribunals are not entitled to acquit a prisoner on one charge and then convict on a less serious offence where no charge in respect of that less serious offence has been laid;[8]
— the criminal burden of proof ('beyond all reasonable doubt') applies to disciplinary charges against prisoners.[9]

Although all these standards were produced by decisions of the English courts, the encouraging influence of the European Court of Human Rights is clear, especially on the issue of legal representation where the Commission's decision in *Campbell and Fell* v. *The United Kingdom* predated the relevant English decision, while that of the Court reinforced the view taken in *R.* v. *Secretary of State for the Home Department, ex p. Tarrant.*

It can be argued that *Tarrant* marked the high-water mark for procedural standards in discipline hearings because it established the criteria for granting legal representation. In a number of cases in following years the courts indicated that they would not scrutinise too thoroughly the results of the discretion exercised by Boards. Boards would not find their decision overturned except when they refused a prisoner legal representation on the most serious charges.[10] Whether, in the wake of the *Campbell and Fell* decision, prisoners had a right to legal representation at all Board hearings was finally answered in the negative by the House of Lords in *Hone* v. *Maze Prison Board of Visitors.* Attempts to establish a right for prisoners to see all statements made by prison officers relating to the case in advance were not wholly succesful.[11] In *R* v. *Frankland Prison Board of Visitors, ex p. Lewis* the court rejected what was, in essence, a challenge to the dual role of Boards of Visitors as both watchdog and disciplinary tribunal. The prisoner in *ex p. Lewis* argued that as one member of the Board of Visitors had sat on a local review committee which had recently refused his parole application, that Board member would have seen prejudicial material against him and might not be entirely unbiased. Woolf J (as he then was) indicated that he did not think a hypothetical bystander – being aware of the dual role of Board members – would regard this as unfair. In addition he indicated that it was a good thing that those who adjudicated on disciplinary offences in prison should have a knowledge of the prison in which the inmate was detained. In his Report he appears to have changed his view (Woolf 1991, para. 14.390).

Decisions on governors' adjudications in Northern Ireland suggest that courts, having established jurisdiction over prison disciplinary proceedings, will not be too anxious to scrutinise the quality of those proceedings. With a four-year start on England and Wales, the Northern Irish courts have built up a lively jurisprudence on the issue of standards in governors' hearings.

Most decisions indicate that similar standards apply to hearings by both Boards and governors, but rather less rigorously for the latter. Thus while *In re Carroll's Application* indicates that a governor must exercise his discretion on whether to grant representation, *In re Reynold's Application* indicates that only where the prisoner is mentally subnormal and clearly unable to conduct his or her own defence will a governor be required to grant it. Only the requirement to allow the calling of witnesses seems to apply with almost equal force. Generally however, the Northern Irish courts have shown themselves more willing to examine governors' hearings (rather than those before Boards) to ensure that, overall, the prisoner had a fair hearing and that no breach of natural justice affected the outcome. They have been reluctant to strike down decisions *per se* for violations of the standards appropriate to a fair hearing in this context.[12]

These reversals for judicial review challenges may explain the decline in judicial review applications brought by prisoners after 1987 (Sunkin 1991). One can also question whether the procedural changes brought about by the successful applications for judicial review significantly improved the quality of justice in disciplinary hearings. In 1991 the average number of disciplinary punishments per male prisoner in England and Wales stood at 1.9, 0.4 up on the figure that prevailed in 1980 before judicial review began to have an impact – although it had declined from 3.3 to 2.7 for women prisoners over the same period (Home Office 1992b). Though figures for acquittals are more difficult to obtain it seems unlikely that the 1990 level of 5 per cent prevailed during this period. Even the number of hearings before Boards of Visitors, which declined to 4.2 per cent of the total disciplinary punishments in 1984 (the year after *ex p. Tarrant*), had risen to 5.5 per cent in 1990, dropping back slightly to 4.7 in 1991. It would appear that more prisoners are being punished for more offences than before *St. Germain (No. 1)*. Certainly when the Woolf Inquiry took evidence in 1990 it did not discover a widespread perception that the complaints against the prison discipline system in the 1970s had evaporated with the impact of judicial review in the 1980s (see Woolf 1991, para. 14.386).

THE LIMITED SCOPE OF JUDICIAL REVIEW

It may be unwise to suggest that judicial review could have had a radical impact on the actual quality of prison justice, as there were many issues outside its scope. First, although it could tighten up the interpretation of prison offences it could not abolish offences such as 'makes any false and malicious allegation against an officer' or 'in any way offends against good order and discipline'. These offences have been criticised by many for their vagueness and as an invitation to arbitrary punishment (Justice 1983). Second, judicial review could not formally do away with the dual role of the Boards of Visitors, though the *ex p. Lewis* case, supported by widespread agreement outside the Home Office, represented an attempt to push in that direction. It looked as if it might be changed after the European Commission on Human Rights indicated in its *Campbell and Fell* decision that Boards were not 'independent' tribunals, as required by Article 6(1) of the European Convention, because the Secretary of State selected them and could remove them. However, the European Court of Human Rights found otherwise regarding this issue. Third, Boards could provide no mechanism for any sort of appeal in respect of a disciplinary hearing. As many cases turned on disputed issues of fact, where a governor or Board might be more likely to believe prison staff at their prison, an independent appeal system could play an important role in ensuring an impartial and thorough consideration of a prisoner's case. Finally, Boards provided no means of ensuring consistency of punishments within their own prisons, let alone between different prisons.

However, if the courts could not do these things the Government could. Stung into action by the Justice Report (1983), by *ex p. Tarrant* and by a fear that discipline hearings would become heavily legalised (a fear that was to prove groundless), the Government appointed a committee chaired by Mr Peter Prior to look into the issue of prison discipline. In its report (Home Office 1985d) the committee recommended, among other things, that the Boards lose their disciplinary function to Prison Disciplinary Tribunals with a legally qualified chair. It also recommended systems of appeal from governors' hearings and from the new Disciplinary Tribunal and further proposed that a number of offences be deleted from Rule 47. By the time the report was published, however, indications were that legal representation was being granted in fewer cases and, when granted, providing less problems than expected (Morgan 1987). Pleading that a new system would give rise to excessive costs the Government decided against making any changes in the structure of discipline proceedings. Rule changes in 1989, however, did remove some offences from the list and reduced the maximum penalty a Board could award to 180 days even on conviction of a number of offences. Since severe loss of remission, whether potential or actual, was often the trigger to judicial intervention, such changes reduced the likelihood of judicial review but were not perceived as having resolved the problems with disciplinary proceedings (Light and Mattfield 1988). Such was the state of affairs at the time of the Strangeways riot.

PRISON DISCIPLINE IN THE WOOLF REPORT AND THE GOVERNMENTS RESPONSE

To a large extent Woolf repeated Prior's criticisms of the existing discipline system, referring to the report as 'the most authoritative source on the prison disciplinary system' (para. 14.363). The Woolf Report strongly criticised the involvement of Boards of Visitors in discipline proceedings, drawing not only on previous criticism but also on a survey of magistrates clerks who had participated in a Home Office experiment to provide legal advice to Boards. The report on this survey indicated 'a closeness between members of the Board and prison staff' and added that

> Those who were ready to state a point of view indicated by a considerable majority that the Board of Visitor[s] did not use the same care in approaching LOR [the penalty of loss of remission] as Justices would have approached imprisonment.
>
> (Woolf 1991, para. 14.394)

Yet, although Woolf agreed with Prior that it was undesirable to mix the Board's disciplinary and supervisory functions, he rejected Prior's solution of replacing Boards with a specialist Prison Disciplinary Tribunal. Instead a more radical separation of disciplinary and criminal offences was recommended, with the former being heard by governors and the latter being referred to the Crown Prosecution Service (CPS) for prosecution in criminal courts. Such an approach, it was thought, would inhibit governors from referring charges to a higher authority when they felt a more severe penalty was appropriate – a practice which Woolf noted led to some Board members apparently feeling 'they were letting down the prison if they did not find a charge proved' (para. 14.377). Moreover, the Woolf Report indicated that the lengthy periods of lost remission that often resulted from Board hearings could not be tolerated without accompanying procedural safeguards, safeguards that were appropriate to a court (paras. 14.392 and 14.405). Loss of remission, if it was to remain a penalty at all, could only be tolerated if the periods of time were relatively short. Indeed the Report expressed the hope that, with an expanding range of opportunities in prison, alternative deprivations could prove a sufficient penalty and loss of remission might be phased out (para. 14.406).

Moving more cases into the criminal courts raises inevitable concerns that this will lead to greater delays before cases are heard, with the likely outcome that prisoners will spend more time in segregation awaiting a hearing. Woolf met this concern by citing Home Office figures which showed that over a nine-month period two-thirds of all disciplinary awards (1,200 of 1,723) in excess of 28 days (i.e. beyond the Governor's maximum penalty) related to absconds, matters which Woolf claimed could more properly be dealt with as disciplinary matters and given lesser penalties. As many of the remaining 500 should also properly be seen as disciplinary offences and could be properly managed within the governors' range of penalties, Woolf concluded that the increase in the number of cases referred to the criminal justice system (220 in 1988) would be 'manageably modest' and that in certain parts of the country a specialised panel of magistrates could be created to deal with them (para. 14.410).

For those cases that remained in the prison disciplinary system, still the overwhelming majority, few changes were recommended. Woolf argued that governors should remain able to give disciplinary awards of up to 28 days' loss of remission and that there should be no legal representation as of right before a governor. The major change Woolf recommended was the setting up of an independent Complaints Adjudicator who would represent the last stage of the appeals process (para. 14.424). Prisoners would thus have the right to appeal against a governor's decisions to the area manager (ie. the governor's boss) and, if not satisfied with the area manager's decision would be able to appeal to the Complaints Adjudicator. Such appeals could be made within seven days of the area manager's decision and both the area manager and Complaints Adjudicator should aim to give a reasoned decision within four weeks.

Virtually all of Woolf's recommendations found favour with the government. In contrast to the resistance to Peter Prior's idea of a Prison Disciplinary Tribunal, the proposal to remove the more serious cases to the criminal courts was quickly accepted in the White Paper *Custody, Care and Justice* (Home Office 1991a) and has since been enacted in the Prison (Amendment) Rules 1992. At the same time the Prison Department has reduced the time that adult prisoners must serve between adjudication and application for restoration of remission from nine to six months; and, for the first time, it is made explicit that governors have a duty first, to allow a prisoner to make a request for legal representation and, second, to consider that representation. The one significant deviation is that no provision exists for prisoners to appeal against the decisions made by the area managers when reviewing the disciplinary findings of governors. However, the White Paper accepts the need for 'an independent avenue of appeal against a disciplinary finding once avenues within the Prison Service have been exhausted' (Home Office 1991a, para. 8.8) and places the idea of a Complaints Adjudicator for the prison system under review (see Postscript). The circular instruction which accompanied the amended rules recognised every prisoner's entitlement to complain to the area manager regarding a disciplinary decision but did not stipulate how soon replies to such complaints should be produced.[13] Woolf had proposed four weeks (para. 14.428) rather than the six weeks allowed in the Grievance Procedures introduced in September 1990 (paras. 14.320–14.325).

As implemented in the Prison Rules these Woolf-inspired changes clearly mark the most significant shake-up of the prison discipline system this century. Prison reformers had consistently pressed for the removal of the adjudicatory function of Boards of Visitors and this has now been achieved. Another reform frequently sought, the introduction of an independent element in the appeals system, now seems attainable. However, the methods chosen to resolve one problem often run the risk of creating others.

ISSUES IN THE NEW PRISON DISCIPLINE CLIMATE

For those who have campaigned for many of the changes in the Woolf Report the advantages are obvious. Where prisoners face serious criminal charges they will now be entitled to legal representation, to trial before an independent tribunal that has no institutional need to maintain good relations with prison staff and to appeal against both conviction and sentence. In terms of the rule of law these are clearly considerable gains.

In addition, the fact that serious charges will now be adjudicated on by outside courts may discourage governors from too readily seeking severe disciplinary punishments as a control tool. As Woolf noted, some members of Boards of Visitors seemed to feel that when a case was referred to them it was because the governor felt a more severe punishment was appropriate. It is unlikely that governors were totally unaware of this perception and may have been tempted to resort to Board hearings, confident that convictions would be obtained, in order to send a signal to a particular prisoner or group of prisoners suspected of certain forms of behaviour. In 1991 around 6 per cent of punishments which were awarded for possessing an unauthorised article or destroying property belonging to another exceeded the maximum that governors may order. Some of these may have been the type of cases Woolf had in mind when he commented that some offences being dealt with by Boards should more properly be dealt with by governors. In terms of affecting the structure and character of discipline hearings a reason for seeking legal representation at discipline hearings was that the presence of an independent lawyer could exercise some scrutiny over the use of disciplinary powers within the prison. An outside court should be in an even better position to examine whether serious charges genuinely arise out of behaviour by prisoners that puts at risk the well being of other inmates and/or officers, or whether they are the product of flawed prison management which seeks to invoke disciplinary powers to deal with the symptoms rather than the causes of problems.

The availability of an appeal from a governor's hearing is obviously important. It was always clear that scrutiny by way of judicial review was a very limited post-disciplinary conviction remedy. Even if prisoners are allowed to call witnesses and cross examine all those who give evidence there are other vital issues outside the scope of judicial review: for example, is the prisoner's evidence properly taken and is his/her defence sufficiently explored? Governors' interests in maintaining internal control may dispose them to upholding an officer's authority in disputed cases. Woolf stressed how crucial justice and fairness were to good order in prison and an appeal system, especially with an independent element, should reinforce that broader view. Prisoners were able to raise issues about adjudications – both their conduct and the level of award – under the old system of petitions to the Home Secretary and, since 1990, they have been able to appeal to their governor's area manager under the new grievance procedures (see Chapter 4). Woolf accepted this avenue but recommended that area managers should be able to quash decisions and to vary penalties by re-hearing cases with the prisoner present (para. 14.422). The independent avenue to the Complaints Adjudicator was also recommended (para. 14.424). The White Paper states that 'the Government [is] attracted . . . to the notion of a Complaints Adjudicator', but assumed this would need primary legislation, and promises further consideration of the proposal that area managers might re-hear cases (Home Office 1991a, ch. 8). The development of a Complaints Adjudicator should enable greater consistency to be established in governors' awards for particular offences. Whether such aspirations are achieved, however, hinges critically on the form which the independent element in complaints and adjudication procedures takes and how the appointees perform their task.

As well as potential advantages there are also potential risks with the new system. Even if Woolf's estimate is correct that considerably fewer than 700 cases will be referred annually to outside courts, his 'manageably modest' number of cases could still be a considerable increase on the number which is currently referred. The delay in hearing these cases in court may be greater than it would have been before the Board of Visitors. This will be particularly disadvantageous to defendants when the governor decides to segregate them from the general prison population prior to the hearing. Changes in the Prison Rules in 1992 were aimed at preventing governors routinely segregating prisoners before hearings by indicating that a governor may only segregate purely in connection with the disciplinary period until the governor's first hearing. Thereafter all segregation must be on the basis of Rule 43 and will be subject to the approval of the Board of Visitors in the normal way. However, given that such oversight appears to have been fairly cursory in the past and that judicial oversight of the exercise of Rule 43 powers was shown to be very limited in the case of *Hague* v. *Deputy Governor of Parkhurst Prison* (1991), this may prove to be less of a protection than it seems.

Once prisoners appear before outside courts there is no guarantee that local panels of magistrates (Woolf's suggestion) will look any more dispassionately on prisoners as a class than Boards of Visitors have done. Perhaps because of this few prison reform groups recommended the outside-court option in evidence to the Prior Committee or to the Woolf Inquiry. In court prisoners face potentially more severe penalties for offences (such as assault) than the 120 days' loss of remission on a single charge that Boards could order. However, in their evidence to Prior the Prison Officers' Association complained that penalties imposed by outside courts were usually light.

How governors will operate the new system also remains to be seen, as their discretion very much remains central to it. Under Standing Order 3D(6) it is for the governor of the prison to decide whether the facts of the alleged offence constitute grounds for criminal prosecution and whether the incident will be reported to the police. Prison Service guidelines indicate which offences should be referred, emphasising offences of violence and concerted action among prisoners designed to undermine security and good order in the prison. Possession of weapons, for example, should only lead to referral when the weapons are guns or explosives, or where there is evidence that the weapons concerned are to be used in an escape or serious assault. Assaults should only be referred where serious injury is occasioned, or is likely, because weapons are involved. Only possession of Class A drugs should automatically be referred, while possession of Class B drugs should be reported when there is evidence of an intent to supply (Teggin 1992). Woolf envisages that governors will both refer 'up' more serious cases for criminal prosecution and refer 'down' some cases that would have gone before Boards to be dealt with within the scope of their own powers. However, as commentators with an inside knowledge have observed, the prison system can be slow to change and its most immediate response may be to seek to continue what it was doing by different means (Quinn 1985). Governors and prison officers may utilise other methods to control prisoners they perceive as problematic. Although fears that removing serious cases to outside courts would be accompanied by an increase in the scale of governors' punishments (Morgan, Maguire and Vagg 1985, p. 221) have proved to be groundless, there remains the possibility that the 'informal' disciplinary system of Rule 43 segregations and 'ghost train' transfers to different prisons will be more widely used. This spectre was raised before both Prior and Woolf. The former found no evidence of an increase in the use of the informal system since judicial review put the formal system under pressure. The latter felt that the requirement to give reasons for all administrative decisions (a recommendation the Government has yet to give formal effect to) should curb abuse of such powers. In any case it is arguable that such mechanisms are less available to governors in overcrowded remand prisons (due to lack of space and the need to keep prisoners close to courts at which they are required) where the greatest rise in the use of disciplinary punishments in the last ten years has occurred.

Nevertheless there is cause for concern. Even in a climate of increased judicial scrutiny, prison administrators had strong grounds for believing they would 'get a result' if they referred a case to a Board. Outside courts look altogether a more uncertain and time-consuming prospect; one does not need to be a conspiracy theorist to see that an institutional temptation to keep things 'in house' exists. In this climate there is a greater responsibility on Boards of Visitors to concentrate their watchdog attention on the use of disciplinary charges and administrative powers to control prisoners, especially since the House of Lords decision in *R.* v. *Deputy Governor of Parkhurst Prison ex p. Hague* is at least ambiguous about the extent of judicial supervision over these powers (Owen 1991). Unfortunately, it is difficult to see how, in the short term at least, removal of the Board's disciplinary role will do anything other than weaken their power within the prison. This removal does not seem to have been accompanied by a serious re-think about the role and powers of Boards, or about the development of an alternative institution, such as the visiting judge in the French system, who may make decisions about how the prisoner serves the sentence and who oversees the extent of disciplinary punishments (Bouloc 1991, pp. 81–109).

As for governors' hearings, the Northern Irish cases tend to indicate that judicial scrutiny of their conduct is likely to remain limited. This may not be too problematic if an effective appeal system is devised. Arguably, judicial review has always been an inadequate substitute for an appeal system. However, the form this appeal system will take, whether it can look at questions of substance as opposed to being limited to procedure, whether it can examine punishments as well as convictions, and what sort of representations prisoners can make to it, all remain to be worked out.

In the end it is unrealistic to assume that prison discipline will ever be more than a relatively rough form of justice. The hope that standards might approximate to those of the criminal law underestimates the effects of the penal context and the role which prison disciplinary punishments play. In civil society the criminal law intervenes relatively infrequently to deter socially threatening conduct. In prison the existence of rules show that prison discipline is designed to intervene regularly to reinforce specific patterns of behaviour amongst prisoners. For example, three disciplinary offences – 'disobeying a lawful order', 'offending against good order and discipline' and 'having an authorised article in one's possession' – account for nearly 40 per cent of all disciplinary punishments. Nowhere is this clearer than in women's prisons, where the rate of disciplinary punishments has consistently been higher than that in men's establishments (as shown earlier, women experience nearly one punishment per prisoner more than men and, for much of the 1980s the annual average number of punishments for women was above 3.0). Most of these punishments are for offences against good order and discipline and many are for forms of behaviour, such as swearing or talking back, that might not be punished in male prisons but which are seen as at variance with the image of the 'normal' woman which the prison seeks to promote. Even self-mutiliation has regularly been defined as suitable for punishment in order to discourage women from behaving in a manipulative and hysterical way (Dobash, Dobash and Gutteridge 1986, pp. 146–58).

In other words, regular disciplinary punishment is built in to the way prisons currently operate. For this reason prison authorities are less able than civil authorities in the wider society to tolerate procedures which check the exercise of disciplinary powers. This is also perhaps why courts, having strongly asserted their jurisdiction over what happens in prison and the reach of the rule of law into prison life, seem unable to exert much control over what actually happens there (Livingstone 1988; Gearty 1991). As Foucault has observed, commenting on a wider notion of disciplinary power, attempts to appeal to the law (or sovereignty as he puts it) to regulate the exercise of disciplinary power are ultimately doomed because law always begins from the premise of the legitimacy of normality, a normality which disciplinary power seeks to maintain and therefore helps to construct. Such attempts fail 'because sovereignty and disciplinary mechanisms are two absolutely integral constituents of the general mechanism of power in our society' (Foucault 1980, p. 108).

Even in the area of criminal law, rule of law notions relating to the legal equality of individuals are substantially attenuated by social-control ideas which emerge when dealing with so-called 'dangerous' offenders. In Roberto Unger's memorable phrase, what courts do in this area is 'supervise the police and the prosecution agencies as they decide which violent members of the underclass to imprison' (Unger 1983, p. 581). When it comes to prison disciplinary 'law' such notions are further attentuated by the context of the defendants already being prisoners, who, by definition, are presumed to be in need of discipline. In these circumstances the rule of law's presumptions of equality before the law will only go so far, as Peter Fitzpatrick puts it, 'law cannot bear too much reality' (Fitzpatrick 1984, p. 127).

This is not to say that change, whether brought about by legal or political intervention, has been useless. Court interventions, domestic and European, have curbed the use of severe disciplinary punishment and increased the visibility of disciplinary practices within prisons. They have also, like all successful litigation, produced moments of empowerment for prisoners sufficient to alter the nature of relationships within prisons (Jacobs 1980). Nor is it to say that disciplinary powers should have no role in prisons. Prisons are more dangerous places than most communities and the extent of violence in many American prisons shows the risks attendant upon an absence of order. It is simply to observe that questions about discipline lead us back to perennial questions about the nature and objectives of the prison enterprise.

POSTSCRIPT

Since this chapter was written two developments have occurred of particular importance in relation to the prison discipline system. First, as a result of the combined effect of section 42 of the Criminal Justice Act 1991 and the Prison Amendment (No. 2) Rules 1992 disciplinary awards of loss of remission have been replaced by a power to award extra days. This is to accord with the changes in remission arrangements brought about by the 1991 Act. As, however, prisoners would expect to be released without any extra days being awarded, it seems that awards of extra days as a result of disciplinary hearing should still be subject to judicial review. Second, the

Government has announced its plans for the Complaints Adjudicator, or Prison Ombudsman as he or she will be known. The Prison Ombudsman will have power to consider both procedure and merits in disciplinary cases but will make recommendations to the Home Secretary rather than having a direct power to overrule decisions taken elsewhere.

NOTES

1 The punishment of unlimited loss of remission was, however, limited to offences of mutiny or of doing gross personal violence to an officer under the old Rule 52.
2 *Lloyd* v. *McMahon* (1987) at p. 702, per Lord Bridge.
3 See *R.* v. *Board of Visitors Hull Prison, ex p. St. Germain (No. 2)* (1979). In *R.* v. *Board of Visitors Nottingham Prison, ex p. Moseley*, (23 January 1981), Glidewell J indicated that failure to allow a witness to be called would render the hearing '*prima facie* unfair'.
4 See *R.* v. *Board of Visitors Blundeston Prison, ex p. Fox-Taylor* (1982).
5 See *R.* v. *Board of Visitors Hull Prison, ex p. St. Germain (No. 2)* (1979).
6 See *R.* v. *Secretary of State for the Home Department, ex p. Tarrant* (1984).
7 See *R.* v. *Board of Visitors Highpoint Prison, ex p. McConkey* (1982).
8 See *R.* v. *Board of Visitors Dartmoor Prison, ex p. Smith* (1986).
9 See *ex p. Tarrant* (1984).
10 See *R.* v. *Board of Visitors Blundeston Prison, ex p. Norley* (1984) and *R.* v. *Risley Remand Centre Board of Visitors, ex p. Draper* (1988).
11 See *R.* v. *Board of Visitors Albany Prison, ex p. Mayo* (1985) and *R.* v. *Board of Visitors Wandsworth Prison, ex p. Raymond* (1985).
12 See *In re Carroll's Application* (1987), *In re O'Hare's Application* (1989).
13 See Circular Instruction 14/1992 'Changes to the Disciplinary System, Implementation (Phase Two).

6

WOOLF AND PRISON STAFF

Still looking for 'good gaolers'

J. E. Thomas

Prison staff, as was typically manifest during the Strangeways and concomitant riots, often feel under siege. Not just from prisoners, but from the public, most of whom would, apparently, be expert at dealing with the problem. But in any discussion of these events or of the prison 'crises', it is important to remember that there have been, and there are, much more serious cases of breakdown in other parts of the criminal justice system. Without doubt, a contemplative member of the British public would hardly single out the events leading to the Woolf Report (Woolf 1991) as being the most unbelievable in the British system.

There is much more reason to be concerned at the behaviour of the courts and the police, especially since the vile treatment associated with some of these has been so chronic and the injustice perpetrated so much less susceptible to analysis and correction than events in prison. The police treatment of alleged terrorists, the refusal of courts to undertake proper reviews until public concern is irresistible, the myopic pronouncements of judges such as Denning and Lawton, the scandals associated with the West Midlands police, all of these, and more, put Strangeways well down any list of officially inspired British criminal justice horrors.

A familiar theme throughout British prison history is the belief that such brutality can be avoided by involving the prison officer in the plethora of reformative initiatives which have characterised penal policy in this century. The Woolf Report is by no means the first to advocate such a role for prisons and there have been several exemplary developments. Until the end of the Second World War, for example, there were schoolmaster officers and clerk officers. The borstal system which, despite every criticism, was the pinnacle of penal reform, depended upon the assumption that officers could play a constructive part in training.

The reasons why the prospect of recreating this role seems remote are manifold. These include the steady erosion of officers' involvement by the growth of professions and consequent specialist activities. Pressure due to overcrowding had an influence, as did the pessimism about 'reformation' which was current in the 1970s and 1980s, not just in academic circles. Yet Woolf is right to remind us that, unless this key relationship between officer and inmate is put right, a prison system cannot work effectively whether in terms of treatment, control, security, or any of the many tasks facing a prison administration.

Dealing then with some of the issues affecting staff as addressed by Woolf, it is difficult because of sheer absence of information to imagine what the present Government thinks about prison staff, their recruitment, their training and more generally their education. Perhaps it will be realised that the quality and attitude of staff, while important in any organisation, is critical in prisons. This is important because the inheritance is not good.

The last major inquiry into prison administration was conducted by a committee chaired by Mr Justice May which reported in May, 1979 (Home Office 1979). Staff figured prominently in this report because of the remarkably undisciplined, often illegal behaviour of prison officers. Examples were plentiful and given on good authority. They included refusing to produce prisoners at court; refusing to allow entry by lawyers, relatives, non-officer staff and contractors; and refusals to staff new or repaired accommodation (King and Morgan 1980). The position did not improve to any great extent in subsequent years; 'Indeed', Woolf points out, 'industrial relations became worse' (Woolf 1991, para. 13.230). In a major attempt to change, the Prison Department negotiated its Fresh Start initiative.

FRESH START

There were several reasons for Fresh Start and some of these will be discussed later. But, *inter alia*, it was in an attempt to put staff disorder right that the scheme was introduced. This was not, at first sight, relevant to the disorder which Woolf investigated, but as he was determined to consider broad issues, he discusses it. As things turned out, this was inevitable, since the subject was raised constantly, notably by representatives of the prison officers. They believed that Fresh Start had not cured their malaise, which they described to Woolf in the same terms as they had done to every inquirer into staff feelings this century:

> evidence would draw attention to the lack of staff, lack of training, a sense of being undervalued, isolation from other staff and the divide between different grades and classes of staff. It would refer also to a lack of leadership within the Service.'
>
> (para. 1.144)

Although the question of what is called in the Report the 'Fresh Start Package' was of primary concern, Woolf does not discuss its workings in great detail. No doubt this was because of the sheer technicality of the subject, and any attempts to analyse it in detail and engage in making recommendations, would have deflected the Inquiry from its main concerns. Nevertheless, any attempt to understand the position of prison staff, most particularly of uniformed officers, must include awareness of the central points in this complex and extraordinary, yet bold attempt to improve the working of the prison system.

Fresh Start was introduced in 1987 after advice from PA Consultants. The Prison Department needed to solve the problem of overtime. Overcrowding had presented an unworkable milieu and overtime appeared equally destructive. There had been earlier attempts to establish an efficient and equitable system which would cope with the simple fact that a prison must be staffed everyday for 24 hours. As Woolf points out, these had failed. They did so because they attempted to improve existing schemes which institutionalised overtime and were technically complex. Whatever was tried, therefore, merely added another level of complexity, and made no impact on overtime. Woolf records (and examples were plentiful) that some officers were working 30 extra hours a week, (para. 13.19).

Some of the likely effects of this are obvious. Engagement in such overtime by anyone is bound to lead to a deterioration in performance at work. Next, guarantees of such extra income would accustom staff to rely on it, so that the ritual pleas by the Prison Officers' Association (POA) to reduce overtime were tempered, not only by the fact that they knew it was impossible, but also by the reality that many would be acutely embarrassed if income suddenly dropped. This is why the 'cultural' response of prison officers to Fresh Start was conditioned by the numerically large numbers of officers located in, for example, large local prisons. But there is another, much more sinister, aspect to the matter. This was that overtime was an important bargaining weapon. Anytime that the POA disapproved of a suggestion for change, the threat to reduce overtime would soon bring back into line a management which realised full well that the organisation would collapse if the threat was carried out, as it almost did in 1986 (see Home Office 1987a).

Despite all this, the officers agreed to accept Fresh Start, but from the outset it ran into controversy. The outcome was that the officers, as the Woolf Report notes, felt betrayed. What should have happened was that their working conditions should have improved. They alleged that they had deteriorated. What had gone wrong?

The first point to be made is that, in composing the 'Framework Agreement' for the scheme, there was little ill will and some optimism that it would be good for all concerned: for the Department considerable savings (see Woolf 1991, paras. 13.35–13.38) and for officers improved conditions. The weakness, and the potential for failure, lay in the fact that few people properly appreciated that this was not, as had been the case in the past, a cosmetic or tinkering exercise, but a transforming one. There were colossal structural problems which were not fully addressed, notably that different establishments started from different bases, and different experiences of manning levels.

It soon became clear that the setting of staff levels was going to be uneven, with a consequent allegation that there was now, in some places, understaffing. It followed that there were a number of possible solutions. The first was to increase the numbers of officers, but this, naturally enough, ran into Treasury resistance. Their attitude was that they had agreed to improve pay and conditions in return for agreed levels of efficiency savings. This in effect set limits on the *global* numbers available to implement the scheme, and required the Prison Department to post staff accordingly. But this was almost impossible because officers do not especially like being transferred, unless it is to a more convivial post, and all establishments would resist losing staff after negotiation had been completed.

The Prison Officers' Association agreed to the scheme because there were many attractions which uniformed staff welcomed. First, everyone, including those who had not worked vast amounts of overtime, received a considerable rise in pay and this, in turn, led to an increase in pension benefits. Second, staff would be allowed to buy their quarters under extremely favourable conditions. There *was* a strong element of inducement and it was particularly attractive to the Treasury because it was consistent with the prevailing Thatcherite philosophy. The disposal of quarters, incidentally, has already proved to be the greatest single mistake in prison administration since the Mountbatten Report (Home Office 1966). Many officers benefited immediately but the impact on the Prison Service was serious and irreparable. Edmund du Cane, the founder of the modern Prison Service in 1877, explained that staff mobility and convenience necessitated the provision of quarters. The consequence of the Fresh Start package is that it is difficult to move staff, and almost impossible to move them to the south. When they are moved, they leave their families and often have to live in what can be called, drawing upon every euphemism, substandard accommodation. There are reliable reports of officers actually having to sleep in their cars.

All these advantages to the generation of officers in post at the time were clear to the POA. But the latter had cause to welcome another change which reversed a practice which had been in place since 1877. This was the abolition of the system of direct entry to the governor grades. They were bound to welcome this, since it had been a source of grievance for at least fifty years. But they were faced with a problem. As part of the restructuring, they had to accept the abolition of the role of the Chief Officer. The Chief Officer had, since Victorian times, been the head of the uniformed staff; a familiar analogy is with the Regimental Sergeant Major. Prison officers always regarded him, as indeed did governors, with great respect. There would now be promotion from

Principal Officer to Governor. It must have seemed extremely unlikely that this would be accepted, but it was, for two reasons. First, it was consistent with the better career prospects described above and, second, some POA activists saw the change as a way of restoring their power, now in danger of disappearing through the abolition of overtime. With the eventual disappearance of the direct entrants, together with their culture of rehabilitation, it was likely that in a unified system all the senior posts would soon be taken up by ex-officers (although the Prison Department reserved an option to recruit directly). Most of these with lengthy service were nurtured in POA tradition and could be relied upon to support POA ambitions and, perhaps, even retain their POA membership. The whole question of direct entry is one to which I shall return.

The results of Fresh Start were, to put it mildly, disappointing. To begin with it was not long before staff felt cheated. Woolf reports that staff felt 'misled' and that 'they do not believe that the Prison Service has delivered what it promised'. This is because additional staff provided in accordance with the Framework Agreement were allocated on a national basis rather than to the individual establishments where identifiable vacancies had been created. The mistake was not to set staffing levels *ab initio,* before any changes. The result, they claim, has been 'still more inadquate staffing levels' (para. 1.162). The Department is trying to put things right by conducting a wide ranging and detailed analysis of the work to be done under the 'Corporate Objectives' exercise. This will lead to new systems of staff attendance to fit the work to be done. Woolf reports that the POA 'are not prepared to be associated with the process', and Woolf urges them to 'rethink' (para. 1.163). Unhappily, this is classic militant POA behaviour, which entirely destroys their credibility. What they are doing instead is to threaten industrial action, unless their manning levels are accepted, and they have found, in at least one prison, in July 1991, such action is effective. This is not new, and was reported by May:

> There is a further point that we have heard in various guises from prison officers, governors, and the Department itself. This is that for whatever reason industrial action has been found to produce results, and that the practice of resorting to such action has developed a momentum of its own. The POA argued that it had been the experience of branches that industrial action produced a response that had not previously been forthcoming, which meant that they would be the more ready to resort to such measures the next time an issue arose.
>
> (Home Office 1979, para. 10.21)

Furthermore:

> The governors are also critical of the policies which management has pursued in the face of industrial troubles. They contend that they

> have felt isolated in the face of trouble and bereft of the support from headquarters which they regarded as their due . . . they claim to receive inadequate support from headquarters in disciplinary cases, and that recommendations for dismissal are not acted upon.
>
> (Ibid., para. 10.19)

Unfortunately, this tradition of declaring institutional independence has begun to affect governors. Both the May and the Woolf Reports reflect the evidence of governors that if they resist the threats of local branches, the Department is likely to undermine their position by entering into some collusive agreement. It would be remarkable if some governors did not themselves collude by allowing the development of local, unofficial practices which are more congenial to staff.

The next complication arose from an integral part of the scheme: Time Off in Lieu (TOIL) was designed to replace overtime. Additional hours have to be worked for a variety of reasons (especially escorts and temporary staff shortages) and the only compensation available is an entitlement to time off at some uncertain, future date. This leads either to undermanning or to officers being tired, and in either event, to inefficiency; so staff will carry out the irreducible minimal part of their contract, such as unlocking, but the more discretionary elements will be put off. By the latter is not meant spending time talking to prisoners but, for example, carrying out regular searches. Some jobs do not have to be carried out at set times and can reasonably be described as 'flexible tasks'. When there is a shortage of staff either additional TOIL has to be accrued (and this will be increasingly difficult to honour) or some of the 'flexible tasks', such as searching, are done less frequently, if at all. In other words, they take chances, and the picture of the prison population of the 1990s which emerges from Woolf is of a kind which underlines the danger of failing to operate properly. This difficulty is compounded by the selling of staff houses. If officers cannot get their TOIL, and they cannot get home, and the financial pressures which have been touched upon increase, then the direction which the stress is likely to take is in the form of sick leave.

Nor are prison officers the only locus of resentment. When Fresh Start was introduced, one of its cornerstones was that it would 'unify' the whole service. The divisions between different sections of staff were keenly felt and were shared by the executive grades of the Prison Department who work at institutional level. These are mainstream civil servants. Many of them have spent all their careers in penal establishments and they supposed, especially in respect of pay, that the clear benefit which would accrue to prison officers would apply to them. They watched the basic pay of prison officers soar but theirs remained static despite considerable expectations. In the case of this sizeable and very influential group of staff, Fresh Start, far from 'unifying', had exactly the opposite effect.

A singular difficulty, and without doubt the most intractable, lies in the dispute over manning levels. The problem precedes Woolf and involves an important principle, namely, who decides staffing levels. It also helps to understand the refusal of the POA to work with the Prison Department on corporate objectives, a refusal which Woolf deplores. In 1986 the POA advanced a case that they should negotiate safe manning levels, subject to a proviso that the Department would have the last word. There are, probably, two reasons why this Department, or any other, cannot agree.

The first is consonant with the historic management view, reinforced by the authoritarianism which is a hallmark of the decade, that the settling of staff levels is a matter for management. The second is that the breakdown between centre and branches of the POA, evidenced in particular by the exploitation of the Disputes Procedure and the history of mistrust, is not likely to inspire the Department with faith in the POA to deliver. Put briefly, the evidence both from the Woolf Report and from other sources is that many prison staff still feel a sense of alienation from the organisation, with the inevitable consequence that prisoners will suffer. But central to any attempt to deal with these colossal problems must be a realisation that serious conflicts of interest remain – between governors and officers, between officers and prisoners, and between other groups. These have to be addressed with resolution and with the certain knowledge that most people in the Prison Service want it to be an effective organisation.

STAFF APPOINTMENTS AND CAREER STRUCTURE

The next important discussion is on the subject of recruitment and training. With regard to the first, the question of recruitment of prison staff has always been of concern to those who wish for a just system. John Howard made the quintessential statement when he wrote 'the first care must be to find a good man for gaoler' (Howard 1929). In absolute terms, for the past few years, recruitment to the prison officer grade has been buoyant, and substantial. In August 1991, for example, there were 650 new officers under training. Woolf (paras. 13.151–13.165) describes the system, applauds the new practice of 'opposite sex working' as beneficial and, contrary to another of Howard's admonitions, this view is commonly held in the system.

Woolf records in this section that 12 per cent of applications are from women, but in August 1991 approximately 20 per cent of trainees were women. He notes that for the Accelerated Promotion Scheme 'the candidates tend to be equally split between the two sexes' (para. 13.174). Woolf did not elaborate upon the position of women staff, nor for that matter women prisoners, and there were apparently two reasons for that. The first is that the Inquiry was concerned with the events of April 1990, none of which occurred in establishments holding female prisoners. The second is that while a wide variety of relevant women's organisations were invited to submit evidence, very few did. In so far as there is evidence, mostly anecdotal, about 'opposite sex working', many people seem to approve, largely because they believe it is a humanising influence.

The Report deals with one major question in recruitment, namely attracting more members of ethnic minorities. They remain under-represented on the staff but overrepresented among the prisoners. Such evidence as was given on the subject led to an observation on the gaps between such minorities and authoritarian organisations. There is a characteristic exhortation to do more, although Woolf points out the efforts that have been made.

There is, however, another general issue, and that is the choice of staff entrusted with the recruitment of officers. It is vital that this is carried out with the greatest care, yet it is commonly observed within the Prison Service that this is not always the case. Some individual recruitment staff have openly expressed prejudice against those considered 'liberal', against ethnic minorities and against women. It goes without saying that the Prison Service does not have a monopoly of such people.

One extremely important change needs to be made, since it was a grave error in Fresh Start and it can be recovered. This is the restoration of direct entry to the governor grades; this would be a major structural change but one which, paradoxically, could be reintroduced as easily as it was abolished. Since it is so important, let us examine it in more detail.

Historically governors could be appointed from outside the Service. During that same period the most senior and suitable chief officers and works officers could also be promoted to governor rank. In the most sophisticated period of recruitment, from the late 1950s to about 1985, governors were appointed through several routes. There was direct entry which attracted a wide variety of professionals (and was open to uniformed officers) and led to an appointment as an assistant governor. Officers could also apply for promotion to assistant governor through 'the limited competition'. Chief Officers could still be promoted to governor.

This is the system which has been abolished. And so a governor arrives either through the unified route – Officer, Senior Officer, Principal Officer, Governor V, or through an accelerated promotion scheme (see Woolf 1991, para. 13.169–13.177) This, it was expected, would attract the calibre of people who in previous generations would have joined as direct entrants. The scheme, which owes a good deal to the methods used in the police, was part of the Fresh Start deal and was supported by the Prisons Board some of whose members at least saw it as just for egalitarian reasons.

Unfortunately, although it may be theoretically just and egalitarian, as Woolf points out 'it has not proved attractive so far' (para. 13.169). In a Report which is notably correct in almost every respect, there occurs an occasional error. It notes that 'it is clearly very important that the accelerated promotion scheme should be successful' (para. 13.175). It will not prove so, and if theory can give way to experience, the reasons are not hard to find.

A system which is essentially unified, whereby promotions are made to a given grade from the next grade below (even allowing for a modest number of accelerated promotions) is called, in crude terms, 'following in dead men's shoes'. The consequences for an organisation which relies on the selection of its senior management in the unified way can be disastrous and the examples are legion. One might be taken from a system common in Australia where, in most states, the appointment of institutional managers relies on people who are variously and mostly, too old, too cynical and in ill health. The British police experience, too, is not felicitous. The 'Hendon' scheme some years ago allowed direct entry to senior posts, but the police now have a unified and an accelerated promotion system. The consequence, in both examples, has been a desperate shortage of people with adequate intellectual ability to occupy senior posts. This is not to say that people who proceed through the ranks do not possess this ability. Nor is it to say that direct entrants have a monopoly of such ability. Indeed, there are plenty of examples to prove the contrary. It is to say, first, that there should be as many entry points to senior command or management as possible. Good examples are to be found in the British armed services where such recruitment is made from A level candidates through the specialised institutions, from graduates and from the ranks. Second, an accelerated scheme will only attract those who are very keen or whose options are limited. This is because, as Woolf points out, the accelerated scheme does not accelerate enough. It takes a well-qualified individual a good deal of patience to serve for four years before achieving the rank of Governor V, the new equivalent of the rank of Assistant Governor Class II (the rank given to direct entrants on appointment under the old system). The fact is that such a scheme does not attract enough people of the right calibre and the Service in using it will be short of that initiative, commitment, principle and imagination which have been the contribution of many of the direct entrants when the English Prison System was at its peak. The direct-entry system should be restored, not for ideological reasons but as a concession to commonly accepted experience within the Prison Service itself. It could co-exist with a variety of appointments schemes, *including* accelerated promotion.

STAFF TRAINING

Woolf recognised the importance of the role of training in the making of an effective organisation, and so did many of the witnesses. Indeed, one of the central figures in the Inquiry, Mr O'Friel, the Governor of Strangeways, wrote to the Director of Personnel and Finance before the riot, expressing his concern that the time allocated for training had, in reality, been reduced. There followed a classic piece of administrative confusion about whether or not this was so (Woolf 1991, para. 13.144). In fact, there is a paradox in the attitude to training in that the Prison Service had been involved in systematic training for a hundred years, has accumulated a good deal of sophisticated experience and spends a good deal of money on it. The Prison Service College is a substantial organisation. In August 1991, for example, some 70 experienced members of staff were engaged, full-time, in training newly joined officers.

In an excellent section of the Report, Woolf touches upon many of the issues which a consideration of training creates. Some of these are detailed proposals, such as the one supporting the Central Council of Physical Recreation's recommendation that people from further education and other sources could be engaged as 'special' prison physical education officers (para. 13.128). Two recommendations will require special recognition during implementation of the Report. First, 'that more attention be paid by the Prison Service to training. A *greater* commitment to training would also help to show that the Prison Service cares about its staff' (para. 13.108). The second is that this has 'resource implications'. The latter is clear enough, and provisional gloom must surround it, if the government maintains its present attitude. An analysis of the questions posed by Mr O'Friel to the Director and the answers he received show that even seven days a year could not be achieved, since officers were denied training because they had to undertake operational duties (paras 13.142–13.146). This is both true and thoroughly unsatisfactory; and Woolf recommends 'ring fencing' fifteen days a year (para. 13.147).

Each days's training for the Service costs £2m. In practice, therefore, this would mean an increase in expenditure on training from about £14m to £30m, or the equivalent of 120 extra officers for each day's training. This would mean one extra officer per establishment.

It is therefore reasonable to ask what 'a greater commitment' might mean, given present substantial overall levels of training. To understand the significance of training and its relationship to the goals of the organisation requires sophistication and commitment. All too often training is held up as evidence that the organisation is serious, or progressive. Training for its part is regarded as being responsible either for everything or for nothing: magical or harmless. The truth is that if training is not fully integrated into the organisation it will be of little importance. There are many indications in the Report that some of this is true of the prison system. For example, training can be cancelled and frequently has been, thus demonstrating to all that its value is peripheral. It is necessary, too, to demonstrate the importance of training by appointing the best staff and at the most senior levels. Yet in establishments training staff are changed far too rapidly. It is impossible to develop a core of shared expertise and experience as long as this is true and visible. There must be engendered a feeling that it is a privilege to work in training and this feeling must be reinforced by senior staff in the Prison Department through their committed recognition that good training is a priority. A healthy commitment to training should be matched by an equal commitment by the staff to the goals of the organisation – a benefit which good organisations recognise and enjoy (see also Woolf's conclusion at para. 13.260). To that end an early objective for the Prison Service should be a systematic, continuous dialogue between the field and training. If this were to be done, the training organisation could ensure that it contributed to emerging and changing practice, and practice could benefit from the trainers' reports about the staff undergoing courses. In this way courses can be 'relevant' to practice, and thus avoid the principal criticism of training.

One special example concerns the training needs of Principal Officers being promoted to Governor V. There is, by common consent, a mammoth problem because there are long-serving officers who are now required to move into senior management positions. Many are quite bewildered so that governors frequently wonder if they should have been promoted. However, the exigency of Fresh Start requires the numbers. Training at this point is more than ever necessary if the system is not to crumble. A major debate is needed to ensure that the experience of such people can be used, modified and transformed to the benefit of the Department and not to further disruption. There must be a studied attempt to consider afresh the role and contribution of training.

MANAGERIALISM, CONTRACTS AND INDUSTRIAL RELATIONS

The problems described in the Woolf Report are formidable and deeply ingrained. A number of major issues have to be tackled and some have been discussed. This final section deals with the biggest of these. It is generally agreed in the Prison Service that a lot of the desperation of staff, especially governors, derives from the new managerialism which underpins organisational practice in this age. It has led to a proliferation of paper work and, far from improving communications, has made things worse. Perhaps the most startling example of this, as Woolf identified, is the failure of the Prison Department and its establishments to agree whether or not there *is* a staff shortage. The nature of this bureaucratic managerialism is badly in need of inspection. Again, one example will illustrate the point. Governors have to agree 'contracts', setting out what they and their establishments should do (see paras. 12.88–12.97). These contracts are agreed once a year. But as has been explained, staff cannot always fulfil what are described as 'flexible tasks' because of other pressures, internal or external. Some flexible tasks are done at other times but some are simply dropped. The inevitable result is that the 'contract' loses its meaning. This is not to say that they should be abolished but that they might perhaps be negotiated more often. And Woolf properly stresses that the Prison Department, through its area managers, must be able to meet its 'reciprocal obligation' (para. 12.97). The Report goes on to recommend contracts between staff and management in each establishment with each side's obligations clearly described (paras. 13.199– 13.203).

There remains the problem of what is euphemistically called 'industrial relations'. Woolf describes the Dispute Procedure but observes that this has not achieved any substantial reduction in industrial action (paras. 13.235–13. 243). 'Indeed neither did the disturbances in April [1990]. Nor did the appointment of this Inquiry' (para 13.239). The Report lists the industrial disputes between 1 January and 3 October 1990 and it is not surprising that the list is described as 'depressingly long', since 70 establishments were involved.

Woolf criticised the POA for its unwillingness to co-operate with the Prison Department in the process of identifying corporate objectives from which appropriate staffing levels could be derived (para. 13.252). Staffing levels have been the cause of so many local disputes since Fresh Start was implemented. Much of the 'dispute' which occurs at an institutional level is not to do with the scheme, 'status quo' is not always maintained and illegal action often follows. The ability of governors to govern is destroyed. The POA is, however, in disarray and its credibility is at an all-time low. Uniformed staff are mainly concerned with their immediate positions and with the fact that they attract little sympathy. The Department should therefore be prepared to dismiss staff who refuse to carry out their duties. Under what circumstances this can be done needs to be considered and tested. The Service cannot operate with staff who disagree with policy and decide what they will and will not do. It has tried to do so for the quarter of a century since the Mountbatten Report and every attempt has failed. It is a failure which has brought the Service into disrepute, heaped misery upon prisoners and drawn public contempt upon officers. It would take courage; without action the anarchy remains and the Woolf Report loses its relevance. The better way is described by Woolf – additional investments by the Department and additional commitments by the staff (para. 13.260).

The other interesting possibility which is consonant with increasing practice in the work place generally, is to employ part-time staff (see para. 13.103). This is complicated because of considerations of security, the need for continuity in handling prisoners and the almost certain opposition of the POA. Nevertheless, it would be interesting to see a working party established to examine its feasibility.

The matters discussed by Woolf in respect of staff are very familiar to those who have read reports made in the past hundred years. There is the notable unhappiness expressed by staff with their conditions, an unhappiness which has increased in the last thirty years. Linked with this is a feeling, well based and documented, that headquarters is not interested in the work of prison officers. Fresh Start was supposed to address some of these problems but, as we have seen, because it was introduced in such an unsatisfactory manner, it created more problems than it solved. This is exemplified by the abolition of direct entry, one lesson which has certainly been learned, since it is highly likely to be restored. The question generally is whether the government will address the problems identified by Woolf, even to the modest extent indicated by official responses. These are very bland, for example, on overcrowding: 'the objective should be that no prisoner should have to be accommodated in overcrowded conditions' (Home Office 1991a, para. 6.11).

Finally, there is the question of the future of Fresh Start. Assuming that in its essentials it remains, the Department should learn some lessons from it. The first is that it was, and is, a transforming exercise, fundamental and radical. The Treasury must understand this, too, and should realise that there needs to be flexibility in the introduction of such a change. Both are hampered by a rigid commitment to limited time scales. Fresh Start was not just an event. As far as the governors are concerned, commitment to a major training programme would show a real recognition of the profundity of the change. A team management approach should be promoted to counter the traditional assumption that governors run prisons hierarchically or by caprice. There is a good case for saying that there should be no major changes in the Service for the next ten years other than those necessary to implement the Woolf recommendations and, perhaps more importantly, to effect a change in the prevailing culture to reflect the underlying philosophy of prison treatment. Some of the observations and suggestions in this chapter may seem harsh. Woolf has reminded us that these are very serious matters in which members of the community have an interest. If there is a half-hearted response, then an excellent report will join others like it, their only function to be used as a text with which to torment students.

ACKNOWLEDGEMENT

I would like to express my appreciation to Mr Gordon H. Lakes, an Assessor with the Woolf Inquiry and formerly Deputy General of the Prison Department, for his considerable help in commenting on this chapter.

7

HEALTH CARE IN PRISONS

Roger A. Ralli

INTRODUCTION

The future provision of health and medical care to prisoners has been clearly addressed in the Woolf Report (Woolf 1991); in the subsequent White Paper *Custody, Care and Justice* (Home Office 1991a); and in the Scrutiny Report into the Prison Medical Service (Home Office 1990e). The various recommendations contained in these official reports, however, must be set in the context of the history of the medical care of prisoners; the reports, investigations and enquiries into medical care undertaken over the last 30 years and their impact; but, above all, the issues related to providing health and medical care in a closed environment to a discrete section of the population.

PRISON MEDICINE

The provision of medical care for prisoners has and always will be a complex and contentious field of specialism. Prisons are the places to which society removes people who break its rules; loss of liberty is their punishment. Whilst prison may provide a chance of rehabilitation it must also be seen as a deterrent to others. In such a setting, the provision of medical care is fraught with practical as well as ethical problems. There are at least seven fundamental questions or dilemmas facing the prison doctor:

1 Are the doctors' primary loyalties to the prisoner-patient or the prison authority? Is this relationship covered by medical ethical codes and do the codes take account of a prison doctor's particular needs and isolated position from the outside medical world?
2 What is the doctor's position in the prison management hierarchy – how does the power of the doctor equate to that of the prison governor, who has ultimate sanction? Should the doctor's performance be assessed by the governor?

3 What is the relationship of the prison doctor to the process of punishment? The line which exists between medication or seclusion for medical reasons and for control purposes is extremely fine.
4 Can medical confidentiality be maintained in the prison environment when disclosure of information in reports is a part of a doctor's work?
5 Is a prison doctor's work open to external scrutiny and professional peer-group audit?
6 If the standard of medical care provided depends, at least in part, upon the quality of the specialist training undertaken by staff, should this be overseen by the medical royal colleges?
7 Should professionally trained prison doctors work with professionally trained prison nurses to form the health-care teams?

Providing medical care is, however, only one part of the whole field of prison health care. Health as defined by the World Health Organisation is 'a state of complete physical, mental and social wellbeing and not merely the absence of disease or infirmity'.

At first sight it might seem that the prison environment is the ideal place to fulfil these criteria, with the potential to provide health care, health education and appropriate treatment to a discrete group, whilst ensuring adequate diet and exercise as well as protection from the use of alcohol and illicit drugs. In reality the environment is often overcrowded and may be unhygienic. Low levels of activity are not uncommon; there is frequent overeating and the use of tobacco is endemic in prison culture (Harding 1987). There are also stresses in detention which emanate from the separation from family and friends, the uncertainty of outstanding criminal proceedings or parole applications, as well as the general problems of adapting to prison life itself. Each of these facets may play a significant part in affecting an individual's state of health. Even with improved conditions and enlightened regimes and programmes, the facts of imprisonment ensure that prison is not a healthy place.

In this setting the need for clear standards and principles of health care is essential. The United Nations standard minimum rules for the treatment of prisoners contains a section on medical services (United Nations 1955). These were revised by the Council of Europe Committee of Ministers and adopted by them in 1973 (Council of Europe 1973). They provide for a basic standard of health care: that this service should work in close relationship with the nation's health service; that suitable facilities should be available for medical and dental care as well as the care of those who are pregnant; and that prisoners may not be subjected to medical or scientific experiments that could result in physical or moral injury. Additionally the medical staff should have an inspectorial role throughout the establishment. These rules form the basis of the ones that govern the provision of health care in prisons in England and Wales.[1]

Responsibility for the provision of health care to prisoners falls to all areas and groups within the prison system: from senior management, through the prison governor, to local management teams; the doctor; the health-care team; and, not forgetting, the individual him- or herself. At the heart of this bureaucracy, however, is the prison doctor. A valuable insight into the doctor's position was provided by Norval Morris who clearly identified the ethical dilemmas that are ever-present in prison medicine.

> The doctor and the attendant medical staff occupy a peculiarly sensitive position in the prison community. It is always a mistake for one in a hurry to ask a prisoner 'How are you?' He will tell you at burdensome length. Hypochondria is chronic and endemic in prison and so is malingering and so I believe age for age is a higher than average incidence of most illnesses. Hence the task of the prison doctor is to meet genuine medical needs without himself becoming cynical, assuming that he is merely the constant butt of the prisoners' efforts improperly to manipulate him, this is no easy challenge. Pressure to debase the healing professions pervades prisons . . .
>
> What underlies this is the sheer sensitivity of the doctor/patient relationship in the penal institution where freedom of choice both for doctor and patient is inexorably limited by the pressures of an unreal social setting. Conflict and hostility tend to replace medical trust and this is true even when medical services are of high quality and facilities adequate to medical needs . . . It is of first importance that the doctor should not confine himself to medical matters. He should be knowledgeable and involved in the whole life of the prison community . . . The doctor has important and sensitive functions in relation to prison discipline and prison punishments.
>
> (Morris 1973, pp. 39–40)

The prison doctors' responsibilities and their professional relationships with their prisoner-patients are exactly the same as in any doctor–patient relationship. But the doctor also has responsibilities to the wider prison community and the community outside prison. In a review of this ethical dilemma Harding (1991) outlines six conditions that need to be met for a prison medical/health-care service to be seen to be ethical:

1 Independence of medical service from prison administration.
2 Freedom of decision-making in arranging specialist consultations and hospitalisation on medical grounds.
3 Equivalence of health care and preventative measures between prison and the community.
4 Freedom of access of prisoners to the medical service.
5 Informed consent to treatment.
6 Confidentiality of medical information and records to only medical staff.

In short, the fact of imprisonment should not be a constraint on the prisoner-patient in seeking care, nor should it constrain the providers of that care in delivering a service which conforms to the same standards and principles as that which would be available to the individual were they not in prison.

THE PRISON MEDICAL SERVICE

The Prison Medical Service is the oldest civilian medical service in England and Wales and was borne out of the work of penal reformer John Howard, whose book *The State of the Prisons in England and Wales* (1929), first published in 1777, described the appalling conditions of prisons in the late eighteenth century. This pioneering work led to an Act of Parliament in 1779 that required a physician to be appointed to each prison and report at the Quarter Sessions on the state of the prisons' health (this requirement continues in the form of an annual report by each prison's managing doctor to the Prison Services Director of Health Care). The first prison rules incorporating instructions for the doctor were made at Shrewsbury Prison in 1794. The doctor was required to visit the patients every day, examine every person on admission and see every prisoner at least once a week and enquire into the state of his body and mind. If he had any reason to consider that one or other was affected by discipline or diet he should, in conjunction with the chaplain, certify this in writing to the governor to persuade him to take appropriate action. The opening of the new model prison Pentonville saw the introduction of specific guidance to tackle health problems, particularly infectious diseases and scurvey

At this time the mentally disturbed, as now, were a considerable cause of concern. By 1836 arrangements were in hand for the transfer from prison of the mentally disturbed to county asylums. None the less, many still remained in prison, mostly at Dartmoor, subsequently being moved to Millbank in 1864. The Criminal Lunatic Asylum Act was passed in 1860 and Broadmoor Hospital opened in 1863 under the management of the Home Office. The Prison Act 1877 unified the responsibility for all prisons in England and Wales under one authority. In 1879 the new Prison Commissioner, Dr Gover, previously medical superintendent at Millbank, drew attention to the continuing large number of mentally disordered in prison and to the high suicide rate. The Gladstone Committee (Departmental Committee 1895) recommended that all prison doctors should have experience in the subject of lunacy and in 1897 arrangements were made for the new Parkhurst Prison to take suicidal prisoners.

There are many further studies from the turn of the century reviewing criminal behaviour and the mentally abnormal. But it was in 1932, when the Departmental Persistent Offenders Committee was established, that a major step forward was taken in the development of mental health facilities for prisoners. The deliberations of the committee led to the appointment in 1934 of the first visiting psychotherapist, Dr W. H. Hubert, at Wormwood Scrubs Prisons. With the medical commissioner, Sir Norwood East, he published a report *The Psychological Treatment of Crime* (1939) which recommended a special institution for the care, study and treatment of selected criminals. This was to become Grendon Prison, which opened some twenty-three years later in 1962.[2]

It can be seen that over the years the mentally disordered offender in custody has been alternately recognised and then ignored. This has been reflected in management policies, as well as in the recruitment strategies of health-care staff. The latest Home Office guidance affirms that prison is not the place for the mentally abnormal and that they are the responsibility of the Health Service.[3] Recent research by Gunn, Maden and Swinton (1991) reveals that there are over 1,100 mentally abnormal offenders in the sentenced prison population, a significant proportion of whom should be accommodated in Health Service psychiatric facilities, given the available resources for them to do so and their willingness to accept them (see Chapter 10).

The establishment of the National Health Service in 1948 set the Prison Medical Service within the Home Office, with all its staff being civil servants. Most prisons by this time had a hospital, which was based on the military sick-bay concept, and was staffed by the prison doctor, who could be either full or part time, and by prison hospital officers. This brand of the prison discipline staff was established in 1899 and originally received only a few weeks training in nursing orderly duties. This grade still exists, though the training has been extended to 6 months. Women's prisons, however, have always employed qualified nurses who have undertaken their professional training prior to joining the Prison Service.

The legislation currently underpinning the provision of prison health care is the Prison Act 1952, which requires every prison to have a medical officer; and the Prison Rules 1964, which underline the doctors' responsibility in the care of the mental and physical health of the prisoners.

RECENT HISTORY

In the last 30 years the Prison Medical Service has been the subject of much comment and criticism, as well as the subject of several inquiries and reports.

In 1962 there was growing concern about the functioning and organisation of the Prison Medical Service and particularly its relationship with the National Health Service. A working party set up by the then Home Secretary, Henry Brook, produced the Gwynn Report (Home Office 1964). The report made 15 recommendations, which included the desirability of establishing a medical advisory committee; the requirement for a systematic review of the needs of establishments; consideration to more work being done by general practitioners; the expansion of the Prison Medical

Service to meet growing demands; improved supervision of doctors by regionally based senior doctors; improved facilities for training; parallel recruitment and training within forensic psychiatry; and the formation of joint Home Office and regional hospital-board consultant forensic psychiatrist posts.

Of all these recommendations only two appear to have been acted on. First, regionally based senior doctors were established, but these have subsequently been centralised in London. Second, the joint appointment of forensic psychiatrist posts was introduced, but this proved not to be a succesful initiative, perhaps because of the conflicting interests of the contract holders and a lack of clarity in setting out exactly what the psychiatrists were to do. Now, 30 years on, many of the other key recommendations are appearing in slightly different guise in the Efficiency Scrutiny Report (Home Office 1990e) which will be discussed later in this chapter.

In 1972 a further committee was established under the chairmanship of Lord Butler to review the law and the powers, procedures and facilities for the treatment of the mentally abnormal offender. The Butler Report (Home Office/Department of Health and Social Security 1975) served to underpin the diversion of the mentally abnormal offender from the penal system and the formation of forensic psychiatry as a specialty, as well as recommending the development of hospital regional secure units. But, as Adrian Grounds notes in Chapter 10, less than a third of the recommended number of places in such units are currently available for use. However, neither the Butler Report, nor the subsequent May Report (Home Office 1979), though expressing concern about the Prison Medical Service, felt able to recommend its incorporation into the National Health Service.

By the early 1980s the Prison Medical Service was receiving considerable criticism in the media concerning the number of deaths and suicides in custody, the alleged use of tranquillizers as a means of control ('the liquid cosh'), and the general standard of prison health care. In 1983 the *British Medical Journal* published a series of articles by Dr Richard Smith, which were subsequently updated and published as a book (Smith 1984), which provided an in-depth and well-balanced view of the provision of medical services for prisoners. He succinctly identified the difficulties in the provision of care and how the care was being delivered:

> No single answer can be given to questions about the quality of the Prison Medical Service, but there is some evidence that it is deficient because of its organisation's invisibility and lack of accountability; it may be difficult for dedicated doctors within the service to do their best by their patients. Prison doctors have to grapple with many difficult problems and close cooperation and better communications with doctors outside the prisons could only benefit prisoners.
>
> (Smith 1984, pp. 100–1)

With the Prison Medical Service under media scrutiny the House of Commons Social Services Committee decided in 1985 to inquire into the Prison Medical Service. The committee, chaired by Mrs Rene Short, reported in 1986 (House of Commons 1986). The committee is noted to have worked closely with the then new Director of the Prison Medical Service, though it is interesting that their appointed specialist advisors were all forensic psychiatrists. They took a considerable amount of evidence both at home and abroad and made 58 recommendations:

> We believe that our recommendations taken together can transform the Prison Medical Service into a prisoners' health service, less doctor dominated, more professional, more primarily concerned with the delivery of multi-disciplinary health care.
>
> (House of Commons 1986, p. 59)

The Government replied to the committee's report in 1987 and broadly accepted 48 of their recommendations (House of Commons 1987). However, reviewing the current situation in relation to the original 58 recommendations: 10 do not relate to prison health care directly and 15 were either rejected at the time or have not been pursued. Of the remaining 33, 20 were implemented shortly after the report was published, including the revision of Standing Order 13, the provision of medical records for every prisoner, the lifting of Crown Immunity, and the publication of the Chief Inspector's medical advisor's report. The remaining 13, which include the undertaking of Medical Audit, setting up contracts for services with health authorities and consideration of the terms of employment of prison doctors, have reappeared as part of the Efficiency Scrutiny Report (Home Office 1990e) and are in the process of being implemented.

The report of the Social Services Committee led directly to the setting up of a working group chaired by the then President of the Royal College of Physicians, Sir Raymond Hoffenberg, to review the recruitment and training of doctors for the Prison Medical Service. Their report reviewed the work of the prison doctor and made 12 recommendations, including the proposal that prison medicine should become a recognised specialty and that an accreditation scheme for training new doctors should be established (Home Office 1990f). They did, however, emphasise that additional finance would be necessary for this training to be implemented. Discussions on the recommendations and the possibility of a recognised qualification in prison medicine are still taking place.

New doctors joining the Prison Medical Service since 1989 have undergone an enhanced introduction to prisons and prison medicine by two senior prison doctors and are provided with an information booklet (Ilbert and Ralli 1989). In October 1991 a diploma course in addictive behaviour, especially designed for prison doctors, was established at St George's Hospital, Tooting, the first qualification developed specifically for prison doctors. A significant amount of other training is now taking place, not only focusing on clinical issues relevant to prisons, but also on management skills for doctors and health-care staff at all levels. This goes some way to meet the specialist training need already identified. However, training programmes established by the medical Royal Colleges are still being developed and have yet to take place.

Efficiency Scrutiny Report

Her Majesty's Chief Inspector of Prisons, Judge Stephen Tumin, in his annual report for 1989 included a chapter specifically on medical services (Home Office 1990g). He described many defects in the provision of health care including low levels of staffing and resources, inadequacies in reception procedures and in suicide prevention, defects in the pharmacy service and problems related to hygiene. As his report was published the next stage in the series of reviews of the Prison Medical Service, the scrutiny of the Prison Medical Service in England and Wales by the Government's Efficiency Unit, was underway, and was subsequently published in October 1990 (Home Office 1990e).

The scrutiny team was required to start from the premise that a separate prison medical service was necessary. The objective of the review was to assess the efficiency and cost-effectiveness of the existing medical and dental services, particularly in relation to their management, and the provision of hospital facilities and staff training. In its 83 recommendations the report, although seemingly recommending radical changes, draws heavily on both the Gwynn Report (Home Office 1964) and the Select Committee Report (House of Commons 1986). The recommendations of the Efficiency Scrutiny Report fall into three key areas:

1 The Prison Medical Service should become a prison health service, emphasising health promotion and the prevention of disease. It should become more clearly aligned with the National Health Service under the supervision of a health advisory committee which would advise the Secretary of State and the Director of Prison Health Care.
2 Clinical practice and medical management should be more clearly distinguished.
3 The Prison Service should become a purchaser of health care and not a provider and should do this by developing contracts for specialist and primary care with health care providers in the NHS. In prisons which need to retain major hospital facilities, full-time medical officers should remain in post to act as clinical managers.

These recommendations were made at the same time as widespread changes were taking place within the National Health Service, including *Working for Patients* (Department of Health 1989), the new general practitioners contract, and the provision of health care on the purchaser–provider model. The Health Service's way forward has now been underlined in the White Paper *The Health of the Nation* (Department of Health 1992). This underpins the latest changes in the provision of health care to prisons and develops the concept of 'healthy prisons' to go along with the already established 'healthy cities' initiatives.

The feasibility and implications of the Prison Medical Service becoming a Prison Health Service have recently been addressed in research by Darkins, a public-health physician (Darkins 1991). He highlights the lack of knowledge about the state of the health of the prison population and underlines the requirement for appropriate resources to be made available to ensure that desired changes can be effectively implemented. Some critics, however, have argued that the review does not go far enough and that the National Health Service should be responsible for purchasing medical services in prisons as well as providing these services (Smith 1992).

Widespread consulation has taken place, both internally and externally, about the Efficiency Scrutiny Report's recommendations. The initial distillation of this by an internal working party concluded that:

1 More use could be made of general practitioners in providing health care, but for more specialist work they will require special training.
2 To attract doctors, work and conditions in prisons need to be improved to create a better health-care climate.
3 Model contracts for general practitioners should be drawn up which clearly specify the service they are required to provide.
4 All specialist mental health care should be contracted-in.
5 Full-time clinicians will continue to be needed in local/remand prisons and in some other establishments.
6 Contracts will need to be sufficiently attractive to encourage current health-care staff as well as outsiders to opt for them.
7 More civilian nurses should be employed in prison health care and the training and qualification of hospital officers should be improved.

There appears to be agreement that change in the provision of health care to prisoners needs to come urgently. The current service and level of resources need to be reviewed and rationalised as much as the health needs of the prison population need to be assessed. However, it is also apparent that a change to a contracted-in service is quite at odds with the Hoffenberg Report (Home Office 1990f) which identified prison medicine as a specialism in its own right. Nevertheless, it does go some way towards increasing the involvement of the National Health Service in prison health care.

Woolf Report

The scrutiny review (Home Office 1990e) and the subsequent work have been taking place in the shadow of the worst prison disturbances in the history of the English penal system. A number of medical and health issues have been highlighted in the report into the April 1990 disturbances by Lord Justice Woolf and Judge Stephen Tumim (Woolf 1991). Following their enquiries they voiced concern that the medical treatment of prisoners was not comparable to that available outside in the National Health Service, and there was an expressed worry that medical treatments were continuing to be used for control purposes, though no evidence was cited to support this. None of Woolf's 12 recommendations, however, was specifically directed to the provision of medical care. Although the Report broadly endorsed the recommendations of the Efficiency Scrutiny Report as being 'in accord with the general approach that we have suggested should be adopted', it concluded that it was not 'in a position to form a detailed judgement on them' (para. 12.134). None the less, the Efficiency Scrutiny Report, and contracts when actioned, should address the concerns identified in the Woolf Report by clarifying the standard of care to be provided for prisoners, which must not only be, but be seen to be, equivalent to that in the National Health Service. But this should not be seen as a panacea for all of the problems surounding the provision of prison health care. It has become clear that across the country NHS standards vary considerably. It is equally clear that those working most of the time in the NHS do not necessarily bring their NHS standards with them when working in prisons. Furthermore, there is little doubt that, in some instances, those working full time in the prison service surpass NHS standards of care.

Although the Woolf Report does not make any recommendations about medical services in general it does make specific proposals on two particular issues concerning the medical care of prisoners: the management of drug users and the management of HIV/AIDS.

In discussing the management of drug abusers, though now much better described as drug users, Woolf details the scale of the drug-user problem in the prison system, drawing on information from research by Gunn *et al.* (1991). However, the Report makes only two proposals:

> The Prison Service should examine the experiences abroad of drug free units and subject to the outcome of that examination, make provision for drug free units in prisons.
>
> (para. 12.350)

> There should be a prison officer responsible for coordinating the service provided within a prison establishment and in the locating of drug and alcohol abusers.
>
> (para. 12.353)

Departmental guidelines on the throughcare of drug users were issued in April 1991,[4] along with the manual *Caring for Drug Users: A Multidisciplinary*

Resource Pack for People Working with Prisoners (Home Office 1991k). These guide-lines address the criticisms raised in the text of the Woolf Report, and also in the research by Gunn *et al.* (1991), and provide a framework for the care of drug users that is on a par with the best available in the National Health Service. They cover problems of identifying drug users; assistance with withdrawal and the appropriate use of medication, including methadone; support and counselling; advice on harm minimisation; and throughcare and liaison with agencies outside. The active involvement of relevant voluntary agencies is particularly encouraged. However, for the policy to be put into practice, there is a requirement for extensive training, some of which is taking place, as well as support and encouragement all along the managerial line. Guidance on this work in prisons is also highlighted in the revised edition of *Drug Misuse and Dependence – Guidelines on Clinical Management* (Department of Health 1991b). Before consideration is given to any further initiatives an opportunity must be given for the new guidelines to be effectively enacted throughout the prison system and for their effect to be reviewed.

It is clear that the proportion of drug users in the prison system is steadily increasing, though perhaps not as rapidly as in some other countries. As a group they present considerable problems for the system which have been highlighted by the advent of HIV/AIDS. These issues were reviewed at a World Health Organisation meeting in 1988, the results of which were published in 1990 (World Health Organisation 1990). Along with the particular medical/health-care needs of the drug user there is the question of drug use itself. Rehabilitative treatment, in essence, aims to modify lifestyles and hence behaviour which, in itself, must entail the development of a positive attitude towards receiving 'treatment' and, thus, a degree of motivation on the patient's part. This motivation is part of the treatment process and may vary considerably over time.

Prison, for the most part, is not a therapeutic environment. If treatment is to take place in prison there is the question as to whether it is voluntary or non-voluntary and, indeed, whether it is ever possible for an inmate to make a free choice in prison. This returns to the issue of the individual's motivation. Research has yet to demonstrate whether detention influences motivation or indeed influences changes in drug-using behaviour. However, studies in Sweden and the Netherlands has suggested that voluntary drug-free (by regular testing) programmes can have positive benefits (World Health Organisation 1990). Thus, in spite of all the complications over motivation, the setting up of similar experimental units in England and Wales must be an option to explore.

In the Woolf Report there is significant discussion of the issues surrounding the management of HIV/AIDS. Three fundamental problems are identified which encapsulate many of the ethical dilemmas discussed earlier in relation to the provision of medical care in prison. The first is the problem of confidentiality – who should be informed if a prisoner is found to be HIV positive? Second, how should the doctor balance the interests of the patient with the interests of the prison population as a whole? Problems have arisen over the policy of placing inmates who are HIV positive under viral infectivity restriction (VIR). Under these restrictions doctors have discretion to place some limitations on the regimes for HIV infected prisoners, such as exclusion from work in the kitchen or in areas where there is a risk of blood spillage. However, the Woolf Inquiry revealed that far too many infected prisoners were being kept in prison hospitals, or in a special wing or unit, effectively segregated from other prisoners. The precise nature of VIR has been left to the discretion of local management and, in consequence, it has varied considerably from one establishment to another. The final problem concerns the confidence which prisoners have in prison medical care. Faced with the possibility of punitive restrictions, it is perhaps not surprising that Lord Justice Woolf received evidence that prisoners who were concerned that they might be HIV positive were reluctant to seek advice and information from the Prison Medical Service.

The Woolf Report has made 6 interlinked proposals which are designed to overcome these difficulties:

> as soon as possible there should be a thorough review of the present policies of the Prison Service in relation to HIV. The review should:
>
> a) subject the present policies in respect of VIR and confidentiality to critical examination with a view to setting them aside;
> b) identify the action which can be taken by establishments to encourage prisoners who feel that they are at risk of being HIV positive to identify themselves and cooperate voluntarily with the carrying out of tests;
> c) draw up a programme of treatment and opportunities for HIV positive prisoners;
> d) examine the best practices which already exist within the Prison Service and the Prison Service in Scotland for training prison officers and then draw up proposals to ensure that the best practices are adopted in all establishments;
> e) consider the best way of achieving close cooperation between prisons and AIDS counselling agencies.
>
> When the review has been completed a new policy on HIV should be announced by the Prison Service and the importance of implementing that policy should be forcefully drawn to the attention of Area Managers and Governors.
>
> (paras. 12.372–12.373)

The need for a full review of policy and of the VIR system had already been recognised by the Prison Department. The interim new policy statement concerning management of HIV/AIDS not only highlights the basic needs for: prevention of spread; protection of the health and safety of prisoners and staff; the provision of support to those infected, but also emphasises the need for this to be undertaken in the framework of total medical confidentiality, with the desirability for those with HIV to be fully integrated into the general prison community (effectively abolishing VIR restrictions).[5]

HIV/AIDS has been defined as a lethal venereal infection whose main modes of spread highlight the issues of drug use in prisons as well as the sexual behaviour of men and women in close confinement. Providing medical care, however, creates an immediate conflict of interest: who should have what information? How large are the boundaries of confidentiality? And what are the doctors' responsibilities for the larger community? In seeking to resolve this conflict the priorities of the system against the individual's care must not come to the fore.

There is still only one weapon against the infection, that is information and education, not only for the prisoner but, equally importantly, for all staff – although this must, as with all other training, compete with other priorities. The Prison Department has developed a clear strategy that has been pursued since the 'epidemic' emerged in the United Kingdom in 1985. It has initiated comprehensive training for all members of staff and prisoners, as well as specific training for medical staff and counsellors and, most recently, training for every prison to establish a multi-disciplinary team to assist in enacting the latest policy. This is supported by a comprehensive manual produced by the AIDS Advisory Committee *HIV and AIDS: A Multidisciplinary Approach in the Prison Environment* (Home Office 19911). Prompted by the Woolf Report, the AIDS Advisory Committee, a committee of experts drawn from within and outside the Prison Service, is currently undertaking a widespread consultation exercise to inform a full review of the current policies and will report in 1993.

As in other health-care issues, there is a clear need for research to be undertaken to consider the size of the 'epidemic', which currently appears to be somewhat smaller than original predictions, and to survey the attitudes and behaviour of prisoners. Funding was successfully obtained for these research projects and they started in April 1993.

That HIV/AIDS has been addressed in a systematic way must be seen to be reassuring. The many issues which are highlighted are directly relevant to all aspects of the provision of health care and, thus, of considerable benefit to the whole prison system. In acknowledging the dilemmas surrounding HIV/AIDS it should not be forgotten that it was the problem of infectious disease in prisons that led directly to the birth of the Prison Medical Service in the eighteenth century.

CONCLUSION

Over the years the medical profession has exerted a significant influence on the penal system, both by those members working from within and by those from outside. This relationship has recently been explored by Sim (1990). It is however clear that it has been the impact of disease or disturbance that has led to change.

Health care for prisoners is a priority area to be addressed and resourced. This at long last seems to be being done. The Health Care Service for Prisoners was launched at an inaugral conference by the Director of Health Care, Dr Rosemary Wool, in May 1992. Those of us within the service do not want to see recommendations made now lying dormant for another thirty years just to be reiterated in a slightly different guise, whilst those attempting to provide care in these difficult circumstances continue to be criticised.

Need is a crucial word. What are the health needs of the prison population? Research into this is essential. What are the staff needs? And, of course, what are the differences between what the prisoners feel they need and what the staff, or indeed society, believe that prisoners need?

How might the seven fundamental questions posed at the beginning of this chapter be answered?

1 If, like doctors outside, the primary duty of the prison doctor is to the patient, should not all medical practitioners in prisons be employees of the National Health Service and not employees of the Prison Service? In order to answer this question we need to consider where the Health Service's priorities lie and review where prisoner care may fall within these. The way in which 'unpopular' specialities are currently resourced by the NHS and treated by other specialities does not suggest that prisoners would necessarily benefit from such a union. It is possible that they would have less priority than now. That said, it may still be preferable for prison doctors to be employed by an organisation concerned primarily with health, and bound by clear ethical principles, rather than one whose key aims and objectives are manifestly not health.

2 Senior doctors within the Prison Service clearly have a management role to play. To underpin this, 'standards' must be set which enable them to make and implement decisions which give priority to health over and above security. There can be no compromises over ethical issues.

3 Clear standards are equally essential to regulate and safeguard doctors' use of medication and seclusion of prisoners.

4 Health care in prisons cannot operate without the umbrella of confidentiality. In order for health care teams to deal successfully with the many sensitive areas which confront them (such as sexual behaviour, drug use and HIV), the co-operation of the patient is of crucial importance.

Without a guarantee of confidentiality the trust and confidence of the prisoner-patient cannot be realistically anticipated.

5 Review and audit is an essential part of any professional's work. For the prison doctor it is essential that standards are set, maintained and monitored by recognised professional bodies.

6 Professionally accredited training, equivalent to that outside prison, is essential for all health-care staff working in prisons.

7 Professionally trained prison nurses supporting the prison doctors should be the mainstay of a high standard, confidential Prison Health Service. The hospital officer grade, with its dual custody and care function, gives mixed messages not only to the prisoners but to everyone else.

The shift from the provision of medical care to the provision of health care reinforces the need for health to be a priority in the whole prison system. This encompasses not only the treatment of illness, but the prevention of disease, health promotion, the need for a healthy and smoke-free environment, healthy diet and adequate, appropriate exercise. It is all embodied in the 'healthy prison' concept. However, medical, nursing and health-care staff must not be diverted from the principles of a high-standard medical service, providing for swift diagnosis and appropriate treatment and management of prisoners' illnesses. Recognised and accredited standards are essential to improve the care given to prisoners and to increase the credibility and professionalism of the carers. It remains to be seen if the lessons from the past have been learnt.

NOTES

1 Standing Order 13, *Health Care* March 1991.

2 This experimental institution has evolved over time but continues to accommodate a difficult section of the prison population within the context of a therapeutic community. The work at Grendon in maintaining control within a humane environment impressed Lord Justice Woolf and Judge Stephen Tumim to the extent that they proposed that a second Grendon should be opened in another part of the country.

3 Home Office instruction 66/1990 *Provision for Mentally Disordered Offenders.*

4 Circular Instruction 12/1991 *Throughcare of Drug Users.*

5 Circular Instruction 30/1991 *HIV/AIDS Organisation and Procedures at Establishment Level.*

Part II

SPECIFIC GROUPS OF PRISONERS

8

AN AWKWARD ANOMALY

Remand prisoners

Rod Morgan

INTRODUCTION

Untried and unsentenced prisoners have attracted little attention historically in the literature on prisons. In his authoritative post-war survey *The English Prison and Borstal System*, Sir Lionel Fox devoted no fewer than fourteen chapters to the training of young and adult sentenced prisoners, a mere two and a half pages to untried prisoners, and a derisory five lines to convicted but unsentenced prisoners. Because they were subject to the presumption of innocence he accepted that the untried had to be protected from conditions of 'undue harshness'. They were, however, an 'awkward anomaly'. They had to be housed in establishments designed primarily for convicted prisoners and it had to be recognised that 'whether or no they have committed the offences currently charged, [they] are not in fact respectable and innocent persons but old hands well known to the prison staffs' (Fox 1952, p. 285–6).

Until very recently the untried fared little better in subsequent official Home Office accounts: neither *People in Prison* (1969) nor *Prisons and the Prisoner* (1977) discussed their condition save to cite the provisions for them in the Prison Rules. Nor have social scientists generally made up the deficiency. Sociologist students of the prisoner culture have invariably focused on sentenced prisoners housed in what the English term training prisons and the Americans call prisons as opposed to gaols (for reviews of that literature see Hood and Sparks 1970, ch. 7; and Jacobs 1983). Even when institutions accommodating remand prisoners have been placed under the microscope, it has been the sentenced on whom the spotlight has invariably fallen. Emery's early study of Bristol Prison made virtually no reference to its remand population (prisoners 'pretty well segregated, and in any case so concerned with their own trial or their special privileges that they present few problems of control' (1970, p. 26)) and Sparks' review of *Local Prisons* had little to say about the untried save to conclude that their presence was 'incompatible with the provision of an adequate regime for men under sentence', a conclusion which led him to recommend their removal to purpose-built remand centres (1971, p.101). Not until King and Morgan's *A Taste of Prison* (1976), was there published a study which looked in detail at the custodial predicament of untried prisoners. The authors found that they were generally held in conditions which in most respects were worse than those for sentenced prisoners, a finding which in the view of later commentators clearly illustrated the principle 'convicted until proved innocent' (Fitzgerald and Sim 1979, p. 38).

King and Morgan's conclusions are now commonplace, part of the orthodox diagnosis of the prison system in the 1980s and early 1990s. Indeed, official reports now employ very much more trenchant language to describe the conditions which many remand prisoners endure than King and Morgan used. Fox's acceptance that conditions of 'undue harshness' should be prevented has not been followed. The Chief Inspector of Prisons was by 1985 describing attempts being made in some local prisons to alleviate the harsh conditions which he recognised most remand prisoners suffered (Home Office 1985c, p. 5). In report after report successive Chief Inspectors chronicled the 'degrading' and 'insanitary' accommodation, the 'enforced idleness', the prolonged daily cellular confinement, and the general lack of access to facilities, to which the untried are routinely subject (see Home Office 1988c; Home Office 1990b; Home Office 1990c for particularly graphic examples). By the 1980s everyone appeared to accept that the conditions in which the untried were kept were 'completely insupportable' (House of Commons 1981, para. 54). They were the 'forgotten people' (Home Office 1989a, para. 4.30), detained in 'the worst conditions the prison system has to offer' (Stern 1987, p. 33). In 1990 the European Committee for the Prevention of Torture and Inhuman or Degrading Treatment or Punishment found that conditions in three local prisons – Wandsworth, Brixton and Leeds – were 'inhuman and degrading' – a judgement which indicated that in the Committee's opinion they breached Article 3 of the European Convention of Fundamental Human Rights (Council of Europe 1991, para. 57). The conditions giving rise to that judgement – crowding three prisoners in cells designed for one without integral sanitation and with scarcely any out-of-cell activities – were most often suffered by remand prisoners. Casale and Plotnikoff's *Regimes for Remand Prisoners* (1990), an examination subsequently matched within the Prison Department by a scrutiny of a 'Model Regime for Local Prisons and Remand Centres' (Home Office 1991c; Home Office 1991f, p. 75), appeared to represent an agreement by critics and administrators alike that the time had come to construct an agenda for urgent action.

Why were remand prisoners for so long neglected and why now is their custody the focus of attention? Four reasons can be identified – their lineage and the linkage between them will be traced in the following sections.

FORGOTTEN PEOPLE

By far the most important factor explaining the historical marginalisation of remand prisoners is to be found in the philosophy and objectives which Parliament has sanctioned and prison administrators have pursued for the prison system. This concerns the *de jure* rise and in recent years the *de facto* demise of the doctrine of 'treatment and training'. The history of and argument about this process has been fully set out elsewhere (King and Morgan 1980; Bottoms 1990) and need be summarised only briefly here. The present Prison Rule 1 – 'The purpose of the training and treatment of convicted prisoners shall be to encourage and assist them to lead a good and useful life'[1] – began to dominate prison administrative thinking in the 1940s when the virtually identical objective comprised Rule 6.[2] From this time onwards prisoners were effectively classified as trainable or untrainable. Those deemed trainable – sentenced prisoners except those serving very short sentences (for whom there was held to be insufficient time) and the recalcitrant (for whom the time had apparently passed) – were to be classified and allocated to the 'training' prison whose regime was best fitted to meet their needs. Untrainable short-term sentenced prisoners (which included most fine defaulters) were to remain in the 'local' prisons where those prisoners morally and legally ineligible for training, the untried and the unsentenced, were also to be housed.

The 'treatment and training' paradigm was never fully operationalised. The management expertise to which it pretended was mythical: for prisoners and prison officers alike it ran contrary to the coercive realities of prison life; and it repeatedly foundered on the symbolic rocks of 'less eligibility' to which, when pressed, most politicians responsible for prisons will defensively cling. Nevertheless, 'treatment and training' did dictate the manner in which the Prison Commission, and after 1962 the Prison Department, allocated resources and distributed the prisoner population.

Not until the building programme begun by the Conservative Government after 1979, and even then somewhat late in the programme, was there built a new local prison. Belmarsh, which opened in 1991, was the first new local prison for over a century. Previously all the new building, with the exception of Holloway which was to serve a multi-functional purpose for women, had been of training prisons or young offender establishments (though the latter included several remand centres built in the early 1960s). With those exceptions all the new building had been of training prisons or young offender establishments.

The old local prisons were also made to bear the brunt of the overcrowding which, from the early 1950s, became a permanent and, until the late 1980s, an ever-increasing problem. It was argued by the Prison Department that overcrowding *had* to be borne by the local prisons, because their larger Victorian cells were capable of multi-occupation to a degree that the newer training prison cells were not. This contention was unsustainable.

The small cells in the modern remand centres were also overcrowded while the Victorian training prisons, many of which had large cells and had formerly been local prisons, were for the most part spared overcrowding.

The local prisons and remand centres were also denied the facilities that might have made their overcrowding bearable. During the 1960s and 1970s the new workshops, educational blocks, sports halls and visiting areas tended to go to the training sector within which the noble mission of treatment and training was allegedly being realised. The local prisons and remand centres became sinks. Their daily regimes became less and less active, particularly for their remand population. The extent of their absolute and relative deprivation, which critics had long argued (King and Morgan 1976; King and McDermott 1989), was eventually graphically illustrated in the regime monitoring data which the Prison Department began to collect and publish. Prisoners in remand centres and local prisons in 1989/90 were on average spending only one-half or as little as one-third as much time (which meant less than two hours per day) engaged in organised activities (work, education, PE, etc.) as their sentenced counterparts in training prisons and young offender institutions (Home Office 1991a, Table 1). Unfortunately, the aggregate data did not yet distinguish untried and convicted prisoners. Had they done so they would have demonstrated that the untried were even worse off.

Second, there were no provisions in either the 1952 Prison Act or the 1964 Prison Rules effectively to prevent the untried being made to bear the brunt of the pressures to which the prison system was subject. The Prison Act 1877 s.39 required that 'a clear difference shall be made between the treatment of persons unconvicted of crime' and the treatment of convicted prisoners, and that special rules be made 'regulating their confinement in such manner as to make it as little as possible oppressive'. Although this provision was not included in the Prison Act 1952, the principle was implicit in the requirement that the Secretary of State make special rules for the treatment of unconvicted prisoners (s. 47(4)(d)). Though successive Home Secretaries failed, contrary to an undertaking given during the parliamentary debate on the Criminal Justice Act 1948, to formulate separate rules for remand centres, the 1964 Prison Rules incorporated nine separate provisions to protect the rights of the untried. They had to be:

Rule 3(2): kept out of contact with convicted prisoners 'as far as this can reasonably be done';
Rule 17(4): provided with the services of their own doctor or dentist 'providing there are reasonable grounds; and at his own expense';
Rule 20(1): allowed to wear their own clothing 'in so far as it is suitable, tidy and clean';
Rule 21(1): allowed to have their own food sent in 'at his own expense, or that of his friends';

Rule 25: allowed 'on payment of a sum' to occupy their own privately furnished and cleaned rooms;
Rule 26 (2): not subject to prison haircut regulations;
Rule 28(5): allowed not to work;
Rule 34(1): allowed as many letters and as many visits as they chose 'subject to such conditions as the Secretary of State may direct';
Rule 41(1): allowed to have sent in books, newspapers, writing materials, etc.

In fact, as King and Morgan's early study demonstrated (1976, ch. 3), these safeguards were either a dead letter (there were no rooms privately to furnish), or were ignored (young remand centre prisoners' own clothes were never judged to be 'suitable, tidy and clean'), or were nugatory (the vast majority of untried prisoners had not the resources to have food and books sent in) or hid an almost cynical reversal of fortune (untried prisoners were not allowed to alter their hirsute appearance, or were not given access to the newspapers received by convicted prisoners *because* they could have their own sent in, or had to stay locked up all day if they chose not to work). Moreover, the Prison Rules served to safeguard the status of the untried less and less as time went on. As overcrowding increased it was found more often to be impracticable to separate the untried and convicted (Morgan and Barclay 1989). There was little or no work on offer for those untried who wanted to work: because convicted prisoners were supposed to be employed, the few remaining jobs went largely to them. Meanwhile the relatively protected training prisons liberalised the amount of contact their prisoners could have with the outside world such that the untried in the remand institutions became relatively worse off. Restrictions on the number of letters convicted prisoners could send or receive were gradually abandoned. Many training prisons were able to allow their prisoners first fortnightly and then weekly visits which might last two hours or more. Open and low security prisons began introducing cardphones. Finally, in 1989, Prison Rule 21 was amended to remove the right of untried prisoners to have food and drink sent in. This was indeed regarded by the Department as an awkward anomaly, a right rarely exercised, administratively inconvenient and allegedly a security hazard. The anomaly was removed.

The net result of all these trends was that the untried, without access to telephones, and restricted to fifteen-minute visits (which in most locals could no longer be had every day but were made longer on selected weekdays so as to add up to the equivalent of fifteen minutes per day) received in crowded and degrading visiting rooms, could no longer be said to be privileged, if ever they were.

Third, there being no legal hindrance, there was no management incentive to change this maldistribution of resources even when the philosophy of treatment and training began to be called into question. From the late 1960s onwards the prison system was regularly disrupted by serious prisoner disturbances, almost all of them in the maximum security 'dispersal' training prisons. Emery's complacency about remand prisoners seemed largely to be justified. Individual remand prisoners might constitute a control problem, but *en masse* they seemed to be relatively quiescent in the face of their intolerable conditions. From a superficial control standpoint there seemed to be good reason to protect the treatment jewels in the crown of the training prison sector and provide more resources, staff and hardware, expanding and stepping up the security quotient of the long-term dispersal prisons.

Fourth, in the immediate post-war period when the treatment and training model was organisationally being developed there were relatively few untried prisoners. Remands made up a relatively high proportion of receptions, but comprised a small proportion – always less than 10 per cent prior to 1960 – of the average daily prison population. Numerically, as well as ideally, the system was geared to the custody and treatment of sentenced prisoners.

MOVING TO CENTRE STAGE

All this changed dramatically during the 1970s and 1980s. First, the philosophy of treatment came increasingly under attack. There was little evidence that the efforts to provide different forms of training or treatment made imprisonment any more effective in terms of post-release behaviour (Brody 1976). As a consequence the paternalism, inequity and lack of due process justice to which all prisoners were subject became increasingly offensive. However, the Prison Department totally failed to fill the philosophical void left by the growing disillusion with the treatment and training approach, and the Department's inertia was scarcely compensated for by the efforts of the official inquiry into the prison services in 1979 under the then Mr Justice May. The May Committee proposed the replacement of Rule 1 by a statement of 'positive custody' (Home Office 1979, para. 4.26). However, the Committee's formulation was no more capable of operationalisation than the 'rhetoric of "treatment and training"' which they argued had 'had its day' (para. 4.27). There was nothing in the statement of 'positive custody' which provided prisoners with entitlements, or assured them of minimum custodial standards, or provided them with a greater voice to determine the choices available to them within the constraints that imprisonment necessarily involves. Moreover, 'positive custody' concerned convicted prisoners: the May Committee formulation made no reference to the untried.

In the absence of either a noble mission or an emphasis on justice and minimum custodial standards, the policies of the Prison Department drifted during the late 1970s and early 1980s. There were considerable pressures, both of overcrowding and staff industrial action. In 1975 the average daily prison population broke through the 40,000 barrier and rose steadily to exceed 50,000 in 1988. By far the largest part of the increase was attributable to the almost three-fold rise during this period of the population of untried prisoners, a phenomenal growth largely explained not by an increase in the number of untried prisoners received, but the longer periods they were spending in custody awaiting trial. The average daily sentenced population changed little. It was only 13 per cent higher in 1988 (the high point) than it had been in 1975. This meant that the remand population now made up a substantial proportion of the daily population. In 1960 remand prisoners comprised 7.7 per cent of the average daily population. In 1970 the figure was 11.9 per cent, in 1980 13.7 per cent and in 1989 21.4 per cent.

Though some training prisons could no longer be spared overcrowding, the bulk of the population increase continued to be borne by the local prisons. During some periods some local prisons were well over 100 per cent overcrowded (Home Office 1988a, Appendix 4). The consequence of this pressure was that the local prisons literally became insanitary, idle and inhumane warehouses. There was still nothing in the Prison Rules to prevent the deterioration and the courts maintained their hands-off posture regarding prison conditions (Richardson 1985a; 1993).

There were three possibilities for reversing this trend. First, alleviation of crowding by expanding the prison estate. Second, reducing the numbers of prisoners remanded in custody and the duration of their custody. Third, redistribution of existing resources within the prison system in favour of remand prisoners.

Following their election in 1979, an election during which the Conservative Party proclaimed a tough 'law and order' message (Conservative Party 1979) and which all the evidence suggested was popular with the electorate (Butler and Kavanagh 1980), the Government first adopted an expansionist solution to the prison overcrowding problem. By the late 1980s their massive building programme began to come on stream. Overcrowding was significantly reduced. However, by the mid-1980s it had become apparent that if the building programme was not accompanied by a vigorous reductionist policy there was a distinct possibility that the additional prison places would do little more than keep pace with the rising prison population. The prospect of an 'end to overcrowding', the Government's proclaimed objective and promise (Home Office 1986b, p. 29), was receding.

The Government therefore embarked on a series of reductionist initiatives, most of them focused on remands. The aim was to increase the proportion of defendants granted bail or, where bail was denied, to reduce the duration of custody pending trial. In the period 1989–91 these initiatives – the development of bail information schemes, the provision of more bail hostel places, more courts, the phased introduction of time limits for bringing cases to trial, and general exhortations to magistrates to use remands in custody more sparingly (see Morgan 1989; Morgan and Jones 1992) – seemed to have some success. During 1989–91 the remand population (as well as the sentenced population) was marginally reduced. Ironically, it was in the middle of this period of optimism that the prison disturbances of April 1990 occurred.

APRIL 1990: STRANGEWAYS AND ELSEWHERE

The disturbances in April 1990 were unprecedented in their ferocity and scale. But they were not without precedent. In 1986 there was a particularly serious spate of disturbances. Forty establishments, including local prisons and remand centres, were involved. What the events of 1986 and 1990 demonstrated was that all establishments were vulnerable to disorder and that remand prisoners were now as likely as sentenced prisoners to participate.

The evidence presented by Lord Justice Woolf's Inquiry into the Strangeways riot was that a demonstration, though not the riot and siege that developed, was planned, mostly by sentenced prisoners who at the time, or previously, were subject to disciplinary measures and held in the segregation unit. Once the disturbance took hold, however, it is clear that prisoners of all types, including remand prisoners, took an active part in the destruction and resistance which went on for over three weeks. The vast majority of prisoners, as is generally the case in prison riots, escaped from the mayhem as soon as they were able. But among the minority of prisoners who held out were remand prisoners, three of them for over two weeks.

Some of the young remand prisoners from Strangeways were transferred to that part of Glen Parva Young Offenders' Institution that is reserved for remand prisoners. One of these prisoners was prominent in the disturbance that took place at Glen Parva on Friday 6 April 1990. Approximately 60 young remand prisoners barricaded and substantially damaged their cell block before surrendering after a few hours. At Cardiff and Bristol Prisons, both traditional Victorian multi-functional local prisons, serious disturbances broke out on 8 April. Both disturbances occurred in wings holding remand prisoners and at Cardiff events appear to have been precipitated by a remand prisoner and engaged in most actively by remand prisoners. At Bristol the riot broke out in a cell block holding a variety of categories of prisoners, including sentenced prisoners from Dartmoor transferred to Bristol following the outbreak there of a riot on 7 April. Nevertheless, once it had started a high proportion of Bristol prisoners, many of them remand prisoners, were all too ready to join in. At nearby Pucklechurch Remand Centre ferocious battles between young prisoners and prison officers took place for nearly 20 hours on 22 and 23 April. The Pucklechurch incident undoubtedly began as a result of the actions of a sentenced prisoner transferred to Pucklechurch to receive accumulated visits but again, once started, the disturbance was joined with alacrity by many of the mostly remand population.

It is significant then that of the many establishments which experienced disorder in April 1990, five of the six most serious disturbances on which Lord Justice Woolf's inquiry concentrated its attention, were remand establishments and that remand prisoners played a leading or contributory part in what happened. Woolf found that these remand prisoners had good reason to feel aggrieved.

At Strangeways, an overcrowded prison in which conditions were generally very poor, the provision for remand prisoners was described by the governor as 'grossly inadequate' (Woolf 1991, para. 3.63). There was no work for them other than a few cleaning jobs and the very limited PE and educational facilities meant that only a few of the young prisoners could be engaged in them on any one day. Most remand prisoners were locked up, two to a cell without integral sanitation, for excessively long periods. As a result 'a large proportion of the inmates in the prison were sympathetic to the instigators of the disturbance and antagonistic towards the Prison Service' (para. 3.432(4)). At Glen Parva Woolf found that the conditions for remand prisoners were significantly poorer than those for sentenced prisoners (paras 4.8–4.13 and 4.48). The overcrowding at Glen Parva was primarily among remand prisoners (72 per cent overcrowded) rather than sentenced prisoners (7 per cent overcrowded). Though they were provided with a regime significantly better than that found at other young remand establishments (Pucklechurch, for example), it was based on an 'opt in' or 'opt out' principle which arguably contravened the spirit of the Prison Rules. Remand prisoners at Glen Parva who chose to work ('opt in') not only received payment but got first choice to take up the limited educational and PE facilities. Those who exercised their right not to work ('opt out') came last for everything else and as a result received little.

At Cardiff the remand prisoners had their own area and were able to spend much of the day out of their cells. This mitigated the gross overcrowding to which they were subject (77 per cent overcrowded). But they had no opportunity to work or attend educational classes or go to the trade training course available to sentenced prisoners (paras. 6.15–6.16). At Bristol, which at the time was not seriously overcrowded, conditions in the wing where the riot took place were found to be particularly 'unacceptable' (para. 7.158(1)). Many of the prisoners had little or no association and were confined for much of the day to cells which, as elsewhere, lacked integral sanitation. At Pucklechurch, a purpose-built remand centre which was 17 per cent overcrowded at the time, there was no workshop or vocational training courses and the limited number of employment places in the kitchen and gardens tended to go to convicted or sentenced prisoners. The education and PE staff were found to have made vigorous efforts to lay on a full programme of activities but prison officer intransigence or staff shortages – it is not clear which factor came first – meant that many activities had to be cancelled for want of escorts with the result that prisoners spent long periods – eighteen and a half hours per day, the regime monitoring data indicated – in small cells without integral sanitation (paras. 8.12–8.26).

THE WOOLF RECOMMENDATIONS

The 1990 disturbances clearly demonstrated that 'it would be quite wrong to assume' (as I have suggested has been the historical tendency of the prison authorities) 'that, because prisoners are on remand, they do not have the potential for creating serious control and security problems' (Woolf 1991, para. 9.6). For Woolf, however, that did not mean the Prison Service had failed to subject remand prisoners to sufficiently secure conditions. The stability of prisons, he suggested, rests on there being adequate attention paid by prison management to the elements of *security, control* and *justice* and there being a balance struck between those three elements (paras. 9.19–9.21). He found no single cause for the riots and no simple solution which would prevent them. It was more a question of establishing an equilibrium between security, control and justice appropriate for each prisoner group. In the case of remand prisoners he found imbalance. They were the object of excessive security. The control measures to which they were subject were inappropriate. And they suffered a grave deficiency of justice. Woolf also doubted whether so many remand prisoners need be held in custody so long (para. 8.188 (47)).

Woolf was circumspect, as his limited terms of reference meant he had to be, about the use made of remands in custody by the courts. It is clear that his inclinations were reductivist, but he aproached the question of whether all remands in custody are necessary by focusing on decision-making. He noted, for example, that the question of bail is procedurally dealt with by the courts in a more casual manner than sentencing. Decisions are sometimes made hurriedly, without adequate information, by one or two rather than three magistrates, and without the benefit of High Court guidelines (para. 10.86). These deficiencies can and should be repaired. Meanwhile he commended current Government initiatives – bail information schemes, the provision of further hostel places, public interest case assessment, etc. – designed to increase resort to bail, or shorten the period that remands spend in custody (paras. 10.88-10.106). Moreoever, his proposal that there be established nationally a Criminal Justice Consultative Council, and parallel local committees, is clearly a mechanism ideally suited to prosecute the development of initiatives designed to reduce the remand population.

With respect to the prison system, Woolf's use of the terms 'security' and 'control' was relatively straightforward. Security referred to the Prison Service's primary obligation to receive those prisoners committed to prison and to keep them there for the period fixed by the court. In the case of remand prisoners that meant until they were due to be tried or sentenced, unless granted bail in the interim. Control referred to orderliness within prison, loss of which may spell – as it did most shockingly at Manchester – loss of security for other prisoners. A failure of control may on occasion lead to a breach of perimeter security.

Woolf's general security and control prescriptions – accommodation units for no more than 50 to 70 prisoners, secure 'firebreaks' between accommodation units, etc. – apply as much to remand as to sentenced prisoners. They have a particular importance for the remand population, however, because of his re-emphasis on separating the convicted from the unconvicted and the high priority he attached to accommodating prisoners as close as possible to their community ties. The development of what Woolf calls 'community prisons' is made more likely by his finding that remand prisoners are currently subject 'to a degree of security and control which is frequently unnecessary' (para. 12.312) and his proposal that they be treated, unless there is good reason to do otherwise, as the equivalent of security Category C rather than B, as is currently the case. He suggested that in the same way that the police, the Crown Prosecution Service, the Probation Service and the courts co-operate to decide on the appropriate level of control needed over defendants granted bail, so those same agencies might assist the Prison Service by marking the files of defendants refused bail who may need to be subject to more than Category C security (paras. 12.316–12.317).

Woolf's use of the term 'justice' is more complex, however. It is arguably too singular a term to encompass the several facets of prison life he wishes to enhance. Justice for Woolf refers to the 'obligation . . . to treat prisoners with humanity and fairness and to prepare them for their return to the community in a way which makes it less likely that they will reoffend' (para. 9.20). Quite apart from the fact that this definition is geared to the convicted – an orientation which Woolf elsewhere corrects by proposing that there be a separate body of prison rules for the untried – it is clear from the body of his report that he means by justice much more than both fairness and due process (paras 14.296–14.297). His recommendations that there be more active regimes for prisoners, access to sanitation at all times, properly paid work, education programmes, improved contact between prisoners and their families, better clothing, etc., indicate that for him justice covers what DiIulio has more accurately described as *amenity* and *service* (DiIulio 1987).

Though the amenities and services available to untried prisoners should be different from those for convicted and sentenced prisoners – for example, the untried, subject to the presumption of innocence, should not be compelled to work and should be given every possibility effectively to conduct their defence – there is no case for denying them access to programmes on the grounds that they have no proven offence to address. The vast majority of persons denied bail, whether or not they are subsequently convicted, are seriously disadvantaged socially and economically. Many have a long record of previous convictions. That is often why they are denied bail. Yet, that is also why they 'should suffer no greater loss of liberty, both in duration and degree, than is necessary to secure the course of justice' (Morgan and Barclay 1989, p. 23) and why it must 'be part of the task of the Prison Service to enable the remand prisoner to spend his time in custody in as constructive a manner as possible' (Woolf 1991, para. 10.61). How this should best be done is the question.

GOVERNMENT PLANS AND THE WAY AHEAD

There are serious difficulties surrounding the achievement of minimum resort to custody for the untried and decent conditions for those refused bail. The presumption of innocence is a legal doctrine belied by a good deal of practice within the criminal justice system. Police tactics and decisions, as recent miscarriages of justice vividly illustrate, are often dictated by an apparent conviction of a suspect's guilt. Bail is most commonly denied because magistrates think there is a likelihood of further offences being committed: the evidence for this usually comprises the defendant's record. We have seen how the unconvicted are treated in prison.

This disjunction between theory and practice is not an exclusively English phenomenon. Repeated surveys of international compliance with the United Nations Standard Minimum Rules reveal that breaches are most often admitted in relation to those rules concerning the untried (United Nations 1985, p. 14) and anyone who has visited remand gaols overseas will be aware that the disadvantages suffered by the unconvicted in England and Wales are as prevalent elsewhere. Indeed, in many jurisdictions, including some noted for their liberal penal systems, either the prosecutor or the court can severely restrict (by limiting visits or access to mass media, for example) the conditions for prisoners awaiting trial on the grounds that the prosecution case will otherwise be undermined (see Council of Europe 1992).

Moreover measures designed to divert the untried from custody can all too easily have 'net-widening' consequences. It was this consideration which, following consultation (Home Office 1988b) led the Home Office (and subsequently Woolf) to abandon the idea of establishing secure bail hostels. There is evidence that existing bail hostels attract residents who would otherwise not be remanded in custody (Lewis and Mair 1989). A similar dilemma surrounds any insistence that the untried be physically separated from the convicted. It could not be achieved without further expanding a system arguably too large already. And yet, as we have seen, the integration of the convicted and unconvicted invariably signals the disadvantage of the latter.

The dilemma is well stated in the Government's response to the Woolf

Report. Competing aims 'may be irreconcilable' (Home Office 1991a, para. 5.5): a 'doctrinaire approach' will not do (para. 5.2). The problem is that the greater the degree to which prisons are specialised, or to which different categories of prisoners are required to be separated from each other – men from women, young from old, the unconvicted from the convicted – the less likely it is that the available estate will be used efficiently, that overcrowding will be prevented and that prisoners will be kept as close to their community ties as possible. Specialisation means tying down resources which are often in the wrong place at the wrong time. There will therefore need to be flexibility, maximising the realisation of competing objectives within a framework far from ideal. What order of priorities and principles should frame the pragmatic judgements which will have to be made?

First, there must be a degree of insulation of the untried from the convicted without which, all experience suggests, the untried will suffer structural disadvantage. This insulation must be both normative – Woolf's proposal, which the Government has accepted, that there be a separate set of Prison Rules for the untried; and physical – untried prisoners must be held in discrete accommodation within prisons if not in separate prisons. Of course, this proposition is more complex than this brief statement suggests. By implication it means that there must also be discrete accommodation for female and for young untried prisoners.

The difficulty of marrying this physical insulation requirement with the idea of the community prison is obvious. Unless there are to be built more new prisons specifically for remand prisoners – a prospect which the White Paper endorses (Home Office 1991a, para. 5.19) but which all the current effort to reduce the use made of custody suggests would be misplaced – prisoners can only be held in institutions proximate to their community ties if many specialised institutions become multi-functional establishments within which different categories of prisoners, including remands, are less than perfectly physically separated.

This is the point at which the battle is joined. The Government suggests, for example, that it is preferable that young offenders and unconvicted prisoners on remand should be located in less crowded conditions with prisoners of a different status, than that they should be held separately in overcrowded conditions (Home Office 1991a, para. 5.14). This assertion is subject only to the proviso that they should never share cells. By the same token the Government considers that women might be accommodated in prisons which also receive men but are close to home, rather than held miles away in prisons solely for females 'providing the accommodation is separate, fully secure and of an adequate size', and that the women have 'satisfactory facilities and regime activities' (para. 5.14).

It is clear that the acceptability of these pragmatic judgements depends on broader assumptions and objectives and the degree to which political will is being exercised to realise them. Have the pressures which create the need to reconcile the irreconcilable to be so great? Is the Government doing all that it can to: reduce the prison population; or to ensure that no juvenile is ever again remanded to a prison; or to prevent defendants being held in custody before trial who, if convicted, are unlikely to receive a custodial sentence? The Government is arguably not doing all that it might to further these objectives. The consequence is a loss of sympathy by the penal pressure groups with the dilemmas confronting the Prison Service and their pragmatic attempts to resolve them.

Of course not all critics of the policies spelt out by the Government in their recent White Paper base their opposition on these contextual grounds. For example, some feminist commentators are more fundamentally opposed to women being accommodated in prisons which also house men. They characterise the proposal as misogynistic, contend that it will encourage more use of imprisonment for women by the courts, and argue that it places women prisoners in danger and will lead to women being deprived of facilities and regime activities. They also doubt that the arrangement will be cheaper (Tchaikovsky 1991, p. 12). These fears need seriously to be addressed, though it should be said that the objective of saving money was never advanced by Woolf as an argument for the creation of community prisons.

The community prison concept is based on the proposition that most prisoners, of all types, are in prison for a relatively short period of time, a few weeks or months. For example, despite the increase in recent years in the average duration of custodial remands, the majority of prisoners are held for less than two months pre-trial. The prison population is for the most part a transitory population whose community ties need to be maintained to the greatest possible extent and whose financial security and social welfare on release need to be assured. Any policy which undermines these objectives is counter-productive in terms of reducing the likelihood of further offences. Community prisons would have two characteristics. They would hold prisoners in the institution closest to their homes. And they would have permeable walls: better visiting arrangements, qualitatively as well as quantitatively, for prisoners and their families; better telephone access; improved provision of legal advice; and greater involvement by those same community groups and statutory agencies with whom prisoners will deal on release.

In areas of low population density, few committals and few institutions, the realisation of the community prison ideal will have to mean multi-functional prisons. In metropolitan areas it will involve clusters of relatively specialised institutions. But whatever the arrangement it will take time to achieve. More training prisons and young offender establishments will have to be re-designated – as a good many were during the 1980s – as local or community prisons in which remand prisoners can be housed. If convicted and/or subsequently sentenced to imprisonment these prisoners can continue to be housed close to home without need for transfer.

This sea change in the distribution of the prison population and in the assumptions on which resources are allocated to that population, will be aided by the Woolf proposal that remand prisoners be security categorised and presumed to be security Category C unless there is evidence that they pose a greater risk. Were that the case many more institutions might house remand prisoners than at present. The Government's response to this suggestion is equivocal. They accept that remand prisoners should be security categorised (Home Office 1991a, para. 5.21) but they ignore the Category C presumption and disparage the thinking that gave rise to it:

> there is no evidence or reason to believe that prisoners remanded in custody by the courts can, as a group, be held securely in Category C conditions. Nor are there at present or in the foreseeable future likely to be sufficient Category C establishments conveniently located for such prisoners.
>
> (para. 5.20).

This is an inflexible and unreasoning response. It ignores the future disposition of most remand prisoners. It implicitly and uncritically accepts the excessively high security rating of some training prisons (see, for example, the Chief Inspector of Prisons' recommendations that Coldingley and Blundeston Prisons be security downgraded (Home Office 1991g; Home Office 1991h)). And it ignores the potential many low security and young offender institutions have, were they modified, to house remand prisoners. Almost half of all unconvicted prisoners (two-thirds of all female unconvicted prisoners) are subsequently found not guilty or receive a non-custodial sentence. Of those who receive a custodial sentence the majority are categorised C or D. There is only one good reason why this low security judgement could not be arrived at while those same prisoners were on remand, and that is lack of information, a deficiency which could be rectified if the other criminal justice agencies gave the matter the highest priority. It is doubtful whether the courts, which have no responsibility for prisons administration, should *determine* the level of security to which a remand prisoner should be subject. That is a matter better left to the prison authorities who *are* responsible for prisoners' security. However, there would be merit in the courts indicating which prisoners – marking their files as Woolf suggested – seem to warrant greater security than normal.

PRISON RULES FOR REMAND PRISONERS AND PRIVATISATION

Woolf recommended, and the Government has reluctantly accepted the recommendation, that there should be a separate body of rules for unconvicted remand prisoners. What should the rules comprise?

Because of the presumption of innocence, unconvicted prisoners cannot justifiedly be deprived of any right, benefit or liberty which is compatible with the fact of custody. Some commentators have proposed that remand prisons should provide a range of services so that those unconvicted prisoners who can afford them can purchase whatever facilities they want (McConville 1987, pp. 234–7). This is right in principle but unrealistic in practice. The vast majority of remand prisoners are impecunious. There is no prospect of the Prison Service earning a profitable return from speculative adaptation of remand accommodation or adding to it. What is required is a steady up-grading of the quality of life that all unconvicted prisoners can expect as of right.

Casale and Plotnikoff (1990) have set out a detailed prospectus of the minimum physical standards of accommodation, duty of care, regime (exercise, skills development programmes, employment, etc.), welfare arrangements, use of time and visiting facilities which remand prisoners should have and which should be incorporated, as specifically as possible, in the prison rules for unconvicted prisoners. They have also highlighted the high priority which the Prison Service should give to ensuring that prisoners get legal advice, information and access to the courts, thereby expediting the likelihood of bail being granted and cases being quickly brought to trial.

Three additional general principles need to be added to the Casale and Plotnikoff prospectus. First, that the provision of money for personal consumption for the unconvicted should be no less than the current minimum allowance awarded by the Department of Social Security for dependent persons. Further, unconvicted prisoners should be entitled to claim whatever benefits (including any unemployment benefit) for which they would normally be eligible, whilst they are in custody. Second, untried prisoners should be held in the remand establishment closest to their community ties and, in the event of their immediate family being distant from the court of committal and receiving prison, prisoners' wishes should be taken into account when deciding where they should be accommodated. This same principle should apply when there is need to 'reconcile the irreconcilable' – for example, women being held in single-sex or mixed establishments. These dilemmas should not be decided by either the Prison Service or dogmatic critics. The prisoner's wishes should count. Third, any prisoner held at a distance from their immediate family (and this distance should be defined) should, unless that arrangement is the prisoner's choice, be the beneficiary of financial assistance to enable partners and children to visit. These three principles, together with others that Casale and Plotnikoff have set out in their 'Charter for Remand Prisoners' (1990, p. 54) should be enunciated in the rules for untried prisoners.

The Government has undertaken to 'prepare a model regime for local prisons and remand centres, taking particular account of the needs of unconvicted prisoners' (Home Office 1991a, para. 7.17). At the time of writing, a first draft of that model regime is in circulation (Home Office 1991c). It is clear that the Prison Service's aspirations are not being pitched at a lower level than that required by the contract for the Wolds, Britain's first prison contracted out for management by a commercial company (Home Office 1991f). The regime at the Wolds is based on prisoners being out of their cells for a minimum of twelve hours on weekdays and ten and a half hours per day over the weekend. Prisoners have an entitlement to six hours per week for education, another six hours for PE, two and a half hours each for visits to the library and the prisoners' shop, and twenty-one hours a week for meals, showers, etc. Further, meals are eaten at the times they are normally taken in the community rather than being compressed into a short day determined by the working convenience of staff. There is the opportunity of a daily change of underwear and convicted remand prisoners are entitled to an hour-long visit each week instead of each fortnight.

This is not the place to debate the arguments for and against contracting out the management of either prisons generally or remand prisons in particular (but see Logan 1990). Woolf avoided pronouncing on this controversial issue. It is clear that the Government intends breaking what many consider to be the monopoly power and restrictive hand of the Prison Officers' Assocation, though it is dubious whether this can be done without incurring higher costs than are currently generated by the Prison Service providing remand accommodation.

Many commentators will find offensive the provisions in the Criminal Justice Act 1991 granting the employees of commercial organisations coercive powers to search, restrain and forcefully remove prisoners (ss. 85–6). Others will entertain doubts about the acccountability of contracted-out arrangements (Sampson 1991, p. 16). Nevertheless, it is clear that the regime for remand prisoners provided at the Wolds (the unconvicted and convicted are not strictly segregated) is vastly superior to that which typically has been long provided in Prison Service establishments. However unfair the comparison, the Wolds provides the flagship regime which the Prison Service is obliged to emulate. However, the Prison Service's *Model Regime for Local Prisons and Remand Centres* (Home Office 1991c) gives no timetable for the realisation of these aspirations and the concept of community prisons is as yet subject only to a consultation paper (Home Office 1992e). That is the issue on which critics and prisoners henceforth will focus their attentions.

CONCLUSION

The prospect of improved conditions for remand prisoners hangs in the balance. The principles enunciated by Lord Justice Woolf have been accepted by the Government and the regime at the Wolds Prison has provided a clear illustration of what can be done. There remain storm clouds, however. Although the prison population, for reasons that are not yet clear, fell substantially in 1992, such that for the first time in almost half a century there was excess capacity in the system – 45,600 places for fewer than 42,000 prisoners – it began to rise again early in 1993. Further, the prison building programme of the 1980s is coming to an end and the latest Home Office projections suggest that the prison population will rise to 57,500 by the year 2000 (Home Office 1992f). By far the largest percentage increase is predicted for the remand population. If this happens there will be prison overcrowding into the twenty-first century and the structural reforms recommended by Woolf seem unlikely to be implemented.

At the time of writing the signs are not good. Since Spring 1992 several police forces have systematically leaked to the press data on the allegedly increasing problem of offences committed while on bail by offenders that the media have dubbed 'bail bandits'. In spite of a careful review of the evidence by the Home Office which suggests that there is no evidence that the problem is significantly worse now than it was a decade ago (Morgan 1992), the Home Secretary has announced measures to 'crack down on bail bandits', measures which seem likely to inhibit magistrates' use of bail (see Morgan and Jones 1992, p. 44). It follows that the foundations laid during the 1980s for the more generous use of bail and the improved treatment in custody of those denied it, has been called into question. There is doubt as to whether there is the political will to build on the foundation.

NOTES

1 SI 1964, No. 388.
2 SI 1949, No. 1073.

9

LONG-TERM PRISONERS

A. Keith Bottomley

One of the most significant features of the profile of the prison population of England and Wales during the last decade has been the increase in the number of adult long-term prisoners.[1] In 1990 the daily average long-term population was 12,149, constituting 42 per cent of the adult sentenced population and 27 per cent of the total population in custody. Five years previously, in 1985, there were just 6,747 long-termers in custody, constituting 25 per cent of the adult sentenced population, and less than 15 per cent of the total in custody. In 1980, long-termers constituted 21 per cent of the adult sentenced population and 13 per cent of the total in custody.

As the daily average prison population is a product of the numbers received into prison (on sentence or before trial) and the average length of time they remain in custody, the increase in the long-term population in recent years could either be due to more being sentenced by the courts, to an increase in the average length of sentence or to an increase in the proportion of their sentences being served before release on parole (or life licence). In fact, it has been due to a combination of all three factors. Receptions of adult long-term prisoners more than doubled in the 1980s, increasing from 1,217 in 1980 to 2,855 in 1990. There was also a significant trend towards longer sentences, with a three-fold increase in the number sentenced to over 5 years up to 10 years (from 490 in 1980 to 1,546 in 1990), and an even greater increase in those given fixed sentences of over 10 years – rising from 55 in 1980 to 254 in 1988, but dropping to 186 in 1990. Not only are the sentences imposed by the Crown Court increasing in length (especially for offences of violence, drug trafficking, etc.) but a larger proportion of a prisoner's sentence is being served in custody before release on parole, particularly as a consequence of the restrictions on parole introduced in November 1983, for those serving over 5 years for offences involving violence, sex or drug trafficking. Thus, in 1983, those sentenced to over 5 years but less than 10 years were released after serving on average 49 per cent of their sentence, whereas by 1985 this had increased to 55 per cent; similarly those serving over 10 years (but excluding lifers) served only 44 per cent on average in 1983, but 59 per cent in 1985. Finally, the number of life-sentence prisoners released on life licence dropped dramatically from over 100 a year in 1982 and 1983 to an average of just under 60 a year in the period 1984–90, following the Home Secretary's announcement in November 1983 of 20-year minimum periods in custody for certain categories of murderers. As a consequence, the lifer population has increased by over 80 per cent from 1,479 in 1980 to 2,689 in 1990.

Particularly as this trend towards an increasingly large population of long-term prisoners continued throughout 1989 and 1990, when there was a significant overall *decline* in the total prison population, it seems almost certain that it is a trend that will continue, or even perhaps gather pace during the 1990s, unless effective measures are taken to shorten sentences, grant earlier parole and/or release life-sentence prisoners at an earlier point in their sentence. Indeed, the Home Office's revised projections of expected trends in the prison population to 1999 not only forecast an increase of 10,000 to 11,000 in the total prison population, but a projected increase of about 7,500 in the sentenced adult male population, being concentrated among those serving longer sentences (Home Office 1991e). These projections were formulated in May 1991, and did not take into account the likely effects of the Criminal Justice Act 1991. However, Home Office speculations on the possible effect upon the prison population of the forthcoming legislation suggested that they could be expected 'to result in a significant reduction in the number of offenders in custody' (1991e, para. 18). This was based on the belief that the new combined probation and community service order should reduce the population by between 400 and 750, and that reduced sentences for theft and non-residential burglary should further reduce it by 800 to 1,600. The new arrangements for parole and supervised early release of short and medium-term prisoners were expected to reduce the population initially by about 500, but it was recognised that this could be offset by a larger increase in those being returned to custody for committing further offences during supervision and the operative period of their original sentence. Account was also taken of the Carlisle Committee's hope that there might be a general reduction of sentence lengths, in view of the fact that their proposals (endorsed by the Government) involved 'restoring meaning' to the full sentence, as imposed by the courts (Home Office 1988e). There is, however, little doubt in most commentators' minds that the emphasis in the White Paper *Crime, Justice and Protecting the Public* (Home Office 1990a) and the Criminal Justice Act 1991 upon the 'twin track' approach of 'just deserts' and 'public protection' may well accelerate the trend towards longer prison sentences for those convicted of violent or sexual offences. As the White Paper clearly stated:

> The Government proposes to take this approach further by giving the Crown Court power to give custodial sentences longer than would be justified by the seriousness of the offence to persistent violent and

> sexual offenders, if this is necessary to protect the public from serious harm. There are a small number of offenders who become progressively more dangerous and who are a real risk to public safety . . . For those convicted of the most serious crimes a sentence of life imprisonment may be justified . . . In these circumstances, the Government considers that an exception should be made to the principle that the length of the individual sentence should be justified by the seriousness of the offence.
>
> (Home Office 1990a, para 3.13)

The Criminal Justice Act 1991 translated this into a more concise but potentially very influential clause 2(2)(b): 'where the offence is a violent or sexual offence, [the custodial sentence shall be] for such longer term (not exceeding the maximum) as in the opinion of the court is necessary to protect the public from serious harm from the offender'.

It seems clear, therefore, that the Prison Service must expect a continued growth in the proportion of those in its custody who will be serving long periods of time out of circulation and removed, to a greater or less degree, from normal contact with their families and friends. What signposts are there in the Woolf Report and the subsequent White Paper *Custody, Care and Justice,* to point the direction into the next decade for the better management and care of this important group of prisoners?

CAUSES FOR CONCERN

Before examining future options and possibilities, it is worth pausing to reflect upon the recent past and trying to identify what appear to have been the particular causes for concern in relation to provision for long-term prisoners, prior to the disturbances of April 1990.

In the mid-1960s and throughout the 1970s, there is little doubt that, apart from a continuing and growing concern about the capacity of the prison estate to accommodate the increasing number of persons being sent to prison by the courts, the major focus of attention was upon the *maintenance of security and control* within the long-term prison system. Following the Mountbatten Inquiry (Home Office 1966) and the Report of the Radzinowicz Sub-Committee (Advisory Council on the Penal System 1968), the dispersal system that was then established was undoubtedly highly successful in preventing the escape of Category A prisoners. Unfortunately, however, and almost it seemed as an inevitable corollary of the achievement of secure containment, the 1970s were marked by a series of violent incidents and disturbances in most of the long-term dispersal prisons, of which the most serious was that which took place at Hull Prison, 31 August to 3 September 1976.

Such examples of the breakdown of order and the loss of control led to a number of Prison Department initiatives, including the short-lived experiment with 'control units' at Wakefield and Wormwood Scrubs Prisons (both of which units were closed in 1975, following a concerted public and professional outcry against their philosophy and practice), and the introduction of the almost equally controversial provision (by Circular Instruction 10/1974 – subsequently revised by CI 37/1990) for the removal of disruptive prisoners for a 28-day 'cooling-off' period.[2] But, despite mounting criticisms and calls for its thorough overhaul, the dispersal system survived throughout the 1970s, and was endorsed, with only minor qualifications, by the May Committee of Inquiry (Home Office 1979).

Nevertheless, the Prison Department remained very concerned about the problems of control in dispersal prisons, so that in September 1983 a special Control Review Committee was set up within the Prison Department 'to review the maintenance of control in the prison system . . . with particular reference to the dispersal system, and to make recommendations'. This was a direct result of a request from the Home Secretary, Leon Brittan, who correctly anticipated that the changes he was shortly to announce to the Conservative Party in October of that year would 'have the effect of redistributing the load between the long-term prisons and the rest of the system' (Home Office, 1984 para. 2) – especially the restrictions on parole for serious violent offenders and the delayed release on life licence of certain classes of murderer, the effects of which have been mentioned above.

The report of the Control Review Committee (CRC), entitled *Managing the Long-Term Prison System* (Home Office 1984), was published in the following year. It provided an authoritative analysis of the existing situation and an impressive agenda for action, which if it had been fully and speedily implemented might have successfully avoided many of the negative effects for long-term prisoners of the changes that were then occurring. As it was, however, a number of the key recommendations of the CRC Report, particularly those relating to the provision of 'a coherent, progressive career for long-term prisoners' (para. 28) based on sentence-planning units and individual career plans drawn up for each prisoner at the start of their sentence, were rejected or deferred by the Home Office, and are only now beginning to take shape in the aftermath of the Woolf Inquiry (see below). On the other hand, among the recommendations of the Control Review Committee which were immediately accepted and have been gradually implemented during the last 5 or 6 years were those relating to the treatment of 'prisoners who present serious control problems', for whom it was proposed that a network of five or six small units should be established to enable them to be taken out of the dispersal system temporarily and located in an environment with which they could cope without recourse to aggressive and disruptive behaviour towards other prisoners or staff. Paradoxically, perhaps, although only four of these special units have so far been opened (at Parkhurst Prison in 1985, Lincoln in 1987, Hull in 1988 and Woodhill in 1993), and without the underpinning of the long-term sentence-planning units and other regime changes recommended by the CRC, they do appear to have been relatively successful in handling the prisoners that have been referred to them, with few serious incidents of inter-personal violence occurring (see Walmsley 1991; Bottomley and Hay, 1991) and with an apparent reduction in incidents of disorder in the English dispersal system during the last 5 or 10 years. Consequently, a review of current causes for concern within the long-term prison system at the beginning of 1990 would probably not have given high priority to the expansion or completion of the initially envisaged programme of special units, but would have emphasised the need for improved regimes in the mainstream (drawing lessons from special units experience), and the reduction of some of the perceived unfairnesses in the parole selection process and the operation of Circular Instruction 10/1974. The question, to which we shall return below, is whether the priorities emerging at the end of the 1980s should be significantly altered in the light of the events and aftermath of April 1990.

THE RELEVANCE OF WOOLF

Even before the riot at Manchester Prison on the morning of Sunday, 1 April 1990, followed by disturbances at many other establishments in England and Wales, it was apparent that the typical location of prison disorder and 'trouble' in the late 1980s had shifted from the dispersal system (where most of the trouble had occurred in the 1970s) to a much wider range of Category B, C and D prisons. Although some of the earlier spates of disorder in 1985 and 1986 coincided with record levels of prison population in England and Wales, it was clear that neither overcrowding nor poor living conditions/facilities *per se* were the simple or only causes of these disturbances (Home Office 1987a). Similarly, although Strangeways was an overcrowded local prison, holding almost 70 per cent more prisoners than its certified normal accommodation (CNA) at the beginning of April 1990, and many of the other serious disturbances that month took place in overcrowded remand centres and local prisons, Lord Justice Woolf certainly did not uniquely highlight overcrowding as the main culprit, with only one of his 12 main recommendations relating to measures to restrict overcrowding, and very few of the other 204 proposals referring directly or indirectly to this aspect of imprisonment.

Furthermore, in view of the fact that only one of the establishments that experienced serious disturbances in April 1990 was a long-term prison (Dartmoor) it was equally clear that Woolf could not point the main finger of blame directly at conditions for *long-term* prisoners. Only half of Strangeways' population of over 1,600 prisoners at the time of the riot were sentenced adults, including 15 Category A and 105 Category B prisoners. These were mainly awaiting allocation to other establishments, but included 10 prisoners who had been returned to Manchester for a six-month period because of the disruption they were causing in their dispersal prisons, and a larger number who had been returned because they did not fit in at their training prison (Woolf 1991, para. 3.40). Although Woolf did not specifically identify the alleged 'ring-leaders', the role of some of these long-term prisoners, including several with records of disruption in the dispersal system, was undoubtedly crucial in the early stages of the planning and instigation of the riot and a small 'hard core' of troublemakers was also blamed by some of the prisoners who submitted written evidence to the Woolf Inquiry. In Woolf's view it was a combination of the perceived grievances and injustices at the way they were treated, plus the generally unacceptable and inhumane conditions in which they were held, that provided the fuel for the riot to take hold and spread in the way it did, amongst an inmate population that was antagonistic towards the prison system in general (para. 3.432).

In view of the scale of the disturbances that took place at Manchester Prison and elsewhere, Woolf was undoubtedly right to take this unique opportunity to examine critically every aspect of the prison system that might have made a contribution to the worst outbreak of disorder in its history:

> The riots which the Inquiry investigated were not isolated incidents . . . They stem from a long history of violent disturbances in the prison system. On the evidence, prison riots cannot be dismissed as one-off events, or as local disasters, or a run of bad luck. They are symptomatic of a series of underlying difficulties in the prison system. They will only be brought to an end if these difficulties are addressed.
>
> (para. 1.142)

Fundamental to Woolf's analysis and his overall objectives for the future direction of the Prison Service was his belief that:

> the Prison Service must set security, control and justice in prisons at the right level and it must provide the right balance between them . . . The April riots occurred because these three elements were out of balance.
>
> (paras. 1.148–1.150)

Security, control and justice arguably affect long-term prisoners' experience of imprisonment more than any other single group of inmates, in view of the considerable length of time they spend in prison, cut off from contact with family, friends and normal community life. Thus the Woolf Report is of central relevance to any consideration of future developments within the long-term prison system. A short essay of this kind cannot hope to cover all aspects of Woolf's many recommendations that might impinge upon the treatment of long-term prisoners, so it will focus upon the two main themes of (a) enhancing the sense of direction and purpose for those serving long sentences; and (b) the future management of 'disruptive' prisoners.

DIRECTION AND PURPOSE FOR LONG-TERM PRISONERS

Apart from the inherent physical and emotional privations and restricted freedoms of any prison sentence, one of the most difficult aspects with which a prisoner has to cope and somehow come to terms is the all-pervasive perception and experience of *uncertainty*. At a day to day level, on the landings and in the workshops, there is the uncertainty and unpredictability of the behaviour of fellow prisoners (and prison staff) in a situation of enforced cohabitation and dependence. Prison subcultures represent one kind of communal 'coping strategy' that has emerged over the years to counter this particular 'pain of imprisonment' (Sykes 1958). Management decisions often appear unpredictable and arbitrary, ranging from responses to minor requests for some small 'privilege' to more important decisions about work allocation, home leave, breaches of discipline, or transfer to another establishment. Probably the worst uncertainty of all for long-termers, and especially for those serving life sentences, is that associated with discretionary release dates, on parole or life licence, where secrecy and arbitrariness often appear to be at their greatest – when arguably openness and consistency should be at a premium.

As noted above, a central theme of the report of the CRC (Home Office 1984) was the need to send the right signals to long-term prisoners, providing them with clear guidelines and 'career plans' for serving their sentences. Similarly, in Lord Justice Woolf's analysis there are a number of interrelated recommendations for enhancing the sense of direction, coherence and justification for much of what happens to prisoners in their state of dependence and uncertainty.

In the evidence presented to Woolf, including the discussions at the public seminars, there was virtual unanimity on the desirability of all prisoners, especially long-termers, having *sentence plans* to provide clear objectives and a sense of purpose, from the induction stage to pre-release planning. It was an issue on which NACRO and the Prison Officers' Association (POA) were in broad agreement, with Paul Cavadino (NACRO) emphasising the importance of the prisoners themselves being involved in the formulation of their own sentence plan, in a process of negotiation with prison staff. In its evidence to Woolf, the Prison Service indicated that the creation of a new Directorate of Inmate Programmes, in the major reorganisation of September 1990, would enable the concept (and hopefully also the reality) of sentence planning to be further extended and progressed throughout the system. Most life-sentence prisoners and all those in young offender institutions (since 1988) already have sentence plans and Brian Emes, the Director of Inmate Programmes, announced that it was intended to introduce sentence planning for all prisoners serving 10 years or more in April 1991. In order to accelerate this programme, Woolf proposed that 'the Prison Service should work towards the time when prisoners serving a sentence of 12 months or more can be given some form of sentence plan' (para. 14.75), in addition to their 'contract', the provision of which was fifth in the list of Woolf's twelve main recommendations. He recommended that there should be a 'compact' or 'contract' for each prisoner setting out the prisoner's expectations and responsibilities in the prison in which he or she is held (para. 1.167(v)). The difference between a prisoner's contract and sentence plan was explained in the following way:

> The 'contract' is the short term document which, as well as setting out the conditions in which he will live, describes what is to happen to the prisoner during the period immediately following the making of the 'contract' . . . The sentence plan, on the other hand, is the long term plan covering the whole period of the prisoner's sentence, be it two years or ten years. It may require variation or amendment. It may have to be replaced. But the new or revised plan would still deal with the whole of the remainder of the prisoner's sentence.
>
> (para. 14.76)

Woolf wanted a greater sense of urgency and higher priority to be given to the extension of sentence planning, and for there to be a greater focus on preparing plans for the prisoner's release – especially in view of the imminent changes to be introduced following the passing of the Criminal Justice Act 1991.

In its White Paper, *Custody, Care and Justice* (Home Office 1991a), the Government reiterated the Prison Service's commitment to the provision and extension of sentence planning. It cited well-developed sentence plan arrangements at adult male prisons such as Full Sutton, Morton Hall and North Sea Camp, and at the women's prison at Drake Hall. Furthermore, and in particular, it promised to:

- introduce and improve sentence plans for all life sentence prisoners . . . centred on offending behaviour and setting programme objectives which will determine progress towards release;
- introduce in 1992 sentence plans for Category A prisoners and for sex offenders;
- move towards providing sentence plans for all prisoners serving substantial sentences as resources allow.

(Home Office 1991a, para. 7.19)

The last commitment is the most important, but (like much in the White Paper) the most vague in terms of a timetable for implementation. Priority will be given to prisoners sentenced to 4 years or more, as the early release of such prisoners under parole supervision remains discretionary under the Criminal Justice Act 1991. But the long-term aim will be to provide an appropriate sentence plan for all but those serving very short sentences.

Woolf's key recommendation of contracts for all prisoners (which, incidentally, the Government did not respond to in its White Paper) is intended to provide a multi-purpose document, outlining a set of mutual expectations and responsibilities between establishment, staff and inmate:

> each prisoner should be offered the opportunity of entering into a 'compact' or 'contract' with the establishment. In that 'contract', the establishment would state, in as precise terms as possible, what it would provide for the prisoner. In return, the prisoner would agree to comply with the responsibilities which the 'contract' placed upon him.
>
> (Woolf 1991, para. 12.120)

'Contracts' would be an essential part of, and have to be compatible with, the overall sentence plan, which would follow a prisoner from establishment to establishment and would be subject to annual review for longer-term prisoners. In Woolf's view, a prisoner would receive progressively more under his contract as he progressed through his sentence and it would therefore be a way of introducing greater incentives into the system. The additional advantages for long-term prisoners were spelled out:

> It could substantially improve the position of the inmate since it would make clear what were his legitimate expectations. It would enable him, if he was being transferred to another establishment which provided a lesser regime, to point out the disadvantage to him of such a transfer. It would assist in providing a structure to an inmate's imprisonment and it would be in accord with the principles of justice which we believe should exist within a prison.
>
> (para. 12.129)

Prisoner contracts were intended to reflect and, hopefully, deliver on the essential principles that informed Woolf's approach to prisoners – many of which were similar to those enunciated by the Scottish Prison Service's important document *Opportunity and Responsibility: Developing New Approaches to the Management of the Long Term Prison System in Scotland* (Scottish Office 1990), which was much quoted in the Woolf Inquiry public seminars. These principles include that of encouraging prisoners to take as full *responsibility* as possible for what happens to them during the sentence, of giving them *opportunities* to make choices (for which they will be then held accountable), of showing and receiving *respect* in relation to all other members of the prison community, and of enhancing *justice* in our prisons – which will only be achieved if prisoners, as well as staff, feel that the system is fair and just (Woolf 1991, paras. 14.11–14.21). In essence, Woolf's hope was that 'a prisoner's time in prison should provide a clear sense of progress from reception to discharge . . . [and] that such progress should provide incentives to prisoners to behave responsibly' (para. 14.22).

The incorporation of incentives and disincentives into 'contracts' and sentence planning was a deliberate attempt on the part of Woolf to integrate them fully into the system and into every prisoner's career plan – very much, and explicitly, following the approach of the Control Review Committee, but extending it to all prisoners, not just the long-termers. For example, the expectation and likelihood of serving their sentence in different establishments not only heightens their uncertainty but is likely to bring them into direct conflict with inconsistent provisions and attitudes. Woolf urges the Prison Service to ensure that there is consistency between what each prison (of the same type) offers, so as to minimise the inevitable disruption and upset caused by transfer from one location to another – which was a factor identified by the Woolf Report as contributing significantly to perceptions of injustice and grievance among prisoners, thereby possibly directly influencing some of the disturbances which were the subject of the Inquiry (paras. 9.24–9.34).

If an integrated package for prisoners, as proposed by Woolf, including 'compacts' and 'contracts', sentence/career planning, purposeful progression through a sentence from induction to preparation for release, and understandable linkage of incentives/disincentives to behaviour, were to be introduced forthwith, and in full, then long-term prisoners would stand to gain considerably. Unfortunately, the indication from the White Paper is that although sentence planning for virtually all prisoners has been accepted *in principle*, its introduction *in practice* is likely to be a long drawn-out process, even for long-term prisoners, despite the fact that it was recommended as long ago as 1984 by the CRC and that the changes to discretionary early release and parole procedures in 1992 make it particularly urgent.

Nevertheless, long-term prisoners' sense of uncertainty and arbitrariness may be slightly reduced by the Government's endorsement of a number of other important principles of Woolf, relating to the need to give reasons, wherever possible, to prisoners for decisions which materially affect them, and a greater openness in discussion and consultations with prisoners about the conduct of their sentence, in line with the new procedures for early release introduced under the Criminal Justice Act 1991. When, or whether, these good intentions will come to fruition in a way that will noticeably affect the experience of the increasing number of long-term prisoners in our prison system remains to be seen.

MANAGING TO CONTROL DISRUPTIVE PRISONERS

Whatever may have been the part played by a small number of long-term prisoners, with a history of disruptive behaviour in other establishments, in the instigation and continuation of the Strangeways riot and the other prison disturbances of April 1990, there seemed to be general agreement (shared by Lord Justice Woolf) on the need to review current policy and practice in the management of so-called 'difficult' or 'disruptive' prisoners, within the long-term prison system.

As noted earlier in this chapter, quite a lot of attention has been paid during the last decade (some would argue too much) to devising an effective strategy for dealing with the very small minority of prisoners within the dispersal prisons who are unable or unwilling to cope with the institutional and/or inter-personal demands and pressures of long periods in custody. This concern stemmed from the post-Mountbatten experiences of the 1970s, during which it seemed that security (from escape) of Category A prisoners had been achieved but at the cost of recurrent, if rather sporadic, outbursts of individual or group violence against people and property in the dispersal system.

The Control Review Committee's strategy for a network of special units, outlined above, was predicated on significant changes occurring within the long-term prison system – particularly in terms of assessment and allocation procedures, sentence-planning units, and enhanced regimes. Their belief was that 'the measures we have proposed . . . should go a long way to preventing serious control problems arising with the great majority of prisoners' (Home Office 1984, para. 41). However, even if all the proposed measures had been accepted and implemented (which, as we have seen, was far from the case) they were in no doubt that 'there will be some particularly difficult prisoners with whom the mainstream long-term prisons simply cannot cope' (para. 42). It was for such prisoners that the strategy of special units was devised, so that the rest of the system could maintain and develop positive and open regimes that would not be put at risk or abused by a few persistently disruptive prisoners. It was, of course, recognised that this minority could not be easily categorised including, as it did, those who behaved aggressively or in a disorderly way themselves, those who encouraged others to misbehave and those who suffered from some form of mental disturbance that might predispose them to violence or make them vulnerable (Home Office 1984, para. 43). The other underlying principle (often subsequently lost sight of) that was at the heart of the CRC strategy was the essentially 'situational' nature of most aggressive and disruptive behaviour:

> Difficult prison behaviour is a function of many things in addition to the prisoner's own character, and it is generally recognised in the prison service that a man who presents intractable control problems in one establishment may be little or no trouble in another.
>
> (para. 44)

Many years later, and with much water having flowed under the bridge (and over prison roofs!), Lord Justice Woolf agreed with the basic premise that whatever improvements might be made in general prison conditions, including those specifically for long-term prisoners, there would remain a minority of potentially disruptive prisoners:

> There are undoubtedly within the prison system of this country a number of prisoners who, given the opportunity and whatever the conditions within the prison, would seek either to escape or to be disruptive. No improvement in the conditions of containment will alter this situation . . . The prison system has to be managed in a way which will enable the required degree of security and control to be provided.
>
> (Woolf 1991, paras. 9.38–9.39)

Woolf also took on board one of the other important lessons of the 1970s that security and control are different issues, that have to be addressed separately:

> The present security categorisation is a poor indication of possible control risks. Many prisoners who attract a high security categorisation, because they may present a risk to the public if they escape, present no appreciable risk of disrupting the life of the prison. Within a secure environment, they could be given a good deal of freedom.
>
> On the other hand, there are some prisoners who present no appreciable risk to the public if they escape, but who present acute control problems within the environment of the prison.
>
> (paras. 9.45–9.46)

To address this distinct problem, suggestions have been made (and were repeated in evidence to Woolf) that 'a control categorisation' system ought to be drawn up, to operate in parallel with the existing system of security categorisation. However, Woolf reached the conclusion that such a system would have problems of its own that could not easily be overcome. In particular, he accepted the crucial points that 'the evidence suggests that a prisoner who creates control problems in one prison may behave with complete propriety in another', and that he knew of 'no objective system for identifying *potentially disruptive* prisoners' (para. 9.48 emphasis added). He did not, for the time being therefore, propose the introduction of any system for control categorisation, but placed the onus firmly back on to establishments to find ways of dealing with prisoners whom they identify as potential control problems: 'An attempt to deal with the cause of the problem – whether it arises from the life of the prison or from outside – may be more effective in deterring disruption than spending time reviewing the prisoner's control categorisation' (para. 9.49).

Having ruled out this particular strategy, Woolf subsequently proceeded, in a later chapter of the report, to address the issue of the management of disruptive prisoners in a very direct and comprehensive way, in view of the part that a group of 'disruptive prisoners' played in the April disturbances.

He drew a distinction between prisoners who are seriously disruptive *without ever being involved in a riot* and those who, whilst not usually disruptive, can become caught up in a disturbance and behave in a most disruptive way (para. 12.223). His analysis addresses the former rather than the latter category – although admitting that it was often very difficult, if not impossible, to anticipate (and therefore ever totally prevent) the causes of such behaviour.

Having reiterated the point that 'however much progress is made to improve conditions within prisons, they will remain places where, if people were to be given the choice, they would prefer not to be held' (para. 12.221), he stated his belief that implementation of his key recommendations for community prisons, with small units offering varied programmes reflected in each prisoner's contract, provided the best foundation for responding to unco-operative prisoners without recourse to force – presumably mainly by making such unco-operative behaviour less likely in the first place.

Woolf accepted that it may not be possible to isolate any single factor, such as overcrowding, which produces disturbances, but on the basis of the evidence before the Inquiry and the experience from visits overseas he came to the conclusion that 'there is a close link between the nature of the regime, in the broadest sense of the word, and the risk of prisoners behaving in a disruptive manner which, in some circumstances, can lead to disturbances' (para. 12.228):

> The best way of reducing the risk of disruption and disturbance is to improve the regime within a prison and to improve the way prisoners are handled within the prison.
>
> (para. 12.231)

I would be surprised if there were many people, either inside or outside the prison system, prisoners or prison staff, academics or administrators, who would wish seriously to challenge that basic proposition. There may, however, be legitimate disagreement about those aspects of a prison regime which, if improved, would have the greatest impact on reducing the likelihood of disruption. Nevertheless, Woolf's main recommendations about regimes and improved quality of life for prisoners are in line with research findings about the factors that are valued by long-term prisoners and appear conducive to non-disruptive behaviour, both at the individual and collective level – particularly bearing in mind the other principle that still needs repeating, as Woolf does: 'Most "disruptive" prisoners are not necessarily disruptive for the whole of their sentence: they are influenced by the conditions in which they are held and by the choice and nature of the prison to which they are allocated' (para. 12.234). Among the key 'situational' elements identified by Woolf are prison location, staff–inmate relationships, incentives/disincentives and effective grievance procedures.

Prisoners are less likely to create trouble if they are in a prison which is located conveniently for their family and friends to visit. Hence the importance of community prisons and the location of prisoners (both remand and sentenced, and short- and long-termers) as near as possible to where their relatives live. One of the most disturbing effects on long-term prisoners is the frequent transfers to which they are subject, whether for security, disciplinary or 'sentence-planning' considerations. Whilst some movement between establishments is always likely to be necessary and appropriate in the course of a lengthy prison sentence, the social and geographical aspects of transfers should always be given the most careful thought and, wherever possible, be fully discussed beforehand with the prisoner concerned.

In this context, it is not without significance that one of the leading participants in the Strangeways riot had been moved between establishments at least six times in the course of the previous 21 months in prison – usually for reasons of maintaining order in the prisons from which he was moved (Woolf 1991, para. 9.26), and other long-term prisoners had resumed disruptive behaviour following transfer and/or recategorisation (paras. 9.27–9.30). Whilst Woolf admitted that 'all this evidence cannot prove that the movement of prisoners is in itself conducive to riot', yet the evidence suggests that it may well be a significant contributory factor for many individuals (para. 9.31). The importance of a stable and predictable environment for prisoners (just as for other people in the outside community, in family, home and neighbourhood) is supported by professional testimony and research evidence from a recent study of Long Lartin and Albany prisons conducted by the Cambridge Institute of Criminology (para. 9.33; see Hay, Sparks and Bottoms 1990).

The importance of getting staff–inmate relationships right, if security and control are to be maintained, was a fundamental principle of the CRC report which Woolf endorsed and was one of the most important reasons underlying his advocacy of small units in prisons, where prisoners and staff could get to know each other better (para. 12.236).

Finally, the introduction of prisoner 'contracts', linked to clear patterns of incentives and disincentives, and effective grievance procedures are essential ingredients for purposeful custody and justice within prisons.

However, despite all the faith and optimism that these proposals, if implemented, should lead to a significant reduction in disruptive behaviour and difficult-to-manage prisoners, it was felt that there would always be a few prisoners who would nevertheless, and perhaps only occasionally, act in such an aggressive or disruptive manner that necessitated additional control or management options. The current options were therefore reviewed by Woolf, and a number of generally very sensible, if rather marginal, proposals were made to improve them and bring them more into line with the overriding principle of justice within prisons.

Perhaps the most controversial option is the power, under the terms of Circular Instruction 37/1990 (which replaced the notorious CI 10/1974), to transfer a prisoner from the dispersal prison to a local prison for a 'cooling off' period of up to one month, in the interests of good order and discipline. There is no doubt that this provision creates a great sense of injustice and often foments bitterness and aggression in those for whom it is used. It is not clear how it could easily be fitted into Woolf's notion of sentence planning or prisoner contracts! The 1990 CI requires that the reasons for the transfer should be recorded on the inmate's record by the governor and that the prisoner must be told the reasons for his transfer 'so far as this is practical and as soon as possible' – although giving the prisoner no absolute right to reasons. Woolf recommends that these reasons should always be given and *in writing*, and that the transfer of disruptive prisoners to local prisons under CI 37/1990 should be used sparingly (paras. 12.252, 12.245).

Reference is made to the policy adopted in some other countries (such as the Netherlands), of a 'carousel' approach, whereby the most difficult prisoners are circulated from one prison to another every few months. Although not admitting that such a practice officially exists in this country (where it is known unofficially, and colloquially, as the 'roundabout') Woolf made it clear that this solution is not acceptable and urged the Prison Service to monitor the operation of CI 37/1990 to ensure that it is not used to the same effect. More radical proposals to reform CI 37/1990, submitted in evidence by Professor Roy King, were carefully considered by the Inquiry but not in the main supported, except in so far as it was recommended that a member of the Board of Visitors should be present at the receiving prison when a prisoner arrives on transfer under CI 37/1990 or should see him as soon as possible thereafter (Woolf 1991, paras. 12.255–12.260).

Segregation of a disruptive prisoner under Rule 43 (GOAD) is perhaps the most commonly used short-term mechanism for the prevention of trouble and the maintenance of order in an establishment, without recourse to a transfer. Not unnaturally it gives rise to considerable feelings of grievance in those for whom it is used. Here again, Woolf recommends that reasons should always be given by the governor, and in writing, either at the time or as soon as possible thereafter (para. 12.271). The Board of Visitors should no longer have authority to extend detention under Rule 43 (GOAD) beyond the governor's initial power to order 72 hours segregation. In future, this authority will be vested in the area manager. Only in exceptional circumstances should there be more than one extension of 28 days (or 14 days in the case of young offenders) (para. 12.270).

The Special Units, as recommended by the Control Review Committee (Home Office 1984), are the most recent option for the management of disruptive long-term prisoners (see above). From evidence to the Inquiry it was apparent that at present the CRC Special Units make only a small contribution to the Prison Service's response to problems of order and control in the long-term prison system – with the three operational units normally holding a total of no more than about 35 prisoners at any one time. These units have been heavily resourced, especially in terms of staffing, and are also the subject of a considerable programme of research and evaluation by Prison Service psychologists, psychiatrists from the Institute of Psychiatry, and a number of independent academic researchers.[3] In the view of some of the researchers, the Special Unit strategy might be seen to be overstating the extent to which control problems in dispersal prisons are the product of 'difficult' or 'disturbed' individuals, rather than of inappropriate or 'disturbing' prison environments. Furthermore, Woolf reported that 'there are indications in the evidence we have received that they may be sending the wrong message to prisoners by apparently placing a premium on bad behaviour' (para. 12.289). It was concluded that: 'Special Units do not provide an easy or complete answer to the problem of dealing with the intransigently disruptive prisoner' (para. 12.290).

However, it was accepted that there was a need for special units in some form in our prison system as it is today, but that they should only be used for a small minority of particularly disruptive prisoners: and the aim of such units should be to return the prisoner to 'normal' prison in the mainstream system before release. If improvements of the kind suggested by Woolf are implemented, there should be little need for many (or any) such special units:

> It is essential that there is as broad a range of regimes within the prison system as is practicable. The small units policy which we recommend, coupled with community prisons, would be important. The aim must be to produce a prison system which can cope with disruptive prisoners in a way which does not allow them to bring the life of a prison to a halt or to be rewarded by specially favourable treatment and conditions for trying to do so.
>
> (Woolf 1991, para. 12.296)

The Government's response to Woolf's recommendations on the management of disruptive prisoners was fairly predictable. Special measures for segregation or control should be used only as a last resort – 'wherever possible . . . each establishment should deal with those who behave in an unco-operative or disruptive fashion from within its own resources and by use of its own accommodation' (Home Office 1991a, para. 5.29). But, it continues, there are likely to be situations and/or prisoners that can only be dealt with by segregation under Rule 43, short-term transfer under CI 37/1990, or re-allocation to a special unit. All these measures should be used sparingly, and reasons given in writing to the prisoners concerned at the time or as soon as possible thereafter. The 'roundabout' should be brought to a halt: 'It should not be the practice for disruptive prisoners to be transferred from one prison to another at frequent intervals in order to control their behaviour or reduce its effects on any particular establishment' (Home Office 1991a, para. 5.31).

The sting in the tail of this section of the White Paper, especially as far as long-term prisoners are concerned, is that the movements of prisoners under CI 37/1990 or to special units will take priority over the general objectives described earlier in the White Paper for the management and allocation of the prison population as a whole, relating to the holding of prisoners in living units in multi-functional community prisons or in groups of prisons near to their homes and families. Such prisoners will therefore be 'double-losers', with even greater cause to feel aggrieved at their treatment by the prison authorities.

One possible ray of hope, or small glimmer of light at the end of the long-termers' tunnel, is the potential role of the 'new generation' prisons. Woolf was impressed by the research evidence from Roy King on Oak Park Heights Prison, Minnesota, and by the visit that was made to it. It was seen as a way of combining the enhanced regime recommendations with an experiment in the handling of actually or potentially disruptive prisoners. It was recommended that the Prison Service should earmark at least one 'new generation' prison for dispersal prisoners, including most of those who would now probably be housed in CRC special units (para. 12.305). This would enable some of the lessons learned from the experimental regimes in the special units in England and Wales, and the range of innovative small units in the Scottish Prison Service, to be applied to a new mainstream long-term prison, rather than used to perpetuate additional 'special units' which create problems of their own, especially in terms of integration with prisoners' sentence plans for preparing them for return to normal location, prior to release. Indeed, when (or if) a greater variety of regimes (and levels of security) are introduced into the community prisons advocated by Woolf (preferably with specialist reassessment and allocation units), many long-term prisoners would be able to move to such community prisons towards the end of their sentence. To the extent that a more integrated, purposive and planned custodial experience can be provided for long-term prisoners, to that extent are they more likely to be re-integrated successfully into the community on release.

NOTES

1 In this chapter, the definition of 'long-term' used will be that of the Prison Department, *viz.* males sentenced to over 4 years, females sentenced to over 3 years, and all life-sentence prisoners.

2 See Circular Instruction 10/1974 *Dispersal Policy – Provision of Cells in Local Prisons,* which was subsequently revised by Circular Instruction 37/1990 *Transfer of Inmates in the Interests of Good Order and Discipline.*

3 For details of the initial research strategy see Home Office 1987b; for pre- liminary research findings see Hay *et al.* 1990; Walmsley 1991; Bottomley and Hay 1991.

10

MENTALLY DISORDERED PRISONERS

Adrian Grounds

THE WOOLF REPORT RECOMMENDATIONS

The Woolf inquiry into the prison disturbances of April 1990 (Woolf 1991) overlapped with the most major review for twenty years of services for mentally disordered offenders in England. This *Review of Services for Mentally Disordered Offenders and Others Requiring Similar Services* was established jointly by the Department of Health and Home Office in November 1990. In November 1991 the first set of reports from this review were published for consultation (Department of Health/Home Office 1991a, b, c, d), and a second group of reports was published in June 1992 (Department of Health/Home Office 1992a, b). The *Final Summary Report* was published in November, 1992 (Department of Health/Home Office 1992c). The conclusions of the Woolf Inquiry in relation to mentally disordered offenders prefigured many of the ideas which have since been developed at length in the Department of Health/Home Office review.

The Woolf Report discusses mentally disordered prisoners in the context of its broader recommendations about limiting the role of the Prison Service. Co-operation between agencies, including the Department of Health, is urged in order to divert remand prisoners and offenders from prison custody, so as to reduce the prison population 'to an unavoidable minimum' (Woolf 1991, para. 10.70). In the interest of avoiding remands in custody, the Report recommends the establishment of further bail information and public interest case-assessment schemes, bail hostels, and specialist hostels for people with mental disorder and those with drug or alcohol related problems. The mentally disordered are included as a specific group, alongside young offenders and fine defaulters, as a category for whom the use of imprisonment should be minimised.

In the main section of the Report dealing with mentally disordered offenders (paras.10.115–10.140) there are two main themes. First, initiatives to minimise the number of mentally disordered people remanded in custody are endorsed. Second, the Prison Department is urged to recognise a special responsibility to the mentally disordered who remain accommodated in prison and, in particular, specific attention should be paid to those with mental handicap (learning disability). The Report welcomed the guidance given by the Home Office to courts, prisons, police and the probation service, summarising the legal powers available to divert mentally disordered offenders from the criminal justice system; and the Report also commended the experimental schemes which were then becoming established to provide a rapid psychiatric assessment service to magistrates' courts.

However the Report was also realistic in acknowledging that the provision of alternative facilities was inadequate and noted that this was also recognised by the Government.

> The Government recognise that action is needed substantially to improve the present situation.
>
> (para. 10.117)

> The Department of Health accepts that, although expanded and developed in recent years, the services that are at present available for the mentally disordered do not work as well as they should in meeting requests for treatment from the Courts and the Prison Service. Nor do they result in the most appropriate placement of offenders.
>
> (para. 10.121)

Following the Woolf Report, the Government published its White Paper *Custody, Care and Justice* in September 1991 (Home Office 1991a). In one important respect the White Paper lacked the realistic and balanced approach that characterised the Woolf recommendations concerning mentally disordered prisoners. The White Paper endorsed the view that whenever possible mentally disordered offenders should be diverted to health or social services, and prisoners requiring psychiatric treatment in hospital should be transferred as rapidly as possible. However, the White Paper was silent in response to the Woolf proposals that the Prison Department should recognise its special responsibility towards the mentally disordered offenders who are accommodated in custody, and that it should ensure that clearer and more specific attention is paid to mentally handicapped prisoners.

The remainder of this chapter will discuss the problems of providing for mentally disordered offenders as highlighted in the Woolf Inquiry, and the prospects for improvement.

HISTORICAL BACKGROUND

Our current difficulties need to be seen in historical context. The practice of remanding defendants in custody for pre-trial diagnosis had become established in a number of London courts by the end of the nineteenth century, and medical remands in custody by magistrates steadily increased during following decades. They were given further impetus in the Criminal Justice Act 1948, which increased the powers of courts to obtain pre-trial and pre-sentence reports. The psychiatric assessment and care of remanded prisoners has traditionally formed a major component of the work of the Prison Medical Service and there has been a long-standing recognition that prison doctors should have training and expertise in psychiatry. However, at the same time this has been combined uneasily with the view that it is undesirable in principle that the mentally disordered should be remanded in custody and their diversion from prison should be the aim.

The difficulty experienced by psychiatric hospitals in coping with mentally disordered offenders also has a long history, and is not merely a recent phenomenon resulting from the advent of community care. This is well illustrated in the evidence given to a Commission of Inquiry established by the Home Secretary in 1880 to enquire into the subject of criminal lunacy (Criminal Lunacy (Departmental) Commission 1882). The Commissioners heard a number of graphic accounts of the objections raised by asylum superintendents to the admission of criminal patients. For example, in giving evidence on 5 August 1880, Dr R. M. Gover, Medical Inspector of Government Prisons, was asked if he was aware of any grievances arising from the detention of lunatics who were dangerous or who exhibited criminal tendencies. He told the Commission:

> I have several friends among the medical superintendents of lunatic asylums and they express themselves unanimously upon that point. They have pointed out to me the extreme inconvenience and in some cases the disastrous effects of the presence of criminal patients among the ordinary patients.
>
> (para. 806)

Likewise, the Honourable Francis Scott, Chairman of the Brookwood, Surrey, Asylum, on being asked whether provision for dangerous lunatics had been included when his asylum was built, replied: 'Certainly not, and as long as I am Chairman I will endeavour to avoid that' (para. 1892). Dangerous lunatics, he argued, are expensive: 'If you have a person requiring a constant attendant to look after him to see that he does not attack others, he is both a dangerous man and an expensive man, and these are both material ingredients' (para. 1848).

The main developments during the last two decades in psychiatric and legal provisions for mentally disordered offenders may be traced back to the report of the Butler Committee (Home Office/Department of Health and Social Security 1975). The Committee drew attention to the problems faced by courts in obtaining hospital orders for mentally disordered offenders who could not be looked after in local hospitals and who, in consequence, were being sentenced to imprisonment. In order to ease both this problem and the problem of overcrowding in special hospitals, the Committee recommended as a matter of urgency that regional units offering a medium level of security should be established with central government funding (Home Office/Department of Health and Social Security 1974). The Committee recommended the development of psychiatric services both in the Health Service and within the prisons, recognising that there may be exceptional circumstances in which a penal disposal could be preferred to a hospital disposal (para. 3.23). New community provision, in particular residential provision, was recommended, together with the retention of the 'asylum' role of local hospitals.

> Hospitals . . . have a role in the continuing care of those who cannot be discharged into the community without serious risk of relapse through self-neglect, . . . The re-introduction to some extent of a sanctuary role would particularly serve those people who are already so damaged that they are unable to take advantage of the rehabilitation measures which hospitals normally pursue.
>
> (para. 6.6)

The Committee also recommended changes in criminal proceedings. There should be more consideration of non-prosecution of the mentally disordered and new powers to remand to hospital for assessment and treatment before trial.

Many of the principal recommendations of the Butler Report have been implemented in the ensuing years, albeit slowly and partially, but their impact has been limited. Regional secure units have been established, but neither the target of 2,000 beds recommended by the Butler Committee, nor the more modest number of 1,000 beds recommended by the Glancy Committee (Department of Health and Social Security 1974) has been met. The current (January 1992) level of provision in England and Wales is approximately 600 beds.

In 1984 new powers for courts to remand mentally disordered defendants to hospital for reports or for treatment came into operation, but their use has been low. The total number of remands to hospital for assessment and treatment has currently reached a plateau of about 300 per year, approximately one-twentieth of the number remanded to prison for medical reports.

In 1987 a further report on mentally disordered offenders in the prison system in England and Wales was produced by an interdepartmental working group of Home Office and DHSS officials (Home Office/Department of Health and Social Security 1987). The working group recommended that further research should be carried out to assess the extent of mental disorder amongst the sentenced and remand populations, that transfer to hospital of mentally disordered inmates should be expedited more rapidly and that health authorities should continue to develop a comprehensive range of provision for mentally disordered offenders. By the time this report was published, evidence of a new gap in secure provision was becoming clear and the working group advised: 'the approach to secure provision has to be further diversified with complementary non-RSU [Regional Secure Unit] facilities, including a range of local hospital accommodation' (para. 8.3).

Despite these various initiatives, concern about mentally disordered prisoners has grown rather than diminished. In contrast to the rather bland conclusions of the interdepartmental working group (Home Office/ Department of Health and Social Security 1987), others have expressed more outraged concern about the unacceptable suffering of seriously mentally ill remanded prisoners. The House of Commons Social Services Committee (House of Commons 1986) advised urgent action to transfer ill prisoners. Coid (1988a, 1988b) described rejection by psychiatric services of chronically disabled men remanded in custody and the Chief Inspector of Prisons has drawn attention to the heavy psychiatric workload and poor facilities at HMP Brixton (Home Office 1990b).

Finally, as described above, a further, comprehensive Department of Health and Home Office Review of services for mentally disordered offenders was established in November 1990. Its content will be further discussed below.

LEGAL AVENUES

The difficulties in achieving the transfer of mentally disordered prisoners to NHS psychiatric services are not due to a lack of legal avenues for transfer. The police have powers to take a mentally disordered person who appears to be in immediate need of care and control to a place of safety, which can include a psychiatric hospital (Mental Health Act 1983 s. 136). Alternatively, if a mentally disordered suspect is taken into police custody a medical assessment can be requested with a view to transfer to hospital and this may provide an alternative to prosecution. Courts can remand to hospital for reports instead of remanding in custody (Mental Health Act 1983 s. 35). Powers to remand to hospital for treatment (Mental Health Act 1983 s. 36) are available only to crown courts. If a defendant is found unfit to plead or not guilty by reason of insanity, a flexible range of disposals is now available (Criminal Procedure (Insanity and Unfitness to Plead) Act 1991). At the sentencing stage two specific medical disposals are available: the hospital order (Mental Health Act 1983 s. 37), and the probation order with a condition of medical treatment, which may be as an in-patient or an out-patient. This order requires the individual's consent.

Although there are deficiencies in some of these legal powers, the difficulties in achieving diversion mainly arise for other reasons. These will be considered in the light of some recent research on mentally disordered prisoners among the remand and sentenced populations.

Remand prisoners

Research carried out at HMP Winchester by Coid (1988a, b) drew attention to the difficulty in securing psychiatric care from NHS consultants when mentally disordered remanded prisoners were referred to them during the remand period. The men rejected for treatment had been remanded on minor charges and were described as typically having chronic psychotic illnesses and socially disorganised lives. Coid's paper argued there was a failure by psychiatric services to look after the people concerned, and he noted: 'During this study I was distressed to see how psychotic and helpless men were ignored by the hospital responsible for their care' (1988a, p. 1782).

However, the commonest reasons cited by NHS psychiatrists for rejecting referred men were that hospital treatment was not appropriate or the diagnosis was disputed. A recent research project carried out at the Institute of Criminology, Cambridge, and the Institute of Psychiatry, London, (Dell, Grounds, James and Robertson 1991; Robertson, Dell, Grounds and James 1992) had similar findings but interpreted them differently. The study was carried out at three prisons, Brixton, Holloway and Risley, and entailed a prospective follow-up of 951 cases from reception in custody to court disposal. The sample consisted of three overlapping groups: first, people with any evidence of past or present psychotic illness, or who were recognised as mentally handicapped; second, all cases referred to outside psychiatric services; and third, all those remanded for psychiatric reports. The sample therefore represented those with conditions which caused, or showed need to cause, some psychiatric intervention in the remand process. Predominantly they were people charged with minor offences and a high proportion (40 per cent in the London samples) were effectively homeless. Most of the people with histories of psychotic disorders were referred to outside psychiatrists. Of these different proportions were accepted following referral. In the Holloway sample, 57 of the 95 women with psychotic disorders (60 per cent) were accepted, and in the Brixton sample 96 out of the 336 men with psychotic disorders (29 per cent) were accepted. Amongst the psychotic men who were rejected for admission or who were not referred, most received non-custodial disposals. If they did receive prison sentences most of these had been served whilst on remand. Most of these people were regarded by the courts as not meriting prison sentences and this, in itself, calls into question whether they should have been remanded into custody.

When prison doctors and visiting psychiatrists took different views about a person's illness and detainability these disagreements could relate to one or more of three issues. First, they sometimes reflected genuine diagnostic difficulties; second, they could reflect different opinions about what treatment was appropriate; third, they could reflect different definitions of the threshold of illness-severity that warrants hospital admission. When there was a disagreement between the prison doctor and the NHS psychiatrist, the prison doctor could seek a second opinion, but this would be at the cost of lengthening the prisoner's period on remand.

The results of the study suggested that NHS psychiatrists may have been acting as gate-keepers, restricting admission to those whom they perceived as requiring in-patient treatment and likely to benefit from it. If this is the case, it indicates that those working in general psychiatric services may have a narrower view than practitioners in the criminal justice system about the criteria for hospital admission and the functions of psychiatric hospitals. In remanding for psychiatric reports, the courts appeared to consider that psychiatric help was needed by a wider range of offenders than were regarded by psychiatric services as requiring psychiatric care. The contrast in expectations between courts and psychiatric services was most marked for those who had non-psychotic mental disorders, for example depression and personality disorders. In these cases requests by courts for medical reports did not usually result in medical disposals. People with personality disorders and mild degrees of mental handicap were unlikely to be seen by visiting psychiatrists as candidates for hospital care, and it may not be realistic to expect that appropriate help will be found as a result of remanding them in custody with requests for reports. People with primary problems of drug and alcohol dependence were also rarely referred to psychiatric services.

A commitment to a policy of diversion should not embrace the simple view that psychiatric hospitals and prisons have equivalent functions and that the hospital constitutes an alternative for the purposes of custody and social control. This may be the case in secure hospital settings for the period of time that someone is thought to require clinical assessment or treatment, but it is not likely to be the case in general psychiatric units. Fundamental differences of this kind in expectations of health and criminal justice agencies need to be recognised, and they may set limits to the degree to which diversion from custody can be achieved.

Sentenced prisoners

A substantial psychiatric study of the prevalence of psychiatric disorder and treatment need in the sentenced prison population has recently been completed by Gunn, Maden and Swinton (1991). A representative 5 per cent sample of the sentenced male prison population and a 21 per cent sample of the female sentenced population were identified. Based on the clinical interviews, the researchers estimated that 3 per cent of the sentenced prison population suffered from psychiatric disorders warranting transfer to hospital beds in the health service (ie. approximately 1,100 prisoners); that 10.5 per cent (approximately 4,000) required treatment of an 'outpatient' kind which could be provided in prison; and that 5.6 per cent (approximately 2,100) required more intensive psychological treatment in a therapeutic community setting, which also, in principle, could be provided within the prison system by means, for example, of an additional prison establishment like Grendon Underwood.

In their discussion, Gunn *et al.* (1991) urged the need for improvements in both the prisons and the National Health Service in order to meet the needs of mentally disordered sentenced prisoners. They emphasised the need for adequate funding for prison health services and adequate training for prison staff. In addition, the Prison Health Service should develop clear policies for the management of psychiatric problems, for example in having guidelines about the degree of mental disorder warranting hospital transfer and about the provision of drug and alcohol services. The authors remark on, 'the failure of the prison medical service to develop an explicit policy on the degree to which it will accept responsibility for managing psychiatric disorder' (Gunn *et al.* 1991, p 96). There should be a principle that inmates suffering from psychotic illnesses should not be contained in prison: as the authors point out, prison 'hospitals' lack the facilities of NHS hospitals.

In relation to the National Health Service, the research pointed to several needs: first, units providing long-term care in conditions of medium security; second, services providing rapid assessment and transfer of acutely ill prisoners; and third, improved district services for chronically ill patients who exhibit problems of social nuisance offending.

THE REED COMMITTEE

The joint Department of Health and Home Office Review of Services for Mentally Disordered Offenders and Others Requiring Similar Services was established in 1990 under the chairmanship of Dr John Reed. The main steering committee of the review delegated examination of specific topics to a series of advisory groups. These advisory groups considered hospital services, prisons, community services, staffing and training, services for people with special needs, research, academic developments and finance. The *Final Summary Report* from the steering committee has now been published (Department of Health/Home Office 1992c).

The reports have as their starting point a commendable set of aspirations. The policy aim expressed in the 1990 Home Office circular[1] that the care and treatment of mentally disordered offenders is the responsibility of health and social services is endorsed, and, as far as possible, services should be provided in the community rather than in institutional settings, in the minimum level of security needed to protect the patient and others, as near as possible to the patient's home, and in a way that promotes rehabilitation and independence (Department of Health/Home Office 1991a).

The *Report of the Finance Advisory Group* (Department of Health/Home

Office 1992a) recommends that district health authorities should be responsible for purchasing a comprehensive range of services for mentally disordered offenders, and that regional health authorities should set performance targets and monitor the achievements of districts in this regard. Regions should work within a framework of objectives set by the NHS Management Executive. However, the reports are less resolute and convincing in considering the financing of their proposals and the feasibility of achieving their recommendations. The reports recommend considerable expansion in services and manpower (Department of Health/Home Office 1992b), a likely doubling of medium secure provision (the exact level depending on the outcome of local needs assessments) (Department of Health/Home Office 1991c), and comprehensive availability of local police and court diversion schemes (Department of Health/Home Office 1991d). However, the funding recommendations of the Finance Advisory Group Report do not include earmarked central funding to enable the development of these services at local level. Without this, the prospects of achieving the goals set by the reports may be poor in the light of current constraints on finance for the health service. Ministers have welcomed the *Final Summary Report* but will decide in due course which recommendations to accept and when to implement them 'bearing in mind the resources available' (Department of Health/Home Office 1992c, p. iii).

The *Report of the Prison Advisory Group* (Department of Health/Home Office 1991b) made a number of positive recommendations for the improvement of services for mentally disordered prisoners. The Report advised that existing powers of courts to remand to prison for psychiatric reports should be examined with a view to amendment or appeal, a step which would be consistent with the principle that care should be provided by health and social services rather than in prison custody. The Report also recognised the need to facilitate more rapid transfers of the acutely ill from prison and advised that a statement of policy should be drawn up in relation to the care and treatment of mentally disordered prisoners, making clear the responsibilities of outside psychiatric services. However, the advisory group also recommended that prison governors should have responsibility for the provision of services for those with psychiatric needs included in their contracts with area managers. There was also endorsement for better discharge planning, involving continuing care for mentally disordered prisoners on release.

EFFICIENCY SCRUTINY OF THE PRISON MEDICAL SERVICE

The Reed Reports endorse the policy that psychiatric and other medical services should be contracted into prisons from the NHS. It is thought that this change should improve the quality of care and enable more rapid psychiatric assessments and continuity of care. This policy was the central recommendation of a *Report on an Efficiency Scrutiny of the Prison Medical Service* published in July 1990 (Home Office 1990e). In Chapter 7 Roger Ralli describes the purpose and outlines the main recommendations of the Efficiency Scrutiny Report. Its most significant recommendation was that the Prison Service should become a purchaser, rather than a provider, of clinical services. Services should be provided through contracts for specialist care and primary care, the latter being undertaken by general practitioners. The report estimated that provision of primary care from general practitioners would result in a financial saving to the Prison Department, but the scrutiny team was unable to cost accurately the provision of specialist services.

The major failure of the report was in not examining thoroughly the feasibility of its proposals. Health authorities, health service managers and their representative bodies do not appear in the list of those consulted by the scrutiny team. This is a remarkable omission in a report whose key recommendation is that contracts should be established with them. In consequence there is no proper assessment of whether the resources and manpower exist to deliver a contracted-in service.

The report also fails to address adequately the issue of clinical standards. The view taken in the Efficiency Scrutiny Report is that the provision of health services through contracts will enable standards of care to be set and monitored, with the Prison Health Service Directorate and the Area Physician contributing to this process (Home Office 1990e, para. 7.35). The report advises that there should be a clear ministerial commitment to a high standard of health care in prisons and that a health advisory committee should be established to advise the Secretary of State and the Director of the Prison Health Service. The committee would receive an annual report from the Health Director on the standards of health care provided.

However, such an arrangement would be unlikely to result in sufficiently close external scrutiny of standards and it is unfortunate that the scrutiny team did not recommend that a body such as the Mental Health Act Commission, or the Hospital Advisory Service should have its remit extended to cover prison hospitals, in view of the fact that these bodies have considerable expertise and experience in visiting secure hospital establishments and bringing poor standards to light. The Mental Health Act Commission, which has a duty to review the care of detained patients, argued in evidence to the Woolf Inquiry that the Commission's remit should be extended to protect the rights and interests of mentally disordered prisoners in prison hospitals. This recommendation was not included in the Woolf proposals, nor in the Government's White Paper, *Custody, Care and Justice* (Home Office 1991a), despite further representations to the Home Secretary by the Chairman of the Mental Health Act Commission following publication of the Woolf Report (Department of Health 1991a).

Reliance has to be placed on such external investigatory bodies rather than the courts to highlight unacceptable standards. In the case of *Knight and Others* v. *The Home Office*, which arose following the death by hanging of a mentally disordered prisoner at Brixton Prison, the High Court held that the standard of care required of the prison was not the same as that required of a psychiatric hospital. Hopes for remedies and more enlightened judgments from the European Commission or the European Court of Human Rights have to face the slowness and infrequency of successful proceedings (Harding 1989).

In response to the *Report on an Efficiency Scrutiny of the Prison Medical Service*, a joint Home Office and Department of Health working party was set up to examine the recommendations in more detail and, in August 1991, the Directorate of Prison Medical Services issued a consultation paper on contracting for prison health services (Home Office 1991m). Whilst accepting the broad recommendations of the scrutiny team, the working party considered that contracting-in of psychiatric services could not be implemented quickly. The proposal would have major manpower and training implications for NHS psychiatric services, and the bodies responsible for accrediting psychiatric training would have to be willing to approve training posts in prisons. The working party advocated 'a step by step approach' (Home Office 1991m, para. 3.20). It recommended the establishment of a small number of pilot schemes, commencing with remand prisoners, the first few of which should be established by the end of 1992.

There have also been external responses to the Efficiency Scrutiny Report. Some initial professional guidance has been issued by the Royal College of Psychiatrists (Royal College of Psychiatrists 1992), which has published an interim report on ethical issues concerning psychiatric care in prison. This commences with the explicit principle that prisoners have a right of access to medical and nursing care of the same standard as that available to other citizens. Medical and nursing staff also have a right to provide this standard of care. The report specifies that where a psychiatric team is responsible for a ward within a prison, admission and discharge decisions should be at the discretion of the psychiatrist. Medical records should be confidential, although prisoners have a right of access to their own health records under the Access to Health Records Act 1990. The report also emphasises that 'whistle-blowing' is not only allowable but may be a duty in situations which clinicians regard as damaging to the standards of care for their patients. As the first pilot schemes for contracting-in psychiatric services become established, it will be important to assess whether they are able to operate with the degree of autonomy envisaged in these recommendations. The *Report of an Efficiency Scrutiny of the Prison Medical Service* anticipated: 'a beneficial pressure from providers in stipulating the standards of the environment and nursing support to be made available by the Prison Service' (Home Office 1990e, para. 7.36). It is to be hoped that such pressure will be applied and will meet with success.

FUTURE PROSPECTS

NHS services for mentally disordered offenders will have to survive and develop in the context of the reformed structure of the National Health Service (Department of Health 1989). These reforms introduced a separation between purchasing health authorities and provider units which are moving increasingly in the direction of becoming self-governing trusts. Under these arrangements it is the responsibility of district health authorities first, to identify health needs and priorities; and second, to purchase the range of services they consider to be required to serve the needs of their population. The future role of regional health authorities is uncertain and could contract so that they primarily become regulators of the NHS internal market. These changes could potentially have harmful consequences for forensic psychiatry services. These services are most wanted by the criminal justice agencies – prisons, courts and the probation service – but these agencies do not have significant powers to purchase medical and social care. Nor are there established structures enabling criminal justice agencies to influence the purchasing decisions of health authorities. Murphy (1992) has argued that two conditions need to be met if the NHS reforms are to benefit mentally abnormal offenders:

> First, districts acquire the necessary knowledge and skill to develop a clear vision of future services for this group of patients; and, second, that regions take seriously their performance monitoring role and set ambitious targets for the service.
>
> (p.23)

Regional health authorities must retain a pro-active role.

In two important respects the response of the Government and of the criminal justice system will also be crucial. First, the area criminal justice committees recommended in the Woolf Report should include health service representation, and this, in turn, should aim to achieve effective liaison and influence by local criminal justice agencies on health authority purchasers and managers of provider psychiatric units. Second, the ideal of community prisons described in the Woolf Report (Woolf 1991, paras. 11.49–11.68) must become a reality if NHS psychiatric services are to care more effectively for their local mentally disordered prisoners and if 'Care in the Community' is to make a significant contribution to resettlement.

NOTE

1 Home Office Circular 66/1990 *Provision for Mentally Disordered Offenders.*

11

THE FUTURE FOR SEX OFFENDERS IN PRISON

Adam Sampson

At 3 p.m. on 3 April 1990, Derek White suffered a fatal heart attack in North Manchester General Hospital. He was a prisoner from A Wing at HMP Manchester and had been admitted suffering from a dislocated shoulder and severe head injuries sustained during the course of the Strangeways riot. On remand, accused of eight sex offences committed against children, he was intending to plead not guilty, and there were indications that the Crown Prosecution Service was preparing to drop seven of the charges. In the meantime he was being held on Rule 43.

Other prisoners held on Rule 43 at Strangeways had similar wounds. By noon on the first day of the riot, the rioters had gained control of the entire prison and, as in previous disturbances, one of their first targets had been sex offenders and others on the Rule. Shouts had been heard: 'We're coming to kill you, beasts.' In desperation, Rule 43s had tried to barricade their doors, to dig their way out through the walls, or even to hang themselves. Many of them had been dragged out of their cells and beaten. One had been stabbed and thrown off the landing into the netting. For days afterwards, the press was filled with stories of castrations and mutilations, sustained by 'eyewitness reports' from prisoners themselves, and it was not until 19 April, more than two weeks after the riot had begun, that Brendan O'Friel, Governor of Strangeways, finally put an end to the speculation that there were dead bodies lying undiscovered in the prison.

Derek White was the first prisoner to die in a prison riot since 1932. However, the violence that he had had to suffer was not unusual; indeed, he was not the first (alleged) sex offender to be murdered in prison. Violent assaults on sex offenders are a staple of prison life and prejudice against them fundamental to the prison ethos. Slashings are administered, using a common prison weapon – a PP9 battery wrapped in a sock – sometimes with the active or passive connivance of prison staff. Sex offenders are served cold or adulterated food. Shouts of 'Beast' or 'Nonce' follow their progress around a prison: an attempt by some prison officers to recover one of the captured Strangeways wings was accompanied by shouts of 'Beast! Beast!' – a reference to the fact that one of the prisoners on the roof had previously been convicted in connection with a rape case. Sex offenders are the natural victims of the prison system.

In part, the victimisation of sex offenders is a product of monotonous, intolerant and oppressive prison regimes. Shorn of dignity, bored and resentful, and roused to heights of frustration and anger by what they perceive as an arbitrary and unjust system, prisoners inevitably look round for targets for their feelings. Sex offenders, together with other prisoners who appear weak or vulnerable, provide a more than adequate target. In some cases too, these feelings are shared by prison staff, who tacitly encourage the creation of a prison pecking order which has sex offenders placed firmly at the bottom.

This prejudice is a very deep-rooted one, as Woolf and Tumim themselves noted: during the open seminar at Lincoln Prison in which prisoners took part, one prisoner who had been making constructive and reasonable contributions to the debate, complained heatedly and repeatedly about the fact that two of the other prisoners at the seminar were on Rule 43 (Woolf 1991 para. 12.187). However, the prejudice against sex offenders is also rooted in a truth. Sex offenders form a uniquely worrying category of offender, many of whom have been offending for many years and in a planned and cold-blooded manner.[1] Their crimes often have appalling consequences for their victims, leaving them with psychological scars which may long outlast the physical scars of the victims of pure violence. The victims of sexual offenders – though 'survivors' is the term which many prefer, emphasising as it does the strength many of them exhibit in seeking to come to terms with what has happened to them – are usually among the more vulnerable members of society: children and women. The sexual abuse of these victims is primarily an abuse of power.

Given the nature of sexual crime, it is therefore, perhaps, not surprising that imprisoned sex offenders should become the targets of abuse and hatred. Indeed, the attitude of many prisoners and staff merely mirrors that of the community outside: both newspaper columnists and Conservative MPs have called for protection for sex offenders to be withdrawn so that 'they will get the kicking they so richly deserve'.[2] However, the presence in our prisons of potentially dangerous offenders who are the objects of loathing on the part of many prisoners and staff poses two particular problems for the prison system. It is these problems that the Woolf Report sets out to consider in its section entitled 'The management of sex offenders' (paras. 12.185–12.220).

First, there is the problem of how best to protect sex offenders and other vulnerable prisoners from attack. The traditional solution to this problem has been to employ Prison Rule 43 (or in the case of young offenders, Rule 46). Rule 43 allows the governor of a prison to 'remove a prisoner from association'; usually this means segregation in a discrete wing or landing of the prison. In 70 per cent of cases, those on Rule 43 are individuals who have been convicted of sex offences (Home Office 1989e).

However, as Woolf and Tumim argue, the use of Rule 43 as a solution has proved to be increasingly problematic. The necessity of running two entirely separate regimes within the one prison places great demands on staff and resources. This is a particular problem at a time when, as J.E. Thomas in Chapter 6 points out, staffing levels are under pressure due to the efficiency savings inherent in the Fresh Start agreement, and when resources are already stretched at many prisons because of the levels of overcrowding they have to endure. Under these circumstances, the necessity of running protected regimes for Rule 43s is an unwelcome irritant.

Moreover the number of prisoners requiring protection has been rapidly increasing: the number of prisoners on Rule 43 or in Vulnerable Prisoner Units (VPUs) increased by 156 per cent between 1983 and 1988; the total prison population showed only a 17.4 per cent increase during the same period (Woolf 1991, para. 12.200). At the time of the Strangeways riot, there were 2,280 prisoners on Rule 43 and 880 in VPUs. In part this is a result of the rise in the number of sex offenders in prison: in 1980 there were 1,654 individuals in prison who had been convicted of sexual offences, 4.5 per cent of the total sentenced population. By 1990, that figure had increased to 3,029, an increase of 83 per cent. Sex offenders now comprise 8.6 per cent of the sentenced population. Given the increasing number of such offenders coming before the courts and the effect of harsher sentencing and parole policies already in existence and signalled in the 1991 Criminal Justice Act, that figure is almost certain to rise.

Part of the reason for the rise in the Rule 43 population can also be put down to the increasing assumption on the part of many solicitors and police, probation and prison officers that Rule 43 is the inevitable destination for sex offenders (Home Office 1989e). However, in part too the rise in the number of prisoners on Rule 43 is itself a product of the resource and overcrowding pressures on the prison system. The consequent poor quality of life for prisoners increases prisoners' levels of frustration and anger, and therefore the likelihood that they will seek scapegoats. Moreover, the pressures on staff and management produced by overcrowding and low staffing reduce their flexibility to find alternative methods of providing protection for vulnerable prisoners other than by segregation.

The growth of the number of prisoners on Rule 43, together with the pressures on resources and staffing, has had a direct impact upon the regimes that could be provided for prisoners in segregation. In many prisons, particularly local and remand institutions, it is extremely difficult to provide work, education or association for prisoners on the Rule. HM Chief Inspector of Prisons has repeatedly commented on the poor quality of life endured by prisoners on Rule 43, and in his report on Parkhurst

Prison he argued that the conditions of virtual solitary confinement endured by the Rule 43 prisoners were beginning seriously to affect their abilities to relate normally to other people (Home Office 1988d)

It is the recognition of the poor quality of life for those on Rule 43 that lies behind the creation of Vulnerable Prisoner Units (VPUs): discrete units sited usually in training prisons, aiming to offer more constructive regimes for longer-term prisoners. However, there is some suspicion that such units were, in part, prompted by a desire to reduce the apparent size of the Rule 43 population – prisoners in VPUs are not officially counted as being on the Rule, despite the fact that they are clearly in protected locations. In addition, there is no little confusion about what is, and is not, a VPU, and in practice, there is little difference between some official VPUs and some long-established Rule 43 units such as Wandsworth's G, H and K wings. Perhaps most important of all, VPUs currently cater only for prisoners who are to be in the system for some considerable period of time and all of the units have long waiting lists. Any sex offender at Wandsworth who has been sentenced to less than four years can have no real hope of transfer to a VPU.

The poor quality of the regimes offered to those on the Rule is also, in part, the result of deliberate policy. Individual prison governors deliberately aim to provide only a very limited regime to those on Rule 43 in order to discourage prisoners from asking for protection; if conditions on the Rule were made equal to those for other prisoners, they believe, many more prisoners would ask to 'go on the Rule'. It is also a policy which has official sanction. The Home Secretary argued in response to Sir James Hennessy's review of Rule 43 in 1986 that: 'Improvements for Rule 43 prisoners should not take place at the expense of conditions for other prisoners in the same establishments' (Home Office 1986a).

However, as Woolf and Tumim argue, the problem with Rule 43 is not simply that it produces a poor quality of life for the prisoners on it. There is also a significant confusion in the very nature of Rule 43. Rule 43 is not simply used to deal with prisoners requiring segregation because they need to be protected from attack; it is also used to deal with prisoners who pose a threat to 'good order and discipline'. In practice, the two functions are distinguished by the use of the terms Rule 43 Own Protection (OP) and Rule 43 Good Order and Discipline (GOAD).

This has two effects. First, the confusion between the disciplinary and administrative functions of Rule 43 produces a quasi-punitive approach to provision for all those on the Rule. It has long been argued that Rule 43 GOAD is used as an informal punishment system to deal with prisoners who are believed to pose a threat but who have not committed any disciplinary offences.[3] In some prisons, all of those who are held on the Rule are held together, and no distinction is made between prisoners on Rule 43 OP and on Rule 43 GOAD. Prisoners on Rule 43 OP therefore suffer regimes that are tantamount to punishment. This is especially true where, as in not a few prisons, prisoners on Rule 43 OP are routinely housed in the punishment block. The confusion between protection and punishment therefore legitimises poor regimes for those on Rule 43 OP.

Second, as Woolf and Tumim point out, the dual function of Rule 43 currently requires it to do two very different jobs. Prisoners who are a genuine threat to discipline may well need to be totally segregated from other prisoners. However, prisoners who need protection do not necessarily require total segregation at all times. In Littlehey, prisoners on A Wing, almost all of whom had previously been on Rule 43, were gradually integrated into the general prison population in carefully structured and controlled settings, such as particular workshops and education classes. The model of semi-segregation on which Littlehey A Wing initially operated (the regime has now gone further down the road towards full integration) provides an interesting example of what is possible. However, the fact that Rule 43 is used to deal with prisoners who require total segregation for control reasons as well as those needing protection has led to it being used as an all-or-nothing measure. The effect has been to discourage governors from taking a more flexible approach to the problem of the protection of vulnerable prisoners. In addition, governors were advised that they could be held personally liable in an action for negligence where a prisoner was injured by another, if they had refused a request for Rule 43 or had failed to consider such segregation.

This all-or-nothing approach of Rule 43 has also had the effect of rendering it extremely difficult to reintegrate a Rule 43 prisoner back into normal prison life. The absence of any halfway house between full segregation and full integration has made it very difficult to get a prisoner off Rule 43. Desperate measures are sometimes taken by the Prison Service: prisoners have been transferred to prisons far from their home bases in an attempt to plant them somewhere where they (and their crimes) are not known. They have also been provided with cover stories to help them to pretend to be a 'normal' offender rather than a 'nonce' (Thornton 1987). Such transfers sit uneasily in the system of community prisons envisaged in the Woolf Report and, as Woolf and Tumim comment, encouraging prisoners to lie about their offences is hardly compatible with a service whose aim is to encourage prisoners to lead law abiding lives inside and outside custody (para. 12.210).

Woolf and Tumim's solution to the problems posed by the need to protect sex offenders and other vulnerable prisoners from attack is admirably direct. They do not flinch from recognising that, for the foreseeable future, sex offenders will require protection. However, they consider that the current Rule 43 does not provide an adequate mechanism to achieve this end. Rule 43 must be redrafted to deal solely with prisoners who require segregation in the interests of good order and discipline. An entirely new Rule should be created to deal with prisoners who require protection (para. 12.203).

The new Rule would place a governor under an obligation 'to take such reasonable steps as he considers necessary for the protection of prisoners whom he considers are vulnerable to attack from other prisoners' (para. 12.203). In many cases, these steps may fall short of 'removal from association': in practice, an adequate level of protection may be provided simply by housing a vulnerable prisoner in a wing with a tolerant and violence-free atmosphere, or in a location where close staff supervision is possible. Governors would also be free to develop the sort of imaginative and flexible alternatives to traditional segregation already in existence at prisons such as Littlehey, Leyhill, Grendon and others. In addition, a 'second Grendon' should be established, to be used as a training ground and a focus for experimental and progressive work with sex offenders (para. 12.211).

However, where there is no alternative to some form of segregation, this should be allowed under the terms of the new Rule, although Woolf and Tumim clearly consider that in most cases this is likely to be only a short-term measure. Removal from association would – as now – be subject to confirmation by the Board of Visitors. This, Woolf and Tumim consider, would guarantee that measures are taken during the period of segregation to develop alternative forms of protection for the prisoner. During the period of segregation, the regime and conditions enjoyed by the prisoner should be comparable with those for all other prisoners.

These plans clearly point the direction towards a more reasoned and imaginative approach to the problem of providing a safe and civilised environment for vulnerable prisoners. The replacement of the blunt instrument of segregation with a more finely tuned tool would result in a more satisfactory response to the problem. However, as Woolf and Tumim themselves note, the schemes which have succeeded in integrating sex offenders into the wider prison population have been largely confined to prisons with liberal regimes and pleasant physical surroundings. The Littlehey scheme for example, has succeeded in part because of an implicit threat to those considering violence towards sex offenders: step out of line and you will be transferred to a nastier prison. That threat would be less effective in an overcrowded local.

Moreover, the success of the new approach is bound up in the success of the Woolf reforms as a package. Small units are necessary to allow staff to keep a careful eye on whether vulnerable prisoners are being bullied. Staff training would need to be improved in order to challenge the unprofessional and macho attitudes exhibited by some prison staff, attitudes which reinforce antipathy towards 'nonces' and 'beasts'. Reception and induction procedures would need to be overhauled to allow initial interviews to take place out of the hearing of other prisoners so that individuals' offences are not generally known,[4] and prisoners' locations and routines would need to be planned more carefully. Finally, the system of justice in prisons would need to be improved along the lines suggested by Woolf and Tumim: assaults against sex offenders should not be tolerated, and if such assaults occur, it is the perpetrator who should be punished by segregation or transfer, not – as often now – the victim.

Nevertheless, if such changes are implemented, it is possible to envisage a time when sex offenders can be safely contained in the prison system and offered equal access to the services and amenities that prisons can offer. However, in many respects, as Woolf and Tumim recognise, that is a very limited aim. Containing sex offenders is all very well, but there will come a time when they are released again into the community. As has been said, some – arguably all – sex offenders will pose a continuing threat to society outside prison.

Woolf and Tumim recognise that the prison system has a wider responsibility to society outside prison to ensure that while sex offenders are in prison, everything possible is done to reduce the risk that they will reoffend after release. This view was urged upon the Woolf team by many of the submissions they received, in particular in evidence from the Suzy Lamplugh Trust and the Prison Reform Trust (1990), and was accepted by the Prison Department, who stressed that treatment was already being provided in 63 prisons.[5] However, even the Home Secretary accepted that the existing treatment provision was uncoordinated and patchy, and that very little of it was adequately monitored for quality and effectiveness.[6] It was also frequently exposed to staffing and resource problems and often dangerously dependent on the enthusiasm and expertise of one or two key individuals.[7]

In arriving at the view that treatment should be offered to sex offenders in a more coordinated and planned manner, Woolf and Tumim were careful not to argue that such offenders should be sent to prison *for* treatment. Nor did they discuss the question of which (if any) treatment programmes would have an impact on reoffending rates, a question about which there is heated academic debate (see Furby, Weinrott and Blackshaw 1989): that, they say, should be a matter for evaluation. Nevertheless, they were adamant that:

> The evidence which we have received, including that from prisoners, strongly indicates that treatment programmes can result in a beneficial change in the attitude of sex offenders. That at least improves their conduct while in prison. Certainly we can confirm from the evidence they provided, that many sex offenders appear anxious to receive and co-operate with treatment.
>
> (para. 12.219)

If efforts are to be made to reduce the likelihood of sex offenders reoffending, that in itself is another reason why the quality of life these offenders have to endure should be improved. Woolf and Tumim argue that the abuse that sex offenders suffer, together with the restricted regimes that they endure, produce in sex offenders a sense that they are somehow victims themselves, rather than perpetrators of crime. Woolf and Tumim argue that if a reduction in reoffending by sex offenders is the aim, their attention needs to be focused on what they themselves have done, rather than on what they are having to suffer (para. 12.215).

On the surface, the Government's response to Woolf's proposal that 'more attention should be given to the treatment of sex offenders and to providing assistance to prevent their reoffending' (para. 15.44) has received a more direct and complete response than almost any other. The Woolf Report was published on 25 February 1991. However, even before the Report had been officially published, the Prison Service had organised a two-day seminar on the treatment of sex offenders at the Prison Service College at Newbold Revel.[8] And on 7 June, the Home Secretary announced that a new treatment programme for sex offenders would be introduced into twenty prisons by the end of the year.[9] The plans themselves were published in the form of a Prison Service document *Treatment Programmes for Sex Offenders in Custody: A Strategy* (Home Office 1991i).

The Government plans as outlined in that paper are for a two-tier system of treatment (see also Prison Reform Trust 1992a). The document specifies that sex offenders sentenced to four years and above will be assessed at one of six specially designated prisons: Wandsworth, Maidstone, Wakefield, Dartmoor, Albany or Full Sutton (Whitemoor has subsequently been added to this list).[10] During the assessment period, offenders' needs and functioning will be determined and they will be assigned to one of two programmes: the core programme or the extended programme. The two programmes will be run either at one of the six (now seven) original prisons, or at one of another eleven. These are mostly male, adult prisons, but include at least one women's establishment and one young offender institution (YOI).

The two programmes differ as to their intensity and length. Both will concentrate on confronting the 'cognitive distortions' which sustain sexual offending – the false belief systems which enable rapists and paedophiles to maintain that their victims consent to and enjoy their assaults. However, the extended programme looks at the functioning of the offender in greater detail, examining social-skill levels, addictions, stress and anger control, and 'deviant sexual arousal'. Both programmes aim to equip offenders with strategies to help them avoid situations which make it likely that they will relapse into offending. The programmes will be closely monitored for effectiveness.

The precise content of what the Prison Department is proposing is still in the planning stage: staff in individual prisons with some experience of working with sex offenders have been asked to supply outlines for individual modules of the programmes. However, it is explicitly based on models used in Canada and various states in the USA and draws on the experience of the programmes in those jurisdictions. Ministers and officials have spoken confidently about the likely effectiveness of the new initiative: in a recent Prison Service Briefing, it was claimed that a reduction of 50 per cent in the recidivism rate was achievable (Home Office 1991n).

The Government's plans have considerable weaknesses. On paper, they appear to form a coherent programme. However, they ignore the context in which they are meant to run. To begin with, Ministers have made it clear that there will be no increase in resources made available to fund the initiative. The programmes will have to be staffed and funded out of existing resources. As Viscount Astor emphasised when challenged on the question in the House of Lords; the only likely increase in resources will come from 'efficiency savings' and the general year-on-year Prison Service allocation in Public Expenditure Survey (PES) round.[11]

The absence of any increase in resources to fund the programmes may not be crucial in the case of prisons such as Littlehey and Grendon because they already have resources directed to work with sex offenders. However, in the case of the seven assessment prisons, which will be required to devote considerable numbers of staff to running the programmes, it may be a very different story. In the main, the programmes are designed to be run by uniformed prison staff, with specialist support from probation officers and psychiatric, psychological and medical back-up. Some aspects of the programmes will need to be performed exclusively by medical or psychology staff – arousal testing using penile plethysmographs is an example.

However, two of the seven assessment prisons – Wandsworth and Wakefield – are prisons with a recent history of industrial disputes over staffing levels.[12] Wandsworth refused to operate as an assessment prison without a substantial increase in resources. Full Sutton too has a history of disputes over staffing levels, in part because of its poor design and the presence in it of a staff-intensive Special Secure Unit. Staff at Maidstone's Thanet Wing are also very doubtful about how they will manage to free up the staff time necessary to run the programmes: at a recent training session given in Maidstone as part of the preparation for the programmes, no uniformed staff were free to attend. There is also some doubt whether Maidstone will be able to fund the building work necessary to convert some of the existing rooms in the wing for the group work required in the programme.

Nor is it just the seven assessment prisons which are affected. Aylesbury YOI has considerable experience of work with sex offenders and has had an informal role as a specialist YOI for sex offenders in the south. However, the Governor of Aylesbury has taken the decision to pull out of the initiative because he feels that he will not be able to spare the staff to run the programmes. Indeed, the result is now that there is an informal ban on any group work with sex offenders at Aylesbury.

Moreover the sex offender initiative, with its new set of obligations on staff time, comes at a time when prisons are already having to cope with the effects of the progressive reductions in staff hours following the introduction of Fresh Start (see Chapter 7). Many regimes, particularly at prisons like Wandsworth, are already limited and under extreme pressure and it is therefore difficult to see how these programmes can be run in such prisons save at the expense of existing activities. The history of attempts to provide specialist programmes in prison for groups such as sex offenders has shown that there is a tendency for them to be cancelled whenever there are security alerts, a higher than normal number of prison escorts, or high levels of staff sickness and leave. There is a risk that these new programmes will go the same way.

Nevertheless, it is possible that staff time will be found to operate the programmes properly even in a prison with very limited resources. However, this will require motivation and flexibility on the part of management and staff to search for solutions to the problem of resources. Again, many of the eighteen prisons participating in the initiative have shown ample evidence of that motivation. However, as Woolf and Tumin commented, there are many staff within the system who share the prisoners' hatred of sex offenders and who deliberately discriminate against them. It will require a special effort at prisons like Wandsworth, Albany and Dartmoor, where the tradition of an anti-sex offender culture has been so strong, particularly if the provision of treatment for sex offenders is to require cuts in the regimes for other prisoners. Indeed, such cuts in regime for 'normal' prisoners may only stimulate further persecution of sex offenders.

This question of culture is vital to the success of the treatment programmes. The programmes which are to be operated crucially depend on staff being able to develop an honest and open relationship with the prisoners with whom they are working. Prisoners have to be encouraged to reveal the full extent of their offending history and to break through the barriers of denial and dishonesty that they have built up over the years. They have to be able to feel secure in the knowledge that this information will not be abused and that staff will treat them as human beings no matter what they have done.

However, the culture in some of the prisons which will be operating the new programmes is far from supportive for sexual offenders. It is doubtful whether many sex offenders will feel able to give their full commitment to programmes run by officers if their colleagues are still calling them 'beasts' and turning a blind eye to abuse from other prisoners. Moreover, if the Woolf reforms to the operation of Rule 43 are successful, and many sex offenders are integrated within the normal prison population, it will be difficult to provide treatment without once again stigmatising the participating prisoners. Prisoners who are participating in the programmes will immediately be identified as sex offenders. As the former governor of

Littlehey has made clear, prisoners are often content to work alongside sex offenders so long as they have no positive evidence that they are sex offenders; however, once they are publicly identified as 'nonces', they are open to abuse (Twinn 1992).

There may also be other disincentives for prisoners to participate actively in the programmes. The Prison Service has said that participation in the programmes will be on a voluntary basis. Woolf and Tumim found that most sex offenders were very motivated towards some sort of treatment, and the evidence from Canada indicates that the initial refusal rate is low. Moreover, there will doubtless be informal pressure put on sex offenders to participate, either by ensuring that the regimes offered to non-participants are of the most basic kind, or by an implicit promise that parole will be easier to obtain for those who can show progress whilst in custody.

It seems clear, however, that sex offenders participating in treatment programmes will form an exception to the Woolf policy of prisoners being located close to home. Although there are seven assessment prisons, four of them are in the southeast; there is one in the far southwest and two in the north. Any participating sex offender from the Midlands will spend a considerable length of time far from home. Participating prisoners can also expect to be moved regularly during the course of the treatment programmes, being shuttled at least twice between the assessment prison and the treatment prison. These difficulties will be compounded for women and young offenders, since there is only one women's prison and two YOIs participating.

Moreover, sex offenders will be faced with a real dilemma when it comes to revealing the true extent of their offending. For the treatment programmes to be successful, prisoners must be honest and open about their desires and offences. However, by revealing just how often they have offended and how ingrained their problems are, offenders may reveal the fact that they pose a far greater danger to society than had been previously thought. Such information could be used as the basis for later parole reports: by participating fully, they may in fact damage their chances of parole. Indeed, it is even possible that they may reveal information in the course of the treatment that could form the basis of further criminal charges.

There are other potential problems with the programmes. Little has been said about the integration of the treatment programmes in prison with the operation of services outside prison. There are no indications that the probation service will receive increased resources to provide aftercare hostels (few probation hostels will accept sex offenders) and increased training for probation officers. The four-year cut-off for treatment, whilst not an absolute, may nevertheless encourage judges to pass sentences of four years and above to ensure that offenders are offered treatment. Disquiet has been expressed about the use of penile plethysmographs to measure arousal. Particular concern has also been raised about the fact that the treatment will be given at the beginning rather at the end of what may be a lengthy prison sentence: by the time the offender has been released, much of the positive impact of the treatment will have worn off.

However, what is possibly most worrying about the Government's initiative is the target that has been set for it. Ministers have been very careful to argue that there is no such thing as a 'cure' for sexual offending and that the best that can be achieved is to equip offenders with skills to enable them to avoid risky situations if they so choose. None the less, the programmes have been developed on the assumption that sexual recidivism can be reduced by half. In private, it is understood, officials have been told that unless such a substantial drop is achieved in the re-offending rate within five years, the programmes may be closed down.

Such expectations of success may be misplaced. Although there is some evidence from Canada and the USA to indicate that some reduction in reoffending rates is achievable, this is by no means universally accepted (Furby *et al.* 1989). Moreover, the use of reoffending rates as the criterion of success is a questionable policy, since very few offences are ever reported, and very few of those reported ever result in convictions. An apparently successful programme therefore, may simply be one that teaches offenders how to offend without being caught.

Most important of all, the impact of such programmes cannot be measured in a short period of time. Research has shown that the longer the follow-up period, the more accurately the effect of treatment programmes can be measured. A five-year probationary period is simply too short to produce any meaningful results: many of those who received treatment in the first wave of the initiative may still be in prison. A far longer commitment is necessary from Government.

If this is not forthcoming, and if Government does not back the initiative with resources, it may be doomed before it is begun. Such a failure would discourage any further efforts to provide treatment for sex offenders and leave them in a worse position than before the Woolf Report. But it is not simply the future of sex offenders that is at risk in this initiative. Woolf and Tumim's proposals for sex offenders are a paradigm for the approach that the Prison Service needs to be taking to many other groups in the system. As they make clear, specialist provision should also be made for drug users and for those with alcohol problems (paras. 12.350–12.353). The same model could be applied to individuals with problems with temper or with authority. The sex offender initiative is a test of the potential for the prison system to adapt to the individual needs of a group of prisoners and to move from simple containment to the more ambitious process of addressing the reasons why individuals are in prison at all. If the sex offender initiative falls, the chances of building a responsive, positive prison system may fall with it.

NOTES

1 When doctors at Oregon State Hospital in the USA arranged an amnesty for 53 sex offenders, they discovered that the men had committed between them some 25,757 offences. Nor is this unique to the USA: on a 1985 edition of the Thames TV programme *TV Eye*, one offender admitted to committing over 2,000 offences.

2 R. Littlejohn, *Sun* 30 November 1989.

3 See *R.* v. *Deputy Governor of Parkhurst Prison, ex p. Hague* (1992).

4 The reception procedures at Armley Prison, Leeds, came in for particular criticism precisely for this reason in the Report to the United Kingdom Government by the European Committee for the Prevention of Torture and Inhuman or Degrading Treatment or Punishment (Council of Europe 1991).

5 This claim was apparently based on the results of research carried out by Malcolm Cowburn of Nottingham Probation Service as part of an M.Phil. thesis. However, that research has not yet been published and the Home Office's use of it is possibly misleading. It seems likely that what is counted by the Home Office as 'treatment' may be of very poor quality or only available to very few prisoners in the establishments concerned.

6 Speech to Prison Governors' Conference, 10 November 1990.

7 Cases in point are the well-documented problems of the Wormwood Scrubs Annexe in 1989, and the decline of Maidstone Prison's Thanet Wing (see Prison Reform Trust 1990).

8 On 30 January and 1 February 1991.

9 Rt Hon. Kenneth Baker MP, speech to the Suzy Lamplugh Trust 7 June 1991.

10 The *Strategy* document gave a list of fourteen prisons to run the core programme. However, this number was rapidly reduced to eleven by the withdrawal of Aylesbury, Featherstone and Feltham. At the time of writing, Swinfen Hall has been provisionally identified as the young offender institution but the identity of the women's prison was still not known.

11 Hansard 1991, 13 November 1991, c. 646.

12 In November 1991, a high-profile dispute at Wakefield over what the Prison Officers' Association regarded as dangerously low staffing levels led to the threat of a lock-out of staff. Industrial action was only averted after a strike vote was narrowly lost.

12

WOMEN'S PRISONS AFTER WOOLF

Elaine Player

The Woolf Report does not inquire specifically into the women's prison system and explicitly excludes 'problems which solely relate to women prisoners' (Woolf 1991, para. 2.18). Its focus of concern is upon issues which potentially contribute to 'fomenting or avoiding disturbances in prisons' and, since none of the riots in April 1990 occurred in female establishments, the specific inclusion of women prisoners was deemed to be beyond the scope of the Inquiry. Curiously, this decision was taken in spite of the fact that a disturbance by women prisoners at Risley Remand Centre had occurred only several months earlier. Whether the causes of this disturbance concerned problems '*solely*' relating to women is unclear; what is clear, however, is that it would be inaccurate to presume that women prisoners do not riot (see Sim 1990). Perhaps the point is that they do not riot badly enough, or publicly enough, to vitalise official concern.

Despite these caveats of exclusion, the Woolf Report undeniably provides the most authoritative and wide-ranging review of prisons in England and Wales this century, and has been heralded as establishing an agenda for change for the next twenty-five years. For this reason its relevance to and impact upon the women's system should be subject to close scrutiny, since, regardless of whether or not Lord Justice Woolf directly inquired into the situation in female establishments, there can be little doubt that many of his recommendations and proposals will affect prisons accommodating women as well as those accommodating men. On the one hand, this may be welcomed as an attempt to treat male and female prisoners equally and to break with a criminological tradition which has medicalised and infantilised women in prison. On the other, it may be resented as the imposition of yet another set of policy initiatives, originally designed for men, to which the women's system will again have to accommodate. What has to be considered in this chapter is how the proposed reforms, which have been designed to resolve the underlying problems of disorder in male establishments, will affect the prison system for women. Three specific areas, central to Woolf's programme for change, will be examined: first, the long-term goal of establishing community prisons; second, the promotion of distinct regimes for remand prisoners; and finally, the development of new systems of accountability and justice.

THE FEMALE PRISON POPULATION

One reason to be cautious about the wholesale applicability of the Woolf Report's recommendations is that the characteristic population of women in prison differs from the male population in a number of important respects.

Criminal profile

Women constitute only a small fraction of the total prison population: on 30 June 1990 there were 1,613 women in prison, less than 4 per cent of the total. Table 12.1 shows that although most men and women have been received into prison following a conviction for a property crime, there are notable differences in the distribution of their offences. Women are considerably more likely than men to have been received for theft, handling stolen goods, fraud and deception, and less likely to have been convicted for offences of burglary and robbery. They are also less likely to have been convicted of an offence of violence, but they are proportionately more likely than men to have been received for drugs offences. The numbers of women who have been received into prison for drugs offences has increased over the past decade[1] and, because many of them serve long sentences, they have come to represent a significant and growing proportion of the female prison population: on 30 June 1980 they accounted for only 6 per cent of all sentenced women but on the same day in 1990 the proportion had grown to 28 per cent.

The sentence lengths of female prisoners tend to reflect the relatively less serious nature of their offences. Table 12.2 shows that in 1990 66 per cent of adult women were received into prison with sentences of 12 months or less, in comparison to 57 per cent of men. Similarly, 8 per cent of male receptions were serving long sentences of 4 years or more in contrast to 6 per cent of female prisoners. Over the last ten years, the gap between the sentences imposed on male and female prisoners has been reduced as sentence lengths have generally increased. In 1980, 84 per cent of women received under sentence were serving a year or less, in comparison to 67 per cent of men; and under 2 per cent of female prisoners were received with sentences in excess of 4 years, in contrast to 4 per cent of male prisoners.

Women prisoners are also likely to have fewer previous convictions than male inmates. In 1990 37 per cent of all sentenced female receptions for whom data were recorded, had two or fewer previous convictions and only 1 in 5 had accumulated 11 or more. In contrast, only 26 per cent of male

Table 12.1 Male and female receptions into Prison Service establishments under sentence of immediate imprisonment by offence 1990

	Males		*Females*	
	No.	*% Total male receptions*	*No.*	*% Total female receptions*
Violence against the person	4,965	14	159	9
Sexual offences	1,872	5	8	0.5
Burglary	5,102	15	73	4
Robbery	1,566	4	30	2
Theft & handling	5,974	17	579	33
Fraud & forgery	1,376	4	132	8
Drugs	2,060	6	240	14
Other offences	7,484	21	316	18
Offences not recorded	4,338	12	197	11
All offences	34,737		1,734	

Source: Home Office 1992a

Table 12.2 Proportions of males and females received into Prison Service establishments under sentence of immediate imprisonment by sentence length, 1980 and 1990

	Males		*Females*	
	1980 (%)	*1990 (%)*	*1980 (%)*	*1990 (%)*
Up to 3 months	22	19	37	25
Over 3 months and up to 6 months	22	19	25	20
Over 6 months and up to 12 months	23	19	22	21
Over 12 months and up to 18 months	11	12	7	10
Over 18 months up to 3 years	15	19	7	14
Over 3 years up to 4 years	3	4	1	3
Over 4 years up to 10 years	3	7	1	5
Over 10 years	(<0.5)	0.5	(<0.5)	(<0.5)
Life	0.5	0.5	(<0.5)	1

Source: Home Office 1992a

receptions had less than three previous convictions and 1 in 3 had 11 or more. Reconviction rates within two years of release from prison show a similarly depressed figure for female inmates. The Woolf Report notes that in 1986 the reconviction rates within two years of release were 63 per cent for male young offenders, 42 per cent for male adult offenders and 34 per cent for female offenders (para. 10.25). In so far as the official statistics are concerned, it would thus appear that, in comparison with male prisoners, women in prison present a relatively less serious and less entrenched criminal profile.

The significance of this becomes apparent when consideration is given to the anticipated effects of the 1991 Criminal Justice Act. This legislation was designed to reform sentencing practice by encouraging judges and magistrates to adopt a 'just deserts' approach, whereby retribution is the primary aim and sanctions are intended to be commensurate with the seriousness of the offence. It has been widely recognised that one reason why judges and magistrates have increasingly imposed custodial sentences is that they lack confidence that non-custodial options have any punitive impact upon adult offenders. In the Criminal Justice Act the Government has attempted to address this problem by introducing a broader and more flexible range of financial and community penalties, designed to facilitate the punishment of offenders in the community. Prison sentences are now explicitly reserved for those who have committed an offence which is so serious that no other penalty could be justified on retributivist grounds (s.1(2)(a)), or for those who have committed a violent or sexual offence and whose detention, it is thought, is necessary to protect the public from serious harm (s.1(2)(b)). The Courts are also empowered to impose a custodial sentence on those who have failed to consent to or comply with the terms of a community penalty (s.1(3), sch. 2, paras. 3(1)(d) and 4(1)(d)). Where serious sexual and violent offences have been committed, however, the judge is free to take into account issues of public safety and, within statutory limits, impose a sentence which is longer than would otherwise be justified in relation to the offence (s.2(2)(b)).The intended bifurcatory effect of this legislation on the prison population is clear: to achieve an overall reduction, by decreasing the numbers of petty property offenders serving short sentences, whilst maintaining the numbers of serious offenders serving long sentences. The extent to which the 1991 Criminal Justice Act will succeed in reducing the prison population is currently a matter of speculation. What is clear, however, is that if these changes in sentencing practice are to be effected then their reductivist impact should be most keenly felt in the women's system, where a higher proportion of the population, by virtue of their less serious offences and fewer previous convictions, would become candidates for punishment in the community. Whilst any diminution of the female prison population must be generally welcomed, it would, as will become apparent in later sections of this chapter, create additional logistical difficulties in running the women's system as it is presently organised, and in facilitating the reforms as specified by Woolf.

Mental disorder

Aside from differences in their criminal profiles there are other differences between the male and female prison populations which should be taken into account when considering the implications of Woolf's recommendations for the women's system. Levels of mental disorder, for example, are assessed as being relatively high in both the male and female prison populations, but a recent survey of 2,042 sentenced prisoners concluded that the incidence of psychiatric disorders is most prevalent amongst sentenced female prisoners (Gunn, Maden,and Swinton 1991). The study revealed that about 1 in 3 (36 per cent) men in prison and young offender institutions were suffering from a mental disorder, in comparison to over half (56 per cent) of all women. Amongst both populations the single most common diagnosis was drug abuse or dependency. However, although this affected 1 in 10 of the adult men they surveyed, and about 1 in 17 male young offenders, it predominated amongst women prisoners to the extent that almost 1 in 4 were classified as suffering from this disorder. In addition, the women were more than twice as likely as the men to be diagnosed as suffering from a neurotic disorder: around 1 in 20 male prisoners in comparison to 1 in 8 of the women. Caution, however, must be exercised in giving meaning to these data. The social construction and attribution of psychiatric diagnoses to women has been critically documented in recent years (Procek 1981; Sim 1990). Precisely how the present survey results should be interpreted extends beyond this brief review. What is indicated, however, is that men and women present different accounts of their experiences and have their problems differentially defined. The 1991 Criminal Justice Act (s. 4) introduces two new requirements in relation to the sentencing of mentally disordered offenders. First, the court is required to obtain and consider a medical report before passing sentence on an offender who is, or appears to be, suffering from a mental disorder. Second, before passing a custodial sentence on such an offender the court must consider the effect which imprisonment could have upon the offender's condition and upon any treatment which might be available for it. As Ashworth (1992) points out, this new section is designed to 'direct sentencers' minds towards the effect of custody on the mentally disturbed' and is a 'step in the right direction' (p.304). However, unless or until this new legislation is accompanied by the provision of new resources in the community it would seem unlikely that the numbers of mentally disordered women in the prison population will be substantially reduced.

Ethnic minorities

The Criminal Justice Act 1991 (s. 95(1)(b)) requires the Home Secretary to publish annually information which might enable those engaged in the administration of criminal justice to perform their 'duties in ways which avoid discriminating against any persons on the ground of race or sex or any other improper ground'. Home Office statistics provide clear evidence that ethnic minority groups are overrepresented amongst the prison population (Home Office 1992a). The reasons for this have been widely debated (Crow and Cove 1984; Moxon 1988; Hudson 1989) but, as Ashworth notes, 'the possibility must . . . be kept in view that sentencing practice tends to exacerbate the effect of racially discriminatory decisions taken in the earlier stages of the criminal process' (1992, p. 174). A comprehensive study by Roger Hood for the Commission for Racial Equality, has provided compelling new evidence which confirms that the sentencing practice of at least some judges is more severe when dealing with ethnic minority defendants (Hood, 1992).

There is, however, a significantly higher proportion of ethnic minorities in women's prisons than in male establishments: 15 per cent of male prisoners in comparison to over 26 per cent of the women. Those of African or Afro-Caribbean origin constitute the largest single minority grouping, forming, on 30 June 1990, 11 per cent of the male population and 21 per cent of all women in prison. In recent years, the prison statistics have revealed differences in the average length of sentence received by each ethnic group (Home Office 1992a). In 1990, for example, adult male prisoners of African or Afro-Caribbean origin were serving sentences 44 per cent longer than comparable white prisoners. The same is true amongst the female population, except the discrepancy is considerably more striking due primarily to the relatively large numbers of foreign nationals imprisoned for drugs-related offences (see Maden, Swinton and Gunn 1992). In 1990 adult women of African or Afro-Caribbean origin were serving sentences 106 per cent longer than adult white women.[2]

The difficulties and deprivations experienced by ethnic-minority women who are foreign nationals and serving medium and long-term sentences are severe. Survey data has revealed that many of them do not speak English; that they have few, if any, opportunities to receive visits; and that their ability to exert any control over the remnants of their outside lives is severely diminished (Posen 1986). It may be that many of these problems are shared by equivalent male prisoners, but the relative scale of the problem within the male and female systems is substantially different. The majority of such women have been convicted of drug trafficking offences and many are poor women who, when recruited as couriers, were unaware of the long prison sentences they could face in this country (NACRO 1991a). Posen's survey revealed that such women were more likely than prisoners normally resident in the UK to have dependent children and to feel that inadequate care arrangements had been made for them. Some of the women she interviewed were unaware of their children's whereabouts and had encountered considerable obstacles in gaining and passing on information about their families. NACRO has argued that 'consideration should be given to other means of dealing with these women' (1991a, p. 8). So long as current methods persist, however, specific policies will have to be designed for this particular group of female prisoners if the objectives of the Woolf Report are to apply to them and if section 95(1)(b) of the Criminal Justice Act is to be realised.

Family ties

The 1991 National Prison Survey (Office of Population Censuses and Surveys 1992) provides compelling new evidence to show that imprisonment has a different impact upon the family ties of male and female prisoners. The national survey is based upon interviews with 10 per cent of all male prisoners and 20 per cent of all women in prison. The final report reveals that just under a third (32 per cent) of male prisoners and almost half (47 per cent) of the women said that they had dependent children living with them immediately prior to coming into prison (Office of Population Censuses and Surveys 1992, p. 13). However, as the Prison Reform Trust has noted, what happens to these children 'is strongly influenced by whether it is their father or mother who is imprisoned' (1991a, p. 3). Nine out of ten male prisoners interviewed said that their children were being looked after by their current or ex-wives or by their partner, and only 2 per cent claimed that their children were in care or with foster parents. In sharp contrast, less than a quarter (23 per cent) of women prisoners said that at least one of their children was being cared for by their husbands or partners. Over half (52 per cent) said that at least one of their children was being looked after by other relatives, and 12 per cent admitted that their children were either in the care of the local authority or with foster parents (Office of Population Censuses and Surveys 1992, pp. 13–14).

Social disadvantage

There are, of course, important similarities in the characteristics of men and women in prison. The national survey shows that both groups tend to be relatively young: 55 per cent of women prisoners and 62 per cent of men were under 30 and more than 80 per cent of both populations were under the age of 40 (Office of Population Censuses and Surveys 1992, p. 6). The survey makes clear that prisoners of both sexes represent a highly disadvantaged sub-group of the general population. Rates of homelessness amongst prisoners were much higher than in the population at large, so too was unemployment (pp. 14–16). Men and women in prison were also significantly more likely than members of the general public to have been taken into local authority care as a child: 21 per cent of female prisoners and 26 per cent of males, in contrast to 2 per cent of the general population (pp. 17–18). Evidence of educational achievements indicates further deprivation. The survey reports that on entering prison over 40 per cent of prisoners had no formal educational qualifications (p. 21). The proportion of women prisoners with no qualifications, however, was slightly lower than in the female population at large but this reflects the overall disadvantaged position of women, whereby 42 per cent have no formal qualifications in comparison to 34 per cent of all men (p. 22). The Prison Reform Trust reports that:

> In the academic year 1984/85, of 28,255 prisoners assessed for literacy, 6.2 per cent had a reading age of eight years or less and 9.4 per cent of 10 years or less. The Home Office has estimated that around one half of all prisoners have functional difficulties with literacy.
>
> (1991a, p. 2)

All of the above underlines the importance of the Prison Service providing facilities to meet the special needs of prisoners. It also indicates that the special needs of women prisoners will not always be the same as those of male prisoners.

COMMUNITY PRISONS

A source of many of the problems experienced by women prisoners is the fact that there are only twelve female establishments, unevenly located across the country, resulting in many women being held at great distances from their home communities. Seven establishments, accounting for over half (52 per cent) of the female accommodation, are in the southeast. There is only one small unit in the southwest, housing fewer than sixty women and no prison facilities at all for women in Wales. The current prison-building programme does not include any new establishments for women.

One of the central recommendations of the Woolf Report, and one which the Government's White Paper *Custody, Care and Justice* (Home Office 1991a) has accepted as a long-term goal, is the development of community prisons:

> where this is practical, prisons should be community prisons sited within reasonable proximity to, and having close connection with, the community with which the prisoners they hold have their closest links.
>
> (Woolf 1991, para. 11.49)

It is evident from the subsequent discussion in the Report that this principle was not destined to be confined to male sentenced prisoners but, if the necessary degree of separation could be organised, was to incorporate young offenders, prisoners on remand and women. On the face of it this seems to provide a straightforward solution to the difficulties of locating women in establishments many miles away from their homes, with all the concomitant problems of maintaining contact with their families and facilitating their reintegration into the community. But is it really that straightforward?

If 1,600 women were to be located in prisons closer to their homes there would inevitably be a larger number of units housing a smaller number of women. These might take the form of separate institutions, similar to secure hostels, or they could be located within existing establishments for men. NACRO has identified four options which could be adopted in an effort to formulate community prisons for women (NACRO 1991a). Option 1 would widen the network of female units by attaching small groups of women to all male local prisons. The fact that female prisoners would constitute such a tiny minority in all of these establishments, however, raises fears that the women would be marginalised and would have last call on any communal facilities.[3] Option 2 attempts to address this difficulty by limiting the location of female units to male establishments in major population centres so that women prisoners might compose between one-third and one-half of the population in any of the chosen establishments. The advantage of this plan is that it would increase the women's accessibility to their visitors by alleviating many of the travel difficulties they presently face, but it would obviously not conform to the principle of a community catchment area. Both of these options, however, imply some sharing of facilities between male and female prisoners and this raises the question of how far the process of sharing communal resources should extend to mixing the populations in certain environments. Opponents of mixing men and women have argued that any advantages for women gained by the provision of wider work, educational and leisure opportunities are outweighed by the detriments associated with such a policy (Tchaikovsky 1991).

Contempory sexual politics in our society ensure that women are typically subordinated to men and that if such power relations were to be reproduced within a prison context, this could only work to the detriment of women prisoners. Many women in prison have suffered abuse from men and it can be argued that, if nothing else, imprisonment provides these women with a welcome respite from male harassment and exploitation. There is also a concern that if there was a degree of integration then prisoners' existing relationships with spouses and partners outside would be placed under intolerable pressure. Maintaining control within such establishments could also become more onerous for staff if sexual jealousies and power struggles had to be contended with. There is, of course, no guarantee that this kind of apocalyptic vision would be fulfilled.

But neither can the potential dangers be dismissed as irrelevant or inconsequential. The experiences of some women admitted to mixed wards in some psychiatric hospitals have not given cause for optimism. Despite an intention to provide a more 'normal' and thus healthier social environment, the shortage of staff and poor ward design have resulted in female patients lacking privacy and, in some instances, suffering physical and sexual assaults by male patients.

The third and fourth options identified by NACRO would require completely separate facilities for women. Option 3 proposes the setting up of discrete community prisons in large population centres. Again, however, this would dilute the principle of keeping prisoners close to home, would demand considerable capital expenditure and would risk a dramatic increase in the numbers of places made available for women. Option 4 moves away from the concept of a large institution in favour of accommodating small numbers of women in their home communities in 'houses set aside for the purpose' (p.19). The impracticality of providing a full programme of activities on site would be resolved by permitting the women access to facilities within the community. It is this option which NACRO believes best serves the interests of women prisoners and is most consistent with Woolf's emphasis on proximity to home and a high degree of permeability between the prison and the community.

NACRO acknowledges that such reorganisation would require 'the greatest leap in perception, policy and practice' (p.19). It will undoubtedly be claimed that such a proposal is 'unrealistic' and that it unfairly distinguishes between the punishment meted out to men and that meted out to women. It is, however, the only option which does not seriously compromise the principles set out by Woolf as fundamental to the development of a secure, controlled and just prison system. The fact that it would appear to depart so substantially from existing arrangements for women prisoners may, however, seem less eccentric and more rational after detailed consideration has been given later in the chapter to the feasibility of providing equality of opportunity for male and female prisoners.

REMAND PRISONERS

Woolf's proposals for remand prisoners fall broadly into two categories: strategies to reduce the remand population and measures to improve custodial conditions.

Reduction of the remand population

The Report calls upon the courts to take a more considered approach to bail decisions and emphasises the importance of co-operation between the various criminal justice agencies in reducing the numbers of defendants who are refused bail and in minimising the length of time they are remanded in custody. Current initiatives, such as bail information schemes, bail hostels and prison bail schemes are applauded for their success in diverting individuals from prisons and police cells. The Report unequivocally states that custodial remands should be used only when absolutely necessary and for the shortest possible time.

The present range of strategies to inhibit the use of custodial remands is clearly relevant to both men and women. Their scope for success, however, must be particularly wide in relation to female defendants. The Bail Act 1976 provides that a defendant may be refused bail only if any of the following conditions are met: the court has grounds to believe that the individual concerned would abscond and fail to turn up for trial; would commit an offence if released on bail; would interfere with witnesses or otherwise obstruct the course of justice; or should be held in custody for their own protection. The most common reason given for refusing bail is the belief that, in the light of the person's previous record, other offences will almost certainly be committed during the remand period. The purpose of remanding a person in custody is thus to enable a degree of surveillance over their behaviour, so that the criminal justice process can proceed unhindered, and to protect the public from further victimisation. Woolf, however, proposes that magistrates 'should attach considerable significance to whether or not the offence . . . if proved, would justify a sentence of imprisonment' (para. 10.84) This is an extremely significant caveat for female defendants since, unlike their male counterparts, the majority of women on remand do not go on to receive prison sentences. In 1989, 63 per cent of men who were received as untried or as unconvicted prisoners were eventually awarded sentences of imprisonment, whereas only 47 per cent of women remanded in custody received a custodial sentence.

It would seem, however, that women are more likely than men to be remanded in custody in order for medical reports to be prepared. Although this is not a relevant criterion under the 1976 legislation it is facilitated under the Magistrates' Courts Act 1980 (s. 30).[4] Between 1 April 1989 and 31 March 1990 the Prison Medical Service prepared a total of 6,812 psychiatric reports which had been requested by the courts.[5] Of these, 801 (12 per cent) were made on female prisoners, despite the fact that women represent only 4 per cent of the total remand population. The Reed Committee, a joint working party of the Department of Health and the Home Office, which was set up to review the health and social services for mentally disordered offenders, has circulated a consultation document by its Prison Advisory Group in which it states:

> There is good research evidence that the courts remand the mentally disordered in custody essentially for psychiatric and social reasons rather than for reasons of public safety or seriousness of offence. In

principle it is wrong that courts should be able to remand to prison for the primary purpose of medical assessment.

(Department of Health and Home Office 1991b, para. 3.3)

The recommendations of this group make clear that a package of schemes should be coordinated to facilitate psychiatric intervention at earlier stages in the criminal justice process. A recent development has been the duty-psychiatrist schemes which now operate in a limited number of courts. These may help to pre-empt the need for a remand period by providing immediate access to medical opinion and, where longer periods of assessment are required, may facilitate a greater use by the courts of appropriate health and social services in the community.

An extension of bail information schemes and the provision of specialist bail hostels should also help to inhibit the imposition of custody for the purpose of gaining a medical assessment. Research has indicated, however, that the provision of hostels may serve to widen the net of the criminal justice system (Lewis and Mair 1989). Inevitably the problem lies in ensuring that such facilities are used to divert defendants from custody, rather than absorbing more residents who would otherwise have been granted bail without this restriction. One solution could be to accept the recommendation made by the Reed Committee's Prison Advisory Group, to prevent the courts from remanding defendants in custody for the purpose of gaining a medical report, by amending or repealing the relevant powers of the Bail Act 1976 and the Magistrates' Courts Act 1980 (para. 3.3). Once this doorway to prison has been closed, they argue, alternative facilities would have to be used.

Improvement of custodial conditions

There can be no disputing the fact that without certain restrictions some defendants would impede the course of justice and that, in a few cases, public safety would be at risk. Such an acknowledgement, however, begs the question as to whether such controls over the unconvicted should take the form of imprisonment. There can be no doubt that prisons effectively neutralise the potential for defendants to undermine the criminal justice process and shield the public from potential harm. Neither can there be any doubt that the *raison d'être* of the prison is to punish offenders for their crimes: they are, first and foremost, institutions of state punishment. Yet the state is not entitled to punish those who have yet to be found guilty of an offence, regardless of how certain the prospect of their conviction may appear. It is for this reason that some distinction has traditionally been drawn between the custodial conditions of remand and sentenced prisoners. The Woolf Report reiterates the need for prison regimes to take account of the special status of the remand population and advocates that a separate Statement of Purpose, setting out the Prison Service's responsiblities to this group, should be established and that untried remand prisoners should be held separately (para. 1.206). It also criticises the high levels of security to which all remand prisoners are subject and proposes the introduction of a system of classification which would start from the presumption of a lower security requirement. The guiding principle, drawn from earlier work by Rod Morgan (Morgan and Barclay 1989), is that prisoners awaiting trial 'should suffer no greater loss of liberty, both in duration and in degree, than is necessary to secure the course of justice' (Woolf 1991, para. 10.59).

Such a perspective would imply that defendants would not be prevented from continuing their legitimate business activities, nor from spending time with their families, if such practices are not thought to jeopardise the course of justice. Facilitating the course of justice, however, would also imply that remand conditions should not impede or disadvantage defendants in the preparation of their case for court. Yet channels of communication in prisons are more restricted and slower than those which exist for defendants on bail. Remand prisoners do not have unfettered access to a telephone, they cannot visit their legal advisers and they are unable personally to investigate or research information relevant to their defence. The reason that untried prisoners are currently denied these opportunities is that the Prison Service lacks the resources to cope with the potential demand. What is deemed to be necessary to secure the course of justice may thus be seen as a relative concept which is currently defined in relation to what the prison system can facilitate.

In Chapter 8 Rod Morgan clearly identifies the operational incompatibility of the various objectives which Woolf sought to achieve in relation to the custody of untried prisoners. In short, the greater the degree of specialisation, in terms of the security and purpose of establishments, the more difficult it becomes to locate prisoners close to their homes. The size of the male service however, provides at least some prospect of establishing community prisons with distinct remand units, which could be run under a separate set of Prison Rules. Accommodating Woolf's proposals in the women's system, however, is considerably more difficult to envisage.

In 1990 the average population of women remanded in custody was less than 400, of which only 300 were untried prisoners.[6] These women were distributed in five establishments described as 'local prisons' which cover very broad catchment areas.[7] It is hard to imagine how this population could be dispersed to community prisons without there being either full integration with sentenced women, with only modest variations in the nature of the regime; or incorporation into discrete remand units which have a separate body of rules but which overwhelmingly accommodate male prisoners.

It does not seem too improbable to speculate that if a system were to be designed from scratch to achieve the purposes which custodial remands are currently expected to serve, the incarceration of women in prison would not be selected as the preferred or expedient option. The costs which are associated with the so-called 'inevitable facts of imprisonment' are not limited to the gratuitous restrictions and unjustified burdens placed upon the prisoner. Remanding a woman in custody has serious implications for the tax payer who, in 1990, had to foot an average bill of £563 per week for each woman held in prison. In addition further expenditure may be required to provide support for her children and to defray the travel costs of her family and her legal representatives who visit her. There can be little dispute that the women's prison system is being asked to fulfil a task for which it is manifestly unsuitable.

The abandonment of women's prisons as remand facilities would not have to mean that serious offenders who pose a significant risk to the public would escape all significant controls upon their behaviour. Bearing in mind that the reason for refusing bail is the need to supervise and monitor behaviour, it should be possible to develop a series of measures, including hostel accommodation of varying levels of security, curfew and even a system of escorts, which would ensure the protection of the public and safeguard the administration of criminal justice whilst respecting the legal status of the defendant. Electronic monitoring might also have a role to play, although recent Home Office experiments have not yielded encouraging results. The Home Office review revealed that the courts were reluctant to use the devices, that there were frequent mechanical failures and that the rate of violation was high (Mair and Nee 1990). Aside from these practical problems there are also principled objections to tagging. It is argued that the wearing of monitoring devices intrudes on the privacy of the individual and violates the principle of equal respect and dignity (see von Hirsch 1990; Ashworth 1992). Despite these major reservations, the future of electronic monitoring as an alternative to a custodial remand should not, at this stage of development, be terminated. Requiring a woman to wear a monitoring device is unlikely to violate her respect and dignity more seriously than remanding her in custody. There is, however, a recognised danger that electronic monitoring, as well as the other measures mentioned, would simply displace less intrusive bail conditions rather than the use of imprisonment. It may also be argued that the overwhelming majority of female remands would not need this level of restriction and that it is therefore unnecessary and unwelcome. But these are concerns which primarily relate to practical difficulties of enforcement and do not undermine the fundamental argument for devising strategies of supervision in the community for those women whom the courts insist are not eligible for unconditional bail.

Periodically, exceptional circumstances must arise in which anything short of high-security incarcaration would be considered inadequate. In these instances extraordinary arrangements could be made with female prisons or with remand centres for men. There is no reason to believe, however, that the overwhelming majority of women charged with serious offences could not be adequately controlled within a system which combined various measures of supervision to provide gradations of surveillance, designed to fit individual circumstances. It is an approach which is consistent with the new sentencing strategies outlined in the 1991 Criminal Justice Act, which advocate the flexible use of community penalties to divert convicted offenders from custody.

It may be suggested that by removing untried female defendants from prison preferential treatment is being extended to women which fuels the dubious presumption that female offenders are not 'real criminals' and should be treated more leniently than men. This is an ill-conceived perspective and wholly irrelevant to the present debate. Providing non-custodial methods of control for women who have been refused bail, is a solution to a structural problem and is geared to facilitating equality of opportunity, both between male and female defendants, and between those currently granted bail and those who require closer surveillance.

CONTRACTS AND JUSTICE

Improving standards

Lord Justice Woolf was unequivocal in asserting that 'Justice refers to the obligation of the Prison Service to treat prisoners with humanity and fairness and to prepare them for their return to the community in a way which makes it less likely that they will reoffend' (para. 9.20). The ways in which inmates are treated in prison have long been criticised as providing a stratum of punishments which extend beyond the deprivation of a person's liberty. The Woolf Report recognised that if control in prisons is to be maintained and if prisoners are to be treated with humanity and justice, efforts have to be made to limit the negative effects which derive from severed family relationships, damaged employment prospects, and the sense of hopelessness which emanates from the devaluation of self-esteem. Woolf recognised that virtually all prisoners will, in time, return to the community and that remedial action has to be taken to limit the deterioration in their abilities to operate effectively and lawfully. A crucial objective is to reduce prisoners' dependency upon the prison authorities by providing them with opportunities to make meaningful decisions, and by holding them accountable for the choices they make. Woolf's recommendation that prisoners should enter into contracts or compacts with the prison in which they are held, the extension of career plans to all prisoners serving 12 months or more, and the proposed changes to the disciplinary and grievance procedures, construct a framework for tackling the collateral punishments of imprisonment and provide prisoners with incentives to co-operate with the system. The question is whether these changes will have a different impact upon the male and female systems.

As Genevra Richardson points out in Chapter 4, the system of prisoner contracts is intended to provide each prisoner with an annual statement of what he or she can legitimately expect from the institution, in relation to standards and conditions of accommodation and regime, and what the establishment can expect from the prisoner in return. It is anticipated that prisoners would receive progressively more under their contracts as they proceed through their sentence, and that they could lose some features of the contract for a period of time should they breach their part of the agreement by offending against prison discipline. Unlike accredited standards, prisoners' contracts would be specific to their current institution and would be liable to vary from one establishment to another. Although the contract does not imbue the inmate with any private law rights, it is intended to provide a vehicle for the prisoner to enforce his or her specific entitlements. If, for example, the prison fails to deliver the contract, or if the prisoner is transferred to an establishment offering a contract which is manifestly less advantageous, the individual concerned may invoke the grievance procedure and ultimately seek judicial review to remedy any unfairness.

Whilst the proposed system of contracts falls short of providing prisoners with substantive rights which are directly enforceable in private law, it is, at least in theory, a step towards a more just prison system. It builds upon the presumption that certain facilities in prisons should be conceived as normal expectations, rather than privileges given out of grace or favour, and thus makes clear the respective responsibilities of the establishment and the prisoner. It also provides a way of raising standards by identifying precise services to be delivered and enabling comparisons to be drawn between the contracts on offer in similar types of establishment. The Report makes clear that 'the aim should be to provide consistency of treatment between different prisoners and different establishments of the same type' and that when a difference of approach does occur, prisoners should be given 'a reasoned explanation for it' (para. 14.39). Finally, it is claimed that contracts between prisoners and establishments which are reviewed every twelve months, and which are geared towards a progressive extension of opportunities and freedom, provide prisoners with a framework which enables them to manage their sentence constructively and increase their sense of autonomy.

The development of sentence plans for all prisoners serving 12 months or more is another strategy designed to achieve these objectives. Sentence plans differ from annual contracts in that they are long-term plans covering the whole period of a prisoner's sentence. Their objective is to give structure and purpose to the time an inmate spends in prison and to focus particularly upon preparing the individual for release and return to the community. Each sentence plan is intended to be tailored to individual needs and circumstances and should be amended and updated over time. Inevitably, however, the content of an inmate's career plan will be affected by the content of the contracts which are available in the establishments to which he or she may be located.

Many of Woolf's proposals for improvements to regimes which could be incorporated into prisoners' contracts are as relevant to women as they are to men. For example, the development of a more collaborative relationship between work and education, the improvement of prisoners' pay, and the introduction of new and extended visiting arrangements and opportunities for home leave, are applicable to both male and female prisoners. Distinctions will inevitably occur, however, in the contracts and sentence plans made available to male and female prisoners. The limited number and uneven geographical distribution of female establishments makes 'career progression' to less secure accommodation more problematic. Special provision must also be made for pregnant women and mothers with babies. The diminutive size of the female system will also determine a more limited range of in-house resources for work and education. The fact that about a third of all prison places for women are situated in establishments which were not built for custodial purposes, ensures that there are wide variations in the nature and organisation of accommodation, both within the female system and in comparison to similar categories of establishment for men. There is, for example, relatively more dormitory accommodation for women and fewer single cells.[8]

Although Woolf intended comparisons to be drawn between establishments in order to facilitate some standardisation of treatment, the Report does not explicitly refer to the possibility of comparing male and female establishments. Yet the system of prisoner contracts could provide an unprecedented opportunity to promote and monitor equal opportunities for male and female prisoners. NACRO has argued that an explicit commitment to equal opportunities should be incorporated into the Prison Service's 'Statement of Purpose' (NACRO 1991a, p. 20). The question, however, is what is meant by 'equality of opportunity'. For reasons already mentioned, it does not mean identical treatment, but implies that different facilities should be provided for men and women to enable them to have an equal chance of limiting the collateral punishments of imprisonment and maximising the opportunities for improving their prospects on release. The concept of treating people differently in order to achieve equality is not a novel idea and is already enshrined in much of the working practice of the Prison Service.

On the basis of recent Home Office data it might be argued that women prisoners already enjoy equal opportunities in relation to education and training facilitities. A profile of inmate occupations for March 1991 revealed that proportionately more women than men were engaged in daytime education or training courses (Home Office 1991a).[9] In recent years there has been a marked shift in some female establishments away from the orthodoxy of domestic training and the reinforcement of gender stereotypes toward the development of specific skills relevant to the job market and the furtherance of the womens' awareness of their rights as citizens (Home Office 1991j). But notwithstanding these important changes, the provision of training for women in prison continues to be dominated by vocational courses in 'womens' subjects' and is considerably more limited in scope than that which is provided for men. If the stated aim of the Prison Service to assist prisoners, regardless of their sex, to 'lead law abiding and useful lives in custody and after release', is to be realised, then the spiral of deprivation within which many women are caught has to be addressed. Opportunities for training must promote the acquisition of skills and qualifications across a spectrum of traditional and non-traditional working roles and enhance the women's competence to deal effectively and legitimately with the difficulties they face in their particular social situations. The Prison Service has explicitly acknowledged the need to broaden the educational and training opportunities for women:

> Some women will be interested in gaining skills in areas in which women have traditionally been employed, such as catering and needle trades. However, others may be interested in learning trades which are widely associated with men, such as car maintenance, bricklaying and carpentry . . . Women might benefit from courses which will enable them to become more self-sufficient on release. Training in this area might vary from courses in establishing and running a small business to painting and decorating . . . Consideration should be given by Governors to the introduction of social/life skills courses which will help women deal with social security and tax and give them an understanding of their legal rights.
>
> (Home Office 1991j, pp. 13–16)

Putting these good intentions into practice across the women's system and facilitating equality of opportunity in this area would inevitably require a fundamental reorganisation in the ways in which education and training are provided for women prisoners. It could entail the sharing of facilities in male prisons and/or the attendance of women prisoners at courses outside the prison. Rarely could equality of opportunity be provided if, as now, some women were permitted to undertake solitary correspondence courses, divorced from an interactive process of learning.

Another area in which prisoners' contracts could promote equal opportunities is in the provision of therapeutic facilities. Despite, or possibly because of, the traditional positivist depiction of female criminals as 'mad' rather than 'bad' (Smart 1977; Carlen 1983) and the dubious history of treatment for women prisoners (Sim 1990), there is a marked lack of therapeutic programmes in contemporary female establishments. Most notable of all is the total absence of any provision equivalent to that provided for male prisoners at Grendon. Each wing of this prison is run as a therapeutic community for inmates who are serving medium-term and long sentences for various offences, and who typically manifest a wide range of attitudinal and behavioural problems. The purpose of the regime is to enable the men to examine their attitudes towards themselves and others, and to question their patterns of behaviour, in an effort to discover alternative and non-criminal ways of adjusting to the dilemmas and difficulties before them. The Woolf Report commented favourably upon the work carried out at Grendon and proposed that a similar prison should be established in another part of the country. The absence of this facility in the female system is particularly anomalous in the light of the recent psychiatric survey of the prison population (Gunn, Maden and Swinton 1991). This revealed high levels of neurotic disorders amongst female prisoners which, the report notes, would be particularly suitable for treatment within a therapeutic community. Ironically, Grendon was originally designed to incorporate a female unit but the accommodation has never been used for this purpose.

In defence of the status quo it may be argued that women prisoners are provided with 'special facilities' which are not available in the male system, such as mother and baby units, and that these services offset or counterbalance the lack of resources for women in other areas. This argument, however, rests upon a double misconception. First, it misconstrues the purpose of the facilities which are provided for women prisoners as mothers of young children. Allowing a woman to keep her child with her in prison is intended to serve the best interests of the child and is not designed to be a reward for the inmate, even though, in practice, it may be (mis)used as a control strategy. Second, it misinterprets the meaning of equal opportunities. Although equality of opportunity critically depends upon treating different groups of people differently, it cannot be achieved by attempting to equate the supply of fundamentally different commodities. Such an equation has been described elsewhere as an 'arithmetical fallacy' (Walker 1991).

Another defence against direct comparisons being drawn between the contracts for male and female prisoners is the 'economy of scale' argument: the women's system is too small to permit the range of facilities which exist for male prisoners. The logic of this argument is indisputable so long as women's prisons operate as a sub-system of the male service. Its reasoning becomes less compelling if one starts from different first principles. The presumption which currently dominates the debate is that policies designed for the male majority can be applied in a scaled-down version to incorporate the minority of women. It is an approach which gives priority to the preservation of a particular organisational system rather than to the principle of equality of opportunity. If the problem is conceived not in terms of how women can be fitted in to a system for men, but in terms of how women prisoners can be afforded an equal opportunity to minimise the unintended pains of imprisonment and to maximise their capacity for self-support outside, then the potential for different strategies and methods of organisation presents itself.

Mechanisms of control

Contracts for prisoners provide not only a means for improving standards in prison they are also mechanisms of control, designed to provide a series of incentives which encourage co-operation with the rules and inhibit disruptive behaviour. Woolf's intention was that prisoners would receive progressively more under their contract as they progressed through their sentence but would lose certain benefits if they broke their part of the agreement by committing a disciplinary offence. Many of Woolf's proposals relating to standards of justice in prisons are relevant to both male and female establishments. An independent element to the disciplinary and complaints procedures; the requirement for prison authorities to give reasons for decisions which materially affect prisoners; and the development of effective lines of communication between inmates and those who manage the Prison Service, are all uniformly applicable. However, the justice of such procedures will be seriously undermined if different disciplinary codes are applied, or if the same code is unevenly applied, and if there is inconsistency in the awarding of punishments. It is well established that the rate of disciplinary offending in women's prisons greatly exceeds that recorded in the male system. In 1991 there were 2.9 offences punished per head of average population in women's prisons, compared with a rate of 1.6 amongst male inmates (Home Office 1992b). Women, however, appear to be punished more frequently for minor infractions of prison rules which would be unlikely to attract formal disciplinary proceedings in male establishments. The triviality of much of the disciplinary offending by women has been noted repeatedly by Judge Stephen Tumin, HM Chief Inspector of Prisons and co-author of Part II of the Woolf Report, in his 1989 inspection reports on Cookham Wood, Styal and East Sutton Park (Home Office 1989b, c, d). Empirical research has also shown that in some female prisons additional, and usually extremely petty, institutional regulations are invoked which do not exist in the male system (Manderaka-Sheppard 1986). The 1991 National Prison Survey confirmed that women prisoners are more likely than male prisoners to find the rules and bureaucracy of prison life 'irritating or annoying' (Office of Population Censuses and Surveys 1992, p. 40).

Other types of injustice associated with the maintenance of control in prison are considerably less common in the women's system. For example, the small size of the service restricts the possibility of sudden transfers ('ghosting') which attracted critical attention in the Woolf Report and prompted a series of proposals and recommendations to inhibit the more egregious features of this procedure (see Chapter 5). There are also fewer women segregated for their own protection in the impoverished and unjustifiably punitive conditions typical of Rule 43 units.[10] However, the delivery of contracts which promote justice and equal opportunities for women prisoners hinge critically on there being a disciplinary system which does not discriminate on grounds of sex. The 'just deserts' approach to sentencing decisions in the courts should similarly guide the decision-making of prison governors when penalising inmates for breaches of prison discipline. Such an approach, however, can only achieve the desired goals if accompanied by a set of disciplinary rules common to both male and female establishments, which are policed consistently throughout the system, and which are not supplemented by unnecessary local additions and amendments.

CONCLUSION

The Woolf Report aims to pave the way for penal reform by detailing changes which would create a new balance between the competing objectives of security, control and justice. The detail of its prospectus, however, has been formulated by reference only to male establishments. The White Paper, *Custody Care and Justice*, (Home Office 1991a) demonstrates that the Government has broadly accepted a number, although not all, of the Report's practical recommendations and proposals. However, the White Paper provides no indication that the delivery of these facilities to *women* prisoners might require different organisational strategies and the creation of different structural arrangements.

The size of the female system and the nature of its population suggests that different policies will be necessary if women are to be incorporated into Woolf's vision of a controlled, secure and humane penal system. Their assimilation, however, hinges critically upon the Prison Service accepting that it has a duty, which is implicit in the achievement of its Statement of Purpose, to provide equal opportunities for female prisoners. The Prison Department has already issued a policy statement acknowledging its responsibility to provide equal opportunities on grounds of race, and has formulated a series of circular instructions which facilitate the differential treatment of ethnic minorities. The scale of the changes that are required if women are to be granted an equal opportunity to benefit from the changes proposed by the Woolf Report is clearly substantial. A major review should be instituted to establish a programme for reform which does not reconstitute a blueprint designed for the male majority, but creates a prototype to fit the exigencies of women's prisons.

The prospect of the women's system breaking free from the dominance of the male service and organising itself to achieve equal opportunities would appear, however, to be increasingly remote. The reorganisation of the Prison Department above establishment level which occured in 1990 has resulted in there being no single division exclusively devoted to the development of a female service. Instead, there is now an integrated structure whereby management responsibilities for both male and female establishments has been divided between the three new directorates, with one of them, the Directorate of Inmate Programmes, incorporating special responsibility for regimes in women's prisons. The Women's National Commission in their report on women's prisons has highlighted concern about this approach:

> The Working Group is concerned that the division of the management responsibilities between Directorates with different areas of policy interest will lead to a lack of coherent policy in tackling the problems that many women share and in developing regimes suited to their particular needs.
>
> (Women's National Commission 1991, p. 20)

It may be argued that Home Office officials are in a no-win situation: if they integrate women's prisons into the mainstream management structure they are criticised for jeopardising women's interests, and if they create a special structure they risk being accused of diverting women into a slipstream, to be by-passed and ignored. The real issue is not whether one management structure is preferable to another, so long as they both function to preserve a single approach. Objectives have to be set for both the male and the female systems, and these will inevitably differ to some extent and be reflected in prisoners' contracts. The fact that the male and female systems vary so greatly in size and in the nature of their populations, and the fact that their respective objectives must vary to some extent, calls for management structures which enable sufficient flexibility in the development and implementation of policies to enable both services to achieve objectives which ensure equal, but not necessarily the same, treatment for men and women in prison.

In many respects Lord Justice Woolf was right to exclude the women's system from his review: it is sufficiently different to warrant separate analysis. Yet he was also right to allude to the fact that many of the fundamental principles informing his recommendations and proposals apply to all prisoners regardless of their sex. A significant opportunity was lost, however, when the Report failed to recommend a separate review of the women's sector, designed to consider how the proposed agenda could be accomplished for female prisoners.

NOTES

1 In 1980 83 women were received into prison for drugs offences but by 1990 the number had increased to 240, having peaked at 480 in 1986, 1987 and 1988.

2 Similar differences are to be found amongst the young offender populations. In 1990 African and Afro-Caribbean male trainees were serving sentences 37 per cent longer than white trainees, and African and Afro-Caribbean female trainees were serving sentences 79 per cent longer than white inmates.

3 See Genders and Player (1988) for a description of the limited regime offered to women lifers and long-termers in H wing, Durham.

4 This section provides that if magistrates trying an accused person for an imprisonable offence are satisfied he or she did the act or made the omission as charged and are of the opinion that an inquiry into his/her physical or mental condition is needed to enable them to decide how to deal with the case, the accused may be remanded in custody for a period up to three weeks in order for reports to be prepared. The remand may take place after the magistrates have convicted the accused, but a conviction is not a precondition.

5 Personal communication from Directorate of Health Care, HM Prison Service.

6 Provisional figures.

7 Holloway in London accommodates women from the south-east and, to some extent, from the Midlands; Pucklechurch in Bristol caters for the south-west (together with emergency accommodation in Exeter, a local prison for men); Risley in Warrington receives women from the Midlands and the north; and Low Newton in Durham and New Hall in Wakefield provide remand facilities in the north.

8 Dormitories account for 45 per cent of certified normal accommodation (CNA) for females but only 18 per cent of CNA for males; and single cells or rooms constitute 44 per cent of the female CNA but 73 per cent of males accommodation.

9 In local prisons and remand centres almost 41 per cent of women were engaged in daytime education or training courses, compared with 22 per cent of male prisoners. In training establishments 27 per cent of women were so employed in comparison with 24 per cent of men in closed training prisons and 36 per cent in young offender institutions.

10 On 30 June 1990 there were 23 women (less than 2 per cent of the total female prison population) and 2,091 men (6 per cent of the male population) segregated for their own protection under Rule 43, or Young Offender Rule 46.

Part III

THE OUTSIDE WORLD

13

THE RELATIONSHIP BETWEEN THE COMMUNITY AND THE PRISON

Jenny Roberts

Of all the different types and degrees of damage caused by the riots at Strangeways and other prisons in 1990, the most persistent and harmful may well be the damage that was caused to public understanding of prisoners and the way that media images of the disorder may have intensified various myths about criminal justice and offenders. These include the belief that the prison population comprises only those defined as dangerous by policy and law; that crime is solely the product of the failure of individual responsibility; that prisons are either neutral in their effects on prisoners, or have a deterrent effect, or are holiday camps – some manage to subscribe to all three of these simultaneously; and that may also have widened the gulf which already exists in the minds of many members of the public, between prisons and the society they serve.

The danger of this position is that criminal justice policy in this country is alarmingly vulnerable to being driven by public opinion. This risk is exacerbated by some characteristics of the system, such as the fragmentation of responsibility for the penal system, and the absence of comprehensive training for those who play key roles in criminal justice administration. Lawyers for example, some of whom become judges – are trained in the law, but not in the consequences of its application; the magistracy are lay people; and civil servants play a dominant role in penal administration. In other European countries where the penal system is more integrated, public opinion is often more informed and moulded by policy makers who are receptive to the findings of research.

Without essaying a comprehensive definition of community, it has to be accepted that 'the community' is not an entity, and that the relationship beween prisons and the communities they serve is at least ambivalent. The normal benefits of community life are an important factor in preventing recidivism; but prisons on the other hand are the expression of society's wish to punish and to exile offenders. The isolation of prisons from the community is a two-way process; and there are many people who would wish to increase the isolation and stigmatisation of prisoners. The notion of investing more public money in prisons is unlikely to be a vote-winner. A closer relationship between prisons and the community could have an impact on attitudes and behaviour on both sides, which might not be entirely for the good.

Although such issues are nowhere directly discussed in the somewhat conservatively styled Woolf Report (Woolf 1991), the effects of its recommendations, if implemented, could do much to address such fundamental issues. Lord Justice Woolf accepted the Home Secretary's invitation to 'interpret' the terms of reference, choosing to examine prisons to a limited extent within their social context, but much more so in relation to the rest of the criminal justice process. Of the main improvements which the recommendations of the Inquiry are designed to achieve, this chapter will be concerned with those which directly influence the relationship between prisons and the community:

— the proposals for community prisons and 'clusters' of prisons;
— improvements in incentives for prisoners which involve contacts with families and outside communities;
— the establishment of a criminal justice consultative structure at national and local level.

The three sets of recommendations are, as I will show, interdependent. None will work properly unless all three are in place.

Since the Woolf Report was so firmly focused on the prison system, it will be necessary first to identify the wider context of these proposals, especially from the perspective of the world outside prisons.

THE ISOLATION OF PRISONS FROM THE COMMUNITY

Although the Inquiry by Lord Justice Woolf and Judge Stephen Tumim avoided the narrow perspectives on the prison system which were evident in some of the evidence offered by the Prison Service itself, and has thus been described as 'wide-ranging', its handling of the position of imprisonment in the wider criminal justice system is fairly cautious, despite the emphasis it places upon a commitment to justice. The overall value and cost-effectiveness of prisons are scarcely mentioned, certainly not critically challenged, and while the extreme isolation of the prison system comes under attack, judgements or speculation about the merits of imprisonment are avoided. There is however a brief reference to the need for all criminal justice agencies to have as their aim the reduction of crime, an aim which prisons are far from achieving.

Within the criminal justice process all agencies which play a part in the regulation of crime are vulnerable to complacency, even to an undue level of moral superiority, because of the simplifications which adversarial criminal justice applies to complex social processes. Offenders are not generally as exclusively or absolutely bad and blameworthy as a finding of guilt might imply. This is not to argue that crime should not be regulated, but that those who are responsible for the system need to remain aware that the process itself can cause harm, albeit indirectly, and that those who punish have a duty to minimise that harm. The Woolf Report acknowledges that 'the natural consequences of a sentence of imprisonment, unless remedial action is taken, will be a deterioration in the ability of the prisoner to operate effectively and lawfully within society' (para. 14.8). The responsibility to mitigate the harm caused by the administration of justice is a principle which should be regarded as equally applicable to the probation service or the courts as to the prison system.

Rightly, Woolf eschewed detailed examination of the harmful effects on offenders of a custodial sentence. But because disorder in prisons is usually connected with the well being of prisoners, many of his proposals are geared to reducing the potential damage which is indirectly caused by imprisonment. Such damage occurs when factors which might encourage a prisoner towards a crime-free future are outweighed by factors which reduce coping skills and encourage further resort to crime. Criminal justice agencies, including prisons, can deliver many positive influences such as training, personal influence and education. But in the long term the most positive influences on offenders and potential offenders are the normal benefits of life in the community. Indeed, this can be deduced from the extent to which prison regimes seek to incorporate as many aspects as possible of normal life in the community. Woolf underlines the scope for improvement in such areas as home leave, contacts with families, giving prisoners the chance to participate in decisions about the way prisons are run, the wearing of personal clothing and improved arrangements for work, education and training.

However, such improvements, while highly desirable as means of providing constructive regimes and reducing discontent, do little to break down the isolation of prisons from the community. That isolation, in Woolf's terms, should be measured by the distance prisoners are removed from their home area and, less explicitly, the degree of ownership that is expressed by local communities for prisoner populations that originate from them.

Since the Mountbatten Report (Home Office 1966) the structure of the prison system has been dominated by considerations of security and control and the effect which this had upon the links between prisoners and their communities has been profound. Directorate and management structures have been superimposed on the map of England and Wales with little regard for local community boundaries or for the importance for prisoners of any roots they may have in those communities. Remand and local prisons allocate prisoners to other institutions in a network which may be very widely dispersed. Unlike the Victorian city gaols, modern prisons are increasingly sited in rural areas, remote from large centres of population. During the 1980s many counties, including the one in which I work, were divided by the Prison Department's quite different regional boundaries, resulting in prisoners being sent to several different remand or local prisons, with the corresponding allocation networks beyond them. In consequence probation officers from the area may at any one time be attempting to maintain contact with prisoners scattered thinly in over fifty different prisons. So too will others who have reasons to maintain such contacts – for example, lawyers, and above all families.

Further dislocation to community ties is caused by transferring prisoners from prison to prison around the system. Transfers take place for many reasons; to allocate prisoners to appropriate regimes, to mark 'progress', to deal with overcrowding and for disciplinary purposes. Again this is a subject outside my scope and expertise, except from the perspective of the outside world. Woolf draws attention to the resentment which transfers can cause and remarks on the positive culture of those local prisons where staff and inmates share common roots in the local area (para. 11.55). Surprisingly, there is no obvious source of monitoring information about the extent of transfers within the prison system. The exercise of power that is involved surely represents a good reason why such information should be included in the Prison Statistics. Nor is there any comment in the Woolf Report about the level of Prison Department resources which are consumed by transferring prisoners in this way. The cost of these transfers must be considerable and could perhaps be more usefully spent by improving regimes and staffing.

THE EFFECTS OF ISOLATION

The depersonalising aspects of custodial regimes also contribute to the loss of contacts with the community. Reception procedures strip away much of the prisoner's links with his or her identity in the community. The prisoner's number becomes as important as his or her name and prison clothing is not only uniform but passed from inmate to inmate. The prisoner's origins are more likely to be described in terms of the prison from which he or she has been transferred; identity in terms of security classification; progress in terms of the stage reached in the sentence. Although people working within prisons acknowledge the reality of the persistent and institutionalised recidivist, the system as a whole does not. Files carrying the prisoner's past institutional history can be tracked down, but there seem to be impenetrable barriers in the way of introducing, within the prison, accounts of the prisoner's identity and prospects which derive from his or her life outside. This can be observed in the deliberations of local review committees considering discretionary release, where the original conviction and the inmate's behaviour within prison can emerge as dominant issues, compared with the individual's prospects and proposals for resettlement which fall into second place.

Agencies in the community are similarly inclined to treat reception into prison as the point at which the individual ceases to be entitled to receive services – and probation services can be as prone as any to 'forgetting' the offender once a custodial sentence has been passed. The families of prisoners also share this depersonalisation and loss of identity. If they are dependent on state benefit or other public services, their entitlement is often defined by the prisoner's status, rather than their own needs. In 'Prison Rule 102: "stand by your man"', McDermott and King (1992) describe their investigation of the demands, stresses and humiliations to which wives and children are exposed when they remain in contact with imprisoned husbands and fathers. They are treated as an additional resource to further the Prison Service objective of resettling prisoners, rather than as people with rights and needs which have been affected by the sentencing of their relative. The prison casts its shadow over their lives too.

The average prisoner does not enter prison with good prospects of resettlement. The incidence of social problems connected with offending among prisoners is well documented – unemployment, addictions, literacy and educational disadvantage, and family breakdown are among the most prevalent (Prison Reform Trust 1991a; Office of Population Censuses and Surveys 1992). They will adversely affect resettlement prospects unless they attract sustained expert intervention. The delivery of relevant services is more likely to be governed by sentence length and security classification than by need (but see Cotgreave 1989).

Those aspects of prison regimes which reduce the prisoner's sense of identity are well understood to affect the prospects of satisfactory resettlement. Large prisons and even large wings or units, where prisoners live and are managed in groups of a hundred or more; the absence for many of a constructive daily programme; and the adverse effects on relationships of staff preoccupation with security, all contribute to the problem. Personal responsibility is correspondingly difficult to maintain and develop when a person's sense of identity is fragile. Even relationships with prison staff are bound to be more fragmented because of the size of the institutions and the nature of the regimes.

The isolation of prisons damages the prospects of offender resettlement in numerous ways. Distancing prisoners from their home communities disrupts family ties to the point where they may be broken altogether. The Nottingham Prisoners' Families Project (Monger and Pendleton 1980) undertaken in 1970–2, studied the effects of imprisonment on prisoners' families; about one-quarter of the marital partnerships broke up (as measured by the prisoner not returning to the family home on the day of release). The proportion of prisoners without a stable family increased with each prison sentence served. The impact of separation on the children of prisoners was less starkly evident, but stress, trauma and loss of trust could readily be inferred. Prisoners became excluded from family decisions which would normally have been taken jointly, wives became more independent and sometimes reluctant to resume shared decision-making. The pressure of visiting distant prisons was enormous, involving complex and exhausting journeys, after which face-to-face contacts were often strained and unsatisfying. Prisoners could easily be 'wound up' into suspicions of infidelity or desertion and these added to the emotional tension of the contacts when they did occur.

After that study, which was completed more than ten years after the first modern account of the effects of imprisonment on the families of prisoners (Morris 1965), another ten years elapsed before further but essentially similar studies were initiated which gained wider public interest. McDermott and King (1992), Shaw (1987) and Light (1989) have again examined the experience of prisoners' families. Shaw (1992) draws together a number of contributions which detail the multiple impact, especially the potentially lasting emotional damage to the children of prisoners, much of which could be alleviated if community prisons were introduced and skilled help and attention provided for this purpose (Richards 1992). Community prisons, with strong links with local services, would offer scope for coordinated and integrated services to be made available to family units, thereby substantially alleviating both the financial and emotional costs of imprisonment.

Other contacts are important for maintaining links with the community. Many public and voluntary services, employers and other potential sources of help in resettlement are unlikely to make the effort which most families make to keep in touch with prisoners held away from their own area. The Nottingham Prisoners' Families Project demonstrated a clear relationship between levels of contact by probation officers with male prisoners and their families during sentence, and the continuation of that contact after release. This is an important finding which may well be equally applicable to other sources of community support. The link between offending and 'social' problems is not readily disentangled, but the level of unemployment, low educational achievement, drug and alcohol abuse and other such problems is very high among offenders in general, so the arguments for promoting continuity in the provision of relevant services to address these needs are overwhelming. In reality, the way prisoners are dispersed away from their home areas makes this extremely difficult. Even where such services are delivered from the outside, this is normally done by seconding staff into prisons (education and probation). On release, even if the ex-prisoner maintains use of the service, a change of delivery point and contact person – which will itself increase the risk of loss of contact – must take place. This hiatus between institution and home probation officer was described in relation to young offenders by the Probation Inspectorate (Home Office 1990d); in addition, a second hiatus was noted between policy and practice. It is reasonable to assume that these problems are not exclusive to the young offender population but exist for women and for adult men.

The institutional nature of prisons discourages more open interaction with outside services. Many probation officers believe that more effective work could be done with prisoners if the services were delivered directly by outside agencies rather than through the secondment system which, they argue, draws them within the institution and vitiates their capacity to deliver relevant services. The Woolf Report is somewhat disappointing on this issue, tending to place emphasis on the importance of rewarding work for prison officers (which is undeniably important) rather than on delivering effective services to prisoners. The recommendation that prison officers should extend their skills to undertake, for example, teaching of basic skills may well be appropriate, but a similar emphasis on the expert services which could be provided from community agencies should not be subordinated to this.

The absorption of community services into the prison system tends to flow from the fact that decisions about the provision tend to be concentrated at national level and, given that most of these services are locally structured, this creates a further difficult interface. No doubt each community agency could cite examples of poor consultation and coordination: the probation services are certainly able to do so. Woolf's exhortation that probation services should work as closely with the Prison Service as they do with the courts (para. 10.161) derives its force from the fact that the two services are contributing to the management of prisoners. The Association of Chief Officers of Probation has been pressing for some years for a probation presence on the Prisons Board, as a means of bringing a community-based perspective to the most senior advisory body of that Service. The difficulty of securing such a modest step in the direction of wider participation in the management of prisons seems remarkable. For probation service managers, there is particular irony in the fact that they are themselves accountable to independent local Probation Committees, composed of lay magistrates, which are likely to be re-structured in order to strengthen representation of local community interests. Coordination needs to take place at both national and local levels, and Woolf's endorsement of the value of devolving key decisions about regime delivery to individual governors, is relevant here. If local establishments were free to arrange the delivery of services from outside sources far more extensively than at present, the creation of a local consultative structure between each prison and relevant local services would be needed. Through such a structure, backed up by quality-based contracts promoting a common concern with the effective resettlement of offenders, there could develop a pluralist system for managing offenders, prisons and crime. Although Woolf's proposals are less radical, what they do make clear is that there is no good reason (including the demands of security) why prisons should not be more open to community participation and ownership.

COMMUNITY PRISONS

The possibility of reducing prison disorder through the design of prisons is Woolf's starting point for firm prescriptions which could radically improve links between prisons and local communities and might evolve towards the type of community ownership described above. First the Report proposes that prisons should accommodate no more than 400 prisoners and should be split into separate units of 50 to 70 prisoners. The level of secure separation between the units would enable different classifications of prisoner to be held in the same prison or on the same site. Where necessary, prisoners could be moved from one unit to another. Alternatively 'clusters' of prisons could be developed to serve a locality, especially in those areas which are currently served by a prison estate located in rural areas many miles from the centres of population. In fact, these recommendations endorse or develop trends that are already happening. Local prisons often do contain 'a cross-section of the entire prisoner population, from those on remand to those serving sentences up to and including life imprisonment. They contain young offenders as well as adult prisoners' (Woolf 1991, para. 11.51). However, this is a product of population pressure on the system and the absence of sufficient secure provision. To achieve such a situation by the purposeful planning of a range of small units would imply substantially greater will and effectiveness than can presently be considered likely. The inclusion of units for women is less common at present, but certainly feasible to my knowledge, having visited a 12-woman unit situated on the top floor of a local prison in a city in the Netherlands. Clusters of prisons are also developing, as new establishments are built alongside older ones (no doubt simply as the easiest means of finding a site). The type of prison being built in 1991 as Woolf reported is somewhat larger than he recommends (the Bullingdon type provides for 650 inmates), and the feasibility of adapting this to the Woolf recommendations is discussed in the Report (para. 11.10).

The White Paper *Custody, Care and Justice* (Home Office 1991a) which sets out the Government's response to the Woolf Report identifies immediate steps to be taken towards achieving these aims:

> identify a number of existing and new local prisons which might be replanned as multi-functional community prisons; consider whether there are existing prisons which could be more directly linked to a local prison so that a prisoner's sentence plan could provide for the prisoner to progress mainly through that cluster of establishments.
>
> (Home Office 1991a, para. 5.16)

It is clear that some aspects of Woolf's proposals for community prisons are less likely to attract a positive response. Woolf saw the necessity, if both overcrowding and unnecessary transfers were to be avoided, to provide for a degree of fluctuation in demand – leaving some places unoccupied when demand is low. The White Paper does not comment on this, nor on the linked recommendation which would prohibit occupancy of a prison above its certified normal accommodation. We must therefore assume only a limited commitment to community prisons and a continuing preference for managing the prison estate as a whole, giving considerations of security, discipline and economy precedence over community links. The following comment in the White Paper most clearly illustrates the limited appreciation of Woolf's proposals for improving both community links and prison regimes: 'Prisoners wanting to benefit from particular regimes – for example the education programme at Sudbury/Foston prison – may have to choose between that or staying nearer their homes' (para. 5.5).

The Prison Department appears wedded to single-purpose prisons and sees the shifts that have occurred in different sections of the population as an obstacle in the way of Woolf's ideas. The reality could be that developing modular prisons would be no more demanding than building new single-purpose prisons – and indeed that smaller units in modular prisons are easier to change.

The White Paper also betrays a lack of interest in community links for remand prisoners. Woolf, proposing a separate Statement of Purpose for remand prisoners, considered that:

> so far as this is reasonable, a remand prisoner's containment should reflect the following considerations:
>
> (a) . . . his custody should contain no more restrictions than those which are necessary to reflect the ground on which he was refused bail. . .
>
> (b) a remand prisoner should be enabled to prepare for his trial and to have access to lawers, probation officers and the Court;
>
> (c) a remand prisoner must be permitted to maintain his links with his family, friends and community;
>
> (d) a remand prisoner should be enabled to attend to business and personal affairs, to preserve his employment and to proceed with any education or training;
>
> (e) a remand prisoner should be encouraged to spend the period on remand constructively in accordance with his wishes . . .
>
> (f) a remand prisoner should have access to welfare bodies, the Social Services and a bail unit.
>
> (para. 10.64)

The White Paper acknowledges none of this, although it does accept the need to establish constructive regimes in remand prisons. It emphasises the need for separate provision for remand prisoners, even separate sites where necessary; whereas in the case of women prisoners 'location as near to their homes as possible' is seen as the first priority (and the possibility of women's units being linked to men's establishments is discussed) (para. 5.14).

There is likely to be something of a gap between community prisons as envisaged by Woolf, and what will be achieved by implementing the White Paper. Almost certainly the timescale will be very long. Some of the advantages that could flow from community prisons have already been identified, at least by implication:

1 Staff and prisoners would have roots in the same area and would have this in common with others who contribute to the running of prisons, such as members of Boards of Visitors. Increased job satisfaction would be a by-product.
2 Services could be delivered as far as possible from the outside; this could include all employment, training and education facilities, health and welfare services. Those staff at present seconded into prisons to deliver such services would no longer be required to work full time in custodial conditions, but could undertake a mix of custodial and community duties.
3 Continuity of services could be maintained during and after sentence; even in relatively minor respects, such as contact with volunteers and prison visitors, which would nevertheless do much to improve resettlement prospects.
4 Prisoners' contact with families, employers and other external resources could be substantially improved, via greater use of home leave, temporary release and day release. This could substantially enhance the range of services which could be made available to prisoners – for example participation in technical education, and skills training.
   Prisoners' community identity would be less likely to be lost as they are received into prison.

Against that brief account of the possible advantages of a prison system committed to a community-based approach, the improvements proposed in the White Paper seem somewhat marginal. Indeed, the provision of telephones, home leave, and family visits facilities all gain greater impact the closer the prison is to the prisoner's home area, especially where access to these facilities has to be purchased by the prisoner or by his or her family.

It is perhaps unsurprising that the centralised, and heavily bureaucratic administration of the Prison Service has given such low priority to Woolf's proposal for community prisons. Despite the efforts of those relatively small groups which have regularly campaigned for such improvements, the virtual absence of informed public opinion demanding that the uncivilised nature of British prisons be improved can be seen as the critical factor.

CRIMINAL JUSTICE CONSULTATIVE COUNCIL AND LOCAL COMMITTEES

The establishment of a consultative process for criminal justice is not a new idea. While the Woolf proposals do not represent either a return to the Advisory Council on the Penal System (1968), or the adoption of Andrew Ashworth's idea of a Sentencing Council (1992), they have two features in common with both: the exposure of the judiciary and the prisons to the influence of other groups involved in the administration of criminal justice; and a permanent and consistent sytem of inter-agency consultation.

The advantages of Woolf's proposal to establish both national and local consultative groups are both political and practical. Effective co-operation between centralised and devolved services is very difficult to achieve. National policy and local ownership are not readily reconciled, either within services or between them. Devolved services are vulnerable to inconsistency of structure and provision, and this makes consensus-based dialogue difficult. On some issues, there can be greater consensus between different services working together at the local level than between operational tiers and central policy makers within a single service. There are also some notorious gaps in communication at national level between government departments. The relationship between the two key bodies involved in criminal justice, the Home Office and the Lord Chancellor's Department, is often described by the press as a power struggle, and that does not bode well for co-operation.

By any measure, and not just for the benefit of the prison system, Woolf's proposed structure is urgently needed and well conceived. There is what might be described as a patchy and variable range of existing networks established to coordinate crime prevention, juvenile crime prevention, the work of court users, juvenile cautioning, responses to mentally disordered offenders and numerous other similar types of work. These groups owe their existence to national directives as well as to local initiatives and vary in the extent of their impact on the criminal justice process itself (although diversion from justice is a key preoccupation for some). What Woolf proposes is centred on the criminal justice process and particularly on the relationship between prisons and courts.

The ground for involving sentencers in this process is carefully laid. The need of courts for more information, especially from prisons, is directly addressed (Woolf 1991, paras. 10.141–10.156). The Report identifies the Prison Service itself as being in need of more effective consultative arrangements: 'The Prison Service is directly affected by any change in sentencing policy . . . by the Courts' approach to bail . . . by changes in the nature and extent of alternatives to imprisonment' (para. 10.158).

However, Woolf is even-handed in his criticism of the insularity of the Prison Service and of the courts (para 10.160). The benefits of better communication and coordination between various other services are identified and although the Report includes Sir Brian Cubbon's opinion that 'it was necessary for sentencers to take greater account of the capacity of the prison system', it stands without comment beyond the need to bridge the gap in communications between 'all agencies in the Criminal Justice System' (para. 10.169). Greater weight is placed on the success of some inter-agency schemes for diverting minor offenders from costly and ineffective sentences of imprisonment, and the encouragement this gives to reduce the prison population 'to an unavoidable minimum'.

It therefore appears very probable that the main aim of this set of proposals is to draw the judiciary into sharing responsibility for the effectiveness of criminal justice, including the way prisons operate. A key element would be the use of local consultative committees to manage prison overcrowding and specifically to ensure that regimes in community prisons are relevant to sentencers' needs and expectations. Perhaps Lord Justice Woolf and Judge Tumim were receptive to the idea that the prison population expands to fill the number of places provided and exploited this alleged principle by encouraging local agencies able to exercise some control to take responsibility for managing the flow of prisoners. Certainly this is compatible with the exhortation that 'the ultimate aim of all those involved should be a reduction in crime' (para 10.188). Although sentencers are obviously the primary group, others, particularly the police, the Crown Prosecution Service and the Probation Service, are capable of much influence, both in relation to the prison population and future crime levels.

This type of consultative structure should be seen as distinct from that suggested earlier, which was directed at sharing with community agencies responsibility for the resettlement of offenders – not the main or proper concern of most criminal justice agencies. But Woolf's proposed structure would complement it, if it were able to ensure that prisons contained only the irreducible minimum of offenders.

The White Paper gave a commitment to the establishment of both the Criminal Justice Consultative Council and the area committees – the former 'as soon as possible' (para. 1.12) and the latter 'in principle' (para. 1.13). The Council was assembled towards the end of 1991, under the chairmanship of the Head of the Home Office and with judicial participation, and an active programme of work was inititated. The area committees began work in 1992 after much debate about judicial participation in these bodies. Prior to the appointment of Lord Justice Taylor as Lord Chief Justice, Woolf's suggestion that judges should chair area committees had not been adopted and Circuit Administrators had been chosen instead. The geographical boundaries of the area committees have also proved a source of controversy. Instead of areas based on county boundaries relevant to existing local criminal justice services (police, Crown Prosecution Service, probation and magistrates' courts), the boundaries proposed are divisions of Crown Court circuits, which sometimes cut across those of existing local sevices.

These departures from Woolf's proposals aroused strong condemnation both from penal reform groups and from representatives of other criminal justice services. The proposed structure neatly modelled the position being taken at that time by the judiciary – maintaining lofty remoteness from dialogue with other agencies, yet controlling through circuit administrators the system by which criminal justice liaison was to be set on a proper footing. The changed nature of the proposals lends weight to the notion of a power struggle between the Home Office and the Lord Chancellor's Department. The area committees as described in paragraph 1.13 of the White Paper are not unlike those discussed in a Green Paper published three years earlier *Punishment, Custody and the Community* (Home Office 1988f) which suggests that there is persistent Home Office interest in this idea. On 1 April 1992, responsibility for magistrates' courts administration passed from the Home Office to the Lord Chancellor's Department. Subsequently, after Lord Justice Taylor had taken up his appointment, the proposals for the consultative structure were modified. Area committees were, after all, to be chaired by judges, and the Consultative Council was to be chaired by a Judge (Lord Justice Farquharson). From the outside one might be forgiven for suspecting that these shifts and modifications bear the hallmark of a trade-off.

The resulting arrangements are far from ideal, and the delay which has occurred in establishing the area committees has been unfortunate, since it has coincided with the critical planning period concerning the practical arrangements for the 1991 Criminal Justice Act (and once again judicial awareness of these arrangements is very limited). Nevertheless, the area committees are the best that can be achieved for the time being, and the complexities which have beset their establishment illustrate why progress in coordinating criminal justice is so slow. It will be important to view the area committees as capable of evolving, in terms of boundaries and membership, as well as remit; and as requiring an authoritative lead to be set by the Criminal Justice Consultative Council.

PROSPECTS FOR THE FUTURE

Woolf's recommendations and proposals to prevent riots in the prisons of the future by establishing links with the communities from which prisoners are transferred were intended to fulfil a number of functions: to reduce overcrowding; to develop community prisons or clusters; to establish constructive regimes; to secure continuity of provision for individual offenders; and to preserve each prisoner's family and community ties. Judging by the appetite for change shown in the White Paper *Custody, Care and Justice* (Home Office 1991a), it will be a long time before this vision is a practical reality.

Woolf's proposals for a consultative structure to deal with the appalling insularity and lack of coordination amongst criminal justice agencies appear more likely to reach fruition, if somewhat diluted, at the local level. It might be argued that these will be talking-shops and achieve little. However, there is a strong case that dialogue between conflicting interest groups, although painfully slow, can in the long term effect more profound change than imposed measures.

Woolf's overall vision of a criminal justice system working together to reduce crime may already have been lost. But, as I have argued, implicit in his Report is an equally important approach which could yet be achieved, and that is to increase participation by community organisations in the resettlement of prisoners. This, if successful, may make a major contribution to the reduction of crime. Yet both prisons and the public seem to accept and even approve of the high level of insulation surrounding prisons and the communities in which they are situated. The price that is paid by those communities, in terms of additional crime, is bound to be considerable. Woolf addressed himself to both issues – riots and the ineffectiveness of prisons as a means of controlling crime. The limitations of the responses to the Woolf Report can ultimately be attributed to the absence of public interest in the issues. But the Woolf Report has set a vision of how prisons might work in the future, against which the reality can be tested and progress measured.

14

THE FUTURE OF THE VOLUNTARY SECTOR AND THE PRESSURE GROUPS

Vivien Stern

In Britain, the tradition of voluntary organisations and charities working to ameliorate the cruelty of society's response to crime has a long and honourable history. The Howard League, for example, was founded in 1866 to campaign for a more humane criminal justice system. NACRO, 25 years old this year, is in fact a phoenix that arose from the ashes of the National Association of Discharged Prisoners Aid Societies, founded in 1886. The Apex Trust was established in 1965 by a progressive business man, Neville Vincent, Chairman of Bovis Builders, to break down the barriers to ex-prisoners finding work. Organisations based on volunteers, such as the New Bridge, and the Society of Voluntary Associates (SOVA), go back to 1956 and 1975 respectively and are well supported. A younger body, the Prison Reform Trust, set up in 1981, has shown how influential and successful an extremely small but well-targeted and professional pressure group can be.

There are also many bodies that provide housing for offenders, ranging in size from the Stonham Housing Association with 3,200 beds, 46 per cent of which are earmarked for ex-offenders, to small organisations running perhaps one hostel. Other bodies provide education, training for work, or counselling help for offenders. Groups such as the Black Female Prisoners Scheme, Women in Prison, PROP and Inquest make an all-important impact on a specific area of concern. It is hard to imagine how public debate would be generated, how change would come about and how offenders would find advocates for their needs and rights without this spectrum of activity.

In this case, however, imagination is not needed. Illustrations are already available in Eastern and Central Europe. The rapid transition to democracy of the countries in Eastern and Central Europe has shed light on the democratic process. Democracy means more than individual citizens voting every few years for a government. Democracy also implies the development of what is called 'civil society', that is a whole range of activities that citizens engage in, as part of their participation in democracy. A democratic society needs a variety of bodies, independent of the state, that exist to provide ways for concerned citizens to further a specific cause, to help fellow citizens and to improve and change their society in ways other than through the party political process.

Such bodies, called voluntary organisations in the United Kingdom but more generally referred to as non-governmental organisations (NGOs), exist across a wide range of social activity but are particularly to be found in areas affecting human rights and freedoms. Criminal justice is, therefore, an obvious area where society needs active, independent, thriving non-governmental organisations. Governments are under pressure from the public to react repressively to crime and ignore the most basic human rights of convicted offenders and unconvicted defendants. NGOs are essential to provide a countervailing force to this pressure, just as they are also needed to mobilise community support for the social reintegration of ex-offenders.

It is thus not surprising that active steps are being taken in countries like Hungary, Czechoslovakia and Poland to bring together academics, practitioners and concerned individuals to create penal reform bodies independent of the government. For example, the Finkey Ferenc Penal Reform Association was established in Hungary on 18 February 1991, at a general meeting attended by over 100 people including government representatives, academics, reformers, non-governmental organisations and church groups. The association aims to work closely with a range of organisations including the Foundation for the Homeless, gypsy organisations and other groups. The Czechoslovak Penal Reform Association was established at the end of 1990. Its chief aims are to promote penal reform and the human rights of prisoners. In Poland the Patronal Penitentiary Association was re-established in 1989. It aims to support prisoners and their families, to reform the prison system and to aid the resettlement of ex-prisoners in society.

What is surprising, when set against the background of this international appreciation of the need for and the legitimacy of NGOs, is the degree of difficulty many voluntary organisations in Britain now face. The independence of voluntary organisations is vital. They are free to argue for a better and more humane system and to be single-minded about this because the achievement of reform is the very reason for their existence. They do not have the dual, and sometimes conflicting, responsibilities of many of the statutory bodies. However, from the late 1980s onwards, the voluntary-sector has faced unprecedented attacks on its basic role. Government funding policies provide mainly short-term grants. These grants are given to voluntary organisations on condition they are used to meet needs as defined by the Government or by statutory bodies. The effect of this is to erode the independence of voluntary organisations and prevent alternative perspectives on offenders' needs being considered.

Against this background, the Woolf Report provided for voluntary organisations a much needed boost to their legitimacy, values and style of operation. First of all, the voluntary sector had three good reasons to welcome the actual process by which the Woolf Inquiry conducted itself.[1] The Inquiry adopted an open and consultative style that reinforced voluntary sector views about the appropriate way to deal with prison questions. There is a natural tendency amongst those responsible for running prisons in any country to keep what goes on behind the walls hidden from public view. Prisons are never, even in the most enlightened of countries, caring, fair and just institutions of which any society can be proud. It is one of the major tasks of pressure groups to resist this tendency to secrecy, to expose, to interest the media and the public in what goes on in prisons and to help create a better informed public opinion that will understand the need for prison reform and support it when politicians have the courage to propose it. The method of approach of the Woolf Inquiry, with public hearings into the events surrounding the disturbances, was a welcome boost to a more open approach.

Second, voluntary organisations try to get a better deal for those at the bottom, those with the least power, namely prisoners. Therefore they welcomed most warmly the fact that, as Rod Morgan, one of the assessors to the Inquiry, has written 'great efforts were made to give a voice to prisoners generally' (Morgan 1991, pp. 720–1). Lord Justice Woolf wrote personally to every prisoner known to be in one of the six 'target prisons' at the time of the disturbances and also wrote a general letter to all other prisoners. The responses sent in by prisoners were analysed and summarised in the Woolf Report. The consideration of the opinions of those whose voices are not often heard added considerably to the depth and impact of the Report.

Third, the voluntary organisations had good reason to welcome the decision of Lord Justice Woolf to hold a series of public seminars where people from voluntary and non-governmental organisations were given an opportunity to contribute and participate on an equal basis with government officials. As Rod Morgan makes clear in the article mentioned above, the system of giving evidence to inquiries, committees and commissions is heavily weighted against non-governmental witnesses. Government departments can afford to assign staff to the task full time and provide statistical and research back-up. They have the resources to produce and publish substantial volumes of evidence and the supporting material. Voluntary organisations have scarcely any research and statistical back-up. For them, providing evidence to inquiries, even when the subject matter goes to the heart of an organisation's *raison d'être*, has to take its place with many other tasks. The freedom for voluntary organisations to adjust priorities is very limited: commitments already entered into and often funded on short timescales with no leeway have to be displaced. Governments are rarely far-sighted enough to provide funding for NGOs to do this work, and private, charitable funders are more interested in funding practical projects that provide immediate help to those suffering from the deficiencies of the system than policy work to make the system better.

The method adopted at the Woolf Inquiry went some way to reducing this great inequality. In the public seminars all participants, non-governmental and governmental, were treated as equals; given an equal chance to participate and listened to with equal respect. The voluntary organisations involved in the process greatly appreciated the opportunity presented by this method and put all their available resources into participating in it. It provided an opportunity that is all too rare in their experience and a model that could be usefully copied elsewhere.

Through the opportunity provided by the seminars, the non-governmental sector had a unique opportunity to exert its influence. Certainly the Report has accepted a diagnosis of the ills of the prison system that accords almost completely with the analyses put forward by voluntary organisations over many years. Its recommendations, too, are familiar. Most of them echoed calls voluntary organisations had been making throughout the 1980s for more justice in prisons, minimum standards, a better coordinated criminal justice system and purposeful and constructive regimes.

Voluntary organisations could also give nothing less than enthusiastic support for the most revolutionary aspect of the Woolf Report, the challenge that it posed to the prison system's view of its task over many years. The most revolutionary aspect of the Woolf Report, which comes as a shock to experienced commentators reading it for the first time, is the way it talks about prisoners as if they were the same as everyone else. It talks about prisoners as if some are decent and brave; some are horrible, cruel and vicious; some are pathetic and frightened; some are unutterably normal. But they are people, just like everyone else, and are entitled to be treated as such. This may not sound very revolutionary. However, we have become accustomed to prison reports that do not describe prisoners as if they were people. They have suggested that they represent a chemical mixture which, when certain elements are mixed together, becomes explosive. They have regretted that they have nothing to do all day because inactivity breeds laziness and this, in turn, may lead to individual deterioration, rather like vegetables that go off if they are not eaten soon enough.

With that starting point, conceiving of prisoners as human beings, it is not surprising that Lord Justice Woolf made the recommendations he did. He found a system based on a series of principles diametrically opposed to those that would guide it if it were set up to meet the needs of people. What the Inquiry team found was a system which had lost its rationale. Since the ideas of treating prisoners and somehow 'curing' them had been discredited, the prison system had operated without any guiding principles, responding to a series of conflicting messages, with no clear focus on how best to carry out its actual task – the custody of human beings.

In constructing his analysis, Woolf did not start from the needs of managers, administrators or system builders. He started from the needs of people that live in a place and people that work in a place. And he concluded that what people living in prison want first of all is to be as near as possible to where they belong, to where they live and to where they have access most easily to what really matters to them – their family, their friends, their community, their chances of building a new life when they come out. Woolf therefore recommended that, wherever possible, prisons should be community prisons so that prisoners could be kept as near to their homes as possible. The whole paraphernalia of local prisons, training prisons, specialised prisons should be more or less dismantled and the basic premise of allocation should be that prisoners normally go to the prison closest to their homes. This is a principle of the utmost simplicity and it is the opposite principle to the one that has shaped the prison system so far.

The second basic need that Woolf identified in prisoners is the need to be treated like a human being. People do not respond well to being treated like commodities, brown paper parcels that can be shipped around from one place to another without explanation or discussion. People respond better when somebody in authority explains, for example, how imperative it is that a move from one prison to another a hundred miles away has to take place; why, therefore, a training course has to be abandoned; and why it is essential that family visits will be made more difficult. As the Report says: 'the Prison Service should adopt the practice as a matter of good and sensible administration and management, of giving reasons to a prisoner for any decision which materially and adversely affects him' (para. 14.300).

Woolf is not calling for a few reforms, a little tinkering with a system which is basically healthy. As the NACRO alternative White Paper, *A Really Fresh Start*, says:

> To regard the prison riots of April 1990 as serious but isolated events that did no more than retard existing developments, or required no more than some slight changes of course, would be to reject the message of Lord Justice Woolf's report . . . . . . The disturbances were symptomatic of serious and long standing difficulties in the prison system.
>
> (NACRO 1991b, para. 2.3)

The NACRO report also concludes:

> That the disturbances were symptoms of a long-standing failure to provide justice and humanity in prisons. It follows that the improvement of physical conditions, and the provision of better facilities, desirable as these are, will not in themselves be enough to heal what must be healed in the prison system.
>
> (para.2.4)

To change the culture of a small organisation with a few years' tradition behind it is difficult. To change one of the biggest organisations in the United Kingdom, with traditions going back at least to 1877, is a frighteningly demanding task. Even if all those responsible believe radical change is required and are totally committed to bringing it about, great imagination and courage will be needed to make it a reality.

Thus, the first clear role for voluntary organisations is to ensure that the Woolf Report is taken note of, that plans are drawn up for its implementation and that these plans are adhered to. Conferences organised by the Prison Reform Trust and others, and publications such as *Who's Afraid of Implementing Woolf* by the Prison Reform Trust and the Howard League (1991) and NACRO's 'alternative White Paper' (1991b), are good examples of basic important work that is appropriate to NGOs. There is no other non-political source of outside pressure to ensure deadlines are kept, new procedures brought in when agreed, pilot schemes set up and evaluated when promised. But the voluntary sector can contribute more to the implementation of Woolf than by simply applying pressure to ensure that reform does not get buried in the press of day to day events in a traditionally crisis-prone service.

It may be that some of the principles and practices which, of necessity, guide and motivate the work of voluntary organisations can also be of use in implementation. In particular, the Prison Service will need to develop a new openness and devise techniques for involving staff at all levels, as well as outsiders. Voluntary organisations have always needed help from all quarters to achieve their objectives and, in order to stimulate discussion and debate, they tend to operate with the greatest possible openness. In the post-Woolf era of change, the Prison Service needs to do the same. Currently it is quite untrammelled by advice from any outsiders. Indeed, the absence of structures for seeking outside advice, support or commitment is quite remarkable. Apart from the two non-Executive members on the Prisons Board there are only two standing Advisory Committees, the Education Consultative Committee and the AIDS Advisory Committee. This inward-looking approach does not help the Prison Service and will certainly not assist the implementation of far-reaching reform. Changing the culture of an organisation like the Prison Service also requires openness and a new view of how staff should be involved in their work. It would greatly aid the process of realising the vision in the Woolf Report if the Government were to establish a consultative group whose duty it would be to oversee the very necessary and far-reaching programme of change. This body could include representatives of a wide range of groups, including people from the voluntary sector, academics and practitioners with experience from the public and private sectors. Its function would be distinct from that of the Criminal Justice Consultative Council.

Widespread discussion with all prison staff, uniformed and otherwise, needs to be generated. Every prison needs to provide at least one day-long opportunity for staff to discuss the Report and its implications in a structured way. Such sessions could be arranged by the Prison Service itself or they could be organised through the involvement of independent organisations. Seminars might be local or regional and should involve prison staff and some interested outsiders with experience of changing organisational cultures. Members of the consultative group proposed above could be drawn into chairing or participating in such seminars.

There also needs to be a new approach to pilot projects. In the past, pilot projects in the Prison Service have usually been one-off attempts by enterprising individuals which have died when the progenitor has moved on. A different view of pilot initiatives needs to be taken. Many of the changes the Woolf Report recommends need to be worked out in practice in particular prisons, or particular parts of the system, before being implemented in all establishments. There should be experiments, for example, in how community prisons might best be set up. No doubt individual governors, granted delegated powers, would want to try out new ideas, but one of the lessons of the past is that experiments must be properly planned, monitored, evaluated and disseminated. The way forward might be for the central consultative group recommended above to devise a series of experiments based in particular prisons and to work out with people in that prison how the experiments should be evaluated and publicised.

The voluntary sector has experience in developing ways of implementing change that should be useful to the process. It also has particular expertise in many of the policy areas relevant to the implementation of the Woolf Report. Certainly, the ideas and experience of the voluntary sector could be drawn upon in devising different ways of turning existing establishments into community prisons, whether the emphasis be on retaining family links or on involving the local community in the work and services of the prison. The experience of the voluntary sector with particular projects shows what can be done. For example, in October 1990 NACRO established a job-club near Holloway Prison exclusively for women prisoners serving sentences there. Women are released on temporary licence to attend four mornings a week. They undergo a job-search programme, apply for jobs and attend job interviews. Women who are successful may start work before release. The results have been encouraging: according to evidence given to the House of Commons Employment Committee, 73 prisoners attended the job-club up to 28 May 1991: 24 gained paid employment; 11 had undertaken voluntary work; 6 had started further education or training; 8 had been released and were awaiting the outcome of job applications; 17 had not yet achieved a positive outcome and 7 had returned to the prison for breaches of discipline.[2]

Another model is the employment activity centre run by the Apex Trust in Pentonville Prison, North London. The centre provides a job-search facility, funded by the Employment Service and run like job-clubs in the community. There is also a training advice service to assist prisoners in identifying their employment goal and the training and education they will need in order to achieve it. The training advisor then links prisoners with the appropriate local training and education provider. Employers such as British Rail and Touche Ross are involved in the centre by assisting prisoners in the development of interview skills. Of the first 60 prisoners dealt with by the centre, 14 have found jobs and a further 16 have gone into further education or training.

General community organisations also have a role. For the past three or four years a worker from a local Citizens Advice Bureau has been visiting the library at Holloway Prison on one day a week for a couple of hours. She holds a 'surgery' for the women, offering confidential advice on a range of problems, including housing benefits, poll tax, social security and debt. Another example comes from East Sutton Park, an open prison for women in Kent, where in June 1991, NACRO's Women Prisoners' Resource Centre, in partnership with the prisoners and prison staff, organised a special day of events called 'Actively Women'. Many organisations providing services for women in prison and in the community participated – including Shelter, the Apex Trust, Women Against Rape and the Hungerford Drug Project. Prisoners could get information and advice on individual problems and, in the afternoon, they took part in workshops covering resettlement, 'mothers behind bars', prisoners' rights, violence against women and other topics.

The voluntary sector also has something valuable to contribute to the debate on what prisons provide for inmates and how prisoners can be given opportunities to take decisions and become more responsible for their own lives. Over the years voluntary organisations that work with ex-prisoners and other offenders have developed a way of working which is distinctive and which derives from the values of the voluntary movement. For example, underlying the work of NACRO and other bodies in the offender field, is a belief that all people have worth, whatever terrible thing they may have done. Therefore, they have a right, in spite of being offenders, to the same access to resources, programmes and facilities as everyone else in the community. The view is strongly held that resources should be made available to offenders and ex-offenders that will make them feel there is a good reason to stay out of trouble in the future – that society actually thinks something of them and values them. Thus, those providing housing try to ensure that hostels for homeless offenders are decent places with reasonable furniture and good living conditions. Training programmes run by voluntary organisations are designed to assess what people are good at and link that to preparation for real jobs in the locality. In all the work of

NACRO and other projects, an attempt is made to start with an individual as a person who has strengths and positive attributes, as well as a lot of problems, rather than the other way around.

NACRO recently carried out an exercise which required those working in projects with offenders to clarify as precisely as possible how they worked; this exercise suggested that certain elements could be defined. For example, NACRO project staff aimed to treat the users with respect. One way of showing respect was to allow people to make decisions, such as signing for a housing tenancy and accepting the responsiblities a tenancy brings. In work training schemes trainees were asked to do a self-evaluation over four weeks and make a commitment to their own progress. Treating each person as an individual was also an element. Plans and programmes were worked out for each resident or trainee. Achievements, however small, were recognised and given value. A fundamental assumption was that everyone has potential skills and talents.

It would be unrealistic to assume that values which are applied to people who are participating in a project in the community from their own choice and because they believe it will help them, can be directly transferred to other people in the coercive setting of custody. Yet some aspects are transferable. Joint seminars between prison staff and voluntary organisations providing services for offenders would benefit the operations of both groups by helping to clarify specific methods of working which could be shared.

As the Woolf Report made clear, the proper treatment of prisoners critically hinges on the attitudes and morale of prison staff. In the Report a letter from one prisoner is quoted as saying:

> I did agree with the riot at Manchester because something had to be done. Because of the inhuman way they treated every inmate; like animals and not like human beings. I keep hearing the prisons are under-staffed but I have spent two years in Long Lartin prison which is the only prison where inmates are treated as human beings, allowed to think for themselves as far as prisons allow. It is not that the prison service wants extra staff, they want retraining to treat people as human beings.
>
> (Annex 2E, para. I.7)

Voluntary organisations have necessarily had to acquire considerable skills in developing shared values in staff and volunteers, in motivating people to work for low financial rewards in difficult circumstances and in mobilising a wide range of people to provide support for a project or a course of action. NACRO's experience since 1985 of training prison officers in providing housing and employment advice to prisoners, shows that these skills are relevant and transferable to the custodial setting. Such expertise could be drawn upon in formulating the staff development plans and programmes that should be an essential component in the implementation of Woolf's recommendations.

It is greatly to the credit of Lord Justice Woolf that he included in his terms of reference a consideration of the role which prisons play in the wider criminal justice system. To ignore the rest of the criminal justice process and simply devise policies for prisons is illogical and unworkable, as experience up till now has shown. Woolf's recommendation for a central Criminal Justice Consultative Council and for local inter-agency machinery, subsequently accepted in the White Paper, are great steps forward. However, they could easily fail. Instead of looking at wider strategic questions, the members could spend their time complaining about the problems they face in their roles and the shortcomings of the other criminal justice services. The subject area could easily be narrowed down to the technicalities and details of managing the system. Disillusionment could set in if members neither aim for nor see positive results following their deliberations. Without considerable input from people committed to success the meetings could degenerate into occasions for protecting territory. The voluntary sector has considerable relevant experience of local and national consultative machinery geared to strategic change and this should be harnessed.

During the 1980s, voluntary organisations played an important role as catalysts in bringing about major changes in ways of dealing with juvenile offenders. In addition to using government grants to set up community-based schemes for offenders, the voluntary sector was able to bring together at a local level senior representatives from criminal justice agencies and social services to develop common policies aimed at reducing levels of crime, prosecution and custody. Experience with juveniles also demonstrates the valuable role which the voluntary sector can play as a national development body in promoting and monitoring the impact of local initiatives and in encouraging consistent policy development (NACRO 1991c). The lessons from the achievements with juveniles are currently being applied in other areas of the criminal justice system, particularly in respect of young adults and mentally disordered offenders. With both groups, the voluntary sector has a substantial contribution to make, both in providing services and in stimulating more effective inter-agency arrangements.

A major role of non-governmental organisations in most countries is the protection of basic human rights. A recent report written by a distinguished group of Commonwealth experts for the meeting of Commonwealth Heads of Government in Harare, recommended:

> The Commonwealth Heads of Government should give explicit recognition to the importance of NGOs in the protection of human rights. They should urge governments not to view NGOs as elements

> hostile to government but as potential allies in the search for human rights to which governments have committed themselves.
>
> (Commonwealth Human Rights Initiative 1991, p. 172)

In the area of respect for basic human rights and adherence to international norms and guidelines the record of the United Kingdom is not impressive. Rule 11.3 of the European Prison Rules says: 'In principle untried prisoners shall be detained separately from convicted prisoners unless they consent to being accommodated or involved together in organised activities beneficial to them.' This rule is not observed in prisons in England and Wales. Among the other provisions of the European Prison Rules which this country has ignored for years are:

> Rule 14, which requires that prisoners 'shall normally be lodged during the night in individual cells';
>
> Rule 17 which requires arrangements for decent sanitation 'to enable prisoners to comply with the needs of nature when necessary';
>
> Rule 71 which requires that useful work or other purposeful activity shall be provided 'to keep prisoners actively employed for a normal working day'.

The Woolf Report makes it clear that justice has been gravely lacking in prisons in the past. It shows how a lack of justice contributes to riots and requires that justice must be acknowledged as a priority alongside security and control in the prison system from henceforth. The White Paper accepts this requirement. Here the contribution of the voluntary sector has yet to reach its full potential. Whilst the Children's Legal Centre, Liberty, Justice and other groups have taken up particular abuses, the range of questions on which important work remains to be done is substantial. The treatment of life-sentence prisoners, the system of additional days for prison offences, the treatment of Category A prisoners, the abuse of confidentiality of medical records, and religious provision for minorities are but a few examples.

Finally, it is incumbent on the voluntary sector to look beyond the Woolf Report, to what it did not cover and to what changes need to be made beyond the scope of the Woolf recommendations. For many proper reasons, the Report did not look at the imprisonment of women. Yet here are many matters which require pressure and change. Women are still the poor relations in the prison system. Many of those imprisoned are in prison inappropriately. They are often held in prisons far from their home area. Visits from families and children are difficult. As Elaine Player observes in Chapter 12, if the Woolf principles were applied to women's imprisonment significant changes would have to follow. Much further discussion on women's imprisonment is needed and the Woolf implementation process must include this.

There are other important post-Woolf questions. For good reasons, integral sanitation is being provided after years of delay and obfuscation.

To end slopping-out is a great step forward. But it is now necessary for reformers to ask 'Should people be required to live, eat and sleep in a lavatory?' It seems to me that the voluntary sector, in its role of stimulator of new and radical thinking, needs to build on the Woolf Report and, in relation to its implementation, to call into question the model of imprisonment currently in force throughout the world. Once people are near home and retaining their family ties, the community is coming in and prisoners are going out to the community, the question will be asked 'Why do we have these expensive, damaging places? We can surely think of something better.'

Vaclav Havel, the former President of Czechoslovakia, spent several years in prison and from there he wrote frequently to his wife, Olga. In one of the letters he managed to get past the very strict censor he wrote:

> I never feel sorry for myself, as one might expect, but only for the other prisoners and altogether, for the fact that prisons must exist and that they are as they are, and that mankind has not so far invented a better way of coming to terms with certain things.
>
> (Havel 1990, p. 270)

It is to be hoped that the Woolf Report will have begun the process of finding a better way of coming to terms with certain things.

NOTES

1 For a description of the methodology adopted, see the Introduction to this volume.

2 Hansard, House of Commons Employment Committee, Session 1990/91, Employment in Prisons and for Ex-Offenders, Minutes of Evidence, Wednesday 5 June 1991, para 35.

REFERENCES

LIST OF CASES

Arbon v. Anderson, [1943] K.B. 252; [1943] 1 All E.R. 154
Campbell and Fell v. United Kingdom (1984), 7 E.H.R.R. 165
Christofi v. The Home Office, The Times, July 31, 1975
Council for Civil Service Unions v. Minister for the Civil Service, [1985] A.C. 374
Davis v. The Prison Commissioners, The Times, November 21, 1963
Egerton v. The Home Office (1978), Crim. L.R. 494
Ellis v. The Home Office, [1953] 2 Q.B. 135
Ferguson v. The Home Office, The Times, October 8, 1977
Fraser v. Mudge, [1975] 3 All E.R. 78, C.A.
Golder v. The United Kingdom (1983), 1 E.H.R.R. 524
H. v. The Home Office, Independent, May 6, 1992
Hone v. Maze Prison Board of Visitors, [1988] 1 All E.R. 321
In Re Carroll's Application (1987), 10 N.I.J.B. 23
In Re Findlay, [1985] A.C. 318
In Re O'Hare's Application (1989), 1 N.I.J.B. 1
In Re Reynold's Application (1987), N.I.J.B. 82
Kiss v. The United Kingdom (1976), 7 D & R 55; 1977 Y.B. EUR. CONV. On HUM. RTS. 156 (Eur. Comm'n on Hum. Rts.)
Knight and Others v. The Home Office [1990] 3 All E.R. 237
Leech v. Parkhurst Prison Deputy Governor, [1988] 1 All E.R. 485 H.L.
Lloyd v. McMahon, [1987] A.C. 625
Middleweek v. Chief Constable of the Merseyside Police and Another, [1990] 3 All E.R. 662
Payne v. Lord Harris, [1981] 1 W.L.R. 754; (1981) Crim. L.R. 838
Pullen v. The Prison Commissioners, [1957] 1 W.L.R. 1186
R v. Albany Prison Board of Visitors, ex p. Mayo, unreported March 18, 1985
R v. Blundeston Prison Board of Visitors, ex p. Fox-Taylor, [1982] 1 All E.R. 646
R v. Blundeston Prison Board of Visitors, ex p. Norley, unreported July 4, 1984
R v. Dartmoor Prison Board of Visitors, ex p. Smith, [1986] 2 All E.R. 651, C.A.
R v. Deputy Governor Camp Hill Prison, ex p. King, [1985] Q.B. 735
R v. Deputy Governor Parkhurst Prison and Others, ex p. Hague, [1990] 3 All E.R. 687, C.A.
R v. Deputy Governor Parkhurst Prison, ex p. Hague, [1992] 1 A.C. 58
R v. Frankland Prison Board of Visitors, ex p. Lewis, [1986] 1 All E.R. 272
R v. Governor of the Maze Prison, ex p. McKiernan, [1985] 6 N.I.J.B. 6

R v. Highpoint Prison Board of Visitors, ex p. McConkey, The Times, September 23, 1982
R v. Hull Prison Board of Visitors, ex p. St. Germain, [1978] 1 Q.B. 678
R v. Hull Prison Board of Visitors, ex p. St. Germain (No. 1), [1979] Q.B. 425
R v. Hull Prison Board of Visitors, ex p. St. Germain (No. 2), [1979] 3 All E.R. 545
R v. Nottingham Prison Board of Visitors, ex p. Moseley, The Times, January 23, 1981
R v. The Parole Board, ex p. Wilson, [1992] 2 All E.R. 576
R v. Risley Remand Centre Board of Visitors, ex p. Draper, The Times, May 24, 1988
R v. Secretary of State for the Home Department, ex p. Anderson, [1984] Q.B. 778
R v. Secretary of State for the Home Department, ex p. Benson, The Times, November 8, 1988
R v. Secretary of State for the Home Department, ex p. Cox, The Times, September 10, 1991
R v. Secretary of State for the Home Department, ex p. Creamer, Independent, October 2, 1992
R v. Secretary of State for the Home Department, ex p. Gunnell (1984), Crim. L.R. 170; (1985), Crim. L.R. 105
R v. Secretary of State for the Home Department, ex p. Handscomb (1987), 86 Cr. App. R. 59
R v. Secretary of State for the Home Department, ex p. Khan, [1985] 1 All E.R. 40, C.A.
R v. Secretary of State for the Home Department, ex p. Leech (No. 2), The Times, May 20, 1993
R v. Secretary of State for the Home Department, ex p. McAvoy, [1984] 3 All E.R. 417
R v. Secretary of State for the Home Department, ex p. McComb, [1991] C.O.D. 415
R v. Secretary of State for the Home Department, ex p. Ruddock, [1987] 2 All E.R. 518
R v. Secretary of State for the Home Department, ex p. Tarrant, [1984] 1 All E.R. 799
R v. Wandsworth Prison Board of Visitors, ex p. Raymond, The Times, June 17, 1985
Raymond v. Honey, [1983] 1 A.C. 1
Ruiz v. Estelle 503 F. Supp. 1265 (S.D. Tex. 1980); affirmed 1982 – 679 F. 2d 1115 (5th Cir. 1982); cert. denied 1983 – 460 U.S. 1042 (1983)
Silver v. The United Kingdom (1983), 5 E.H.R.R. 347
Thynne, Wilson and Gunnell v. The United Kingdom (1991), 13 E.H.R.R. 135
Weeks v. The United Kingdom (1988), 10 E.H.R.R. 293
Williams v. The Home Office (No. 2), [1981] 1 All E.R. 1211; [1982] 2 All E.R. 564, C.A.
X v. The United Kingdom (1982), 4 E.H.R.R. 188

BIBLIOGRAPHY

Adams, R. (1992) *Prison Riots in Britain and the USA*, London: Macmillan.

Adler, M. and Longhurst, B. (1991) 'The Future of Imprisonment in Scotland: A Great Leap Forward?', unpublished paper.

Advisory Council on the Penal System (1968) *The Regime for Long-Term Prisoners in Conditions on Maximum Security* (Radzinowicz Report), London: HMSO.

Aldous, G. and Alder, J. (1985) *Applications for Judicial Review,* London: Butterworth.

American Correctional Association (1981) *Standards for Adult Correctional Institutions,* 2nd ed., January.

Andrews, G. (ed.) (1991) *Citizenship,* London: Lawrence and Wishart.

Ashmore, Z., Creamer, M., Evans, R., MacLean, M. and Readman, M. (1988), *Functional Information About Unconvicted Prisoners,* London: Home Office, Directorate of Psychological Services Report, Series II, no. 163.

Ashworth, A. (1992) *Sentencing and Criminal Justice,* London: Weidenfeld and Nicolson.

Atholl, J. (1953) *Prison on the Moor*, London: John Long Ltd.

Austin, C. and Ditchfield, J. (1985) 'Internal ventilation of grievances: applications and petitions', in M. Maguire, J. Vagg and R. Morgan (eds) *Accountability and Prisons: Opening up a Closed World*, London: Tavistock.

Baker, K. (1991) 'The Woolf Report: an agenda for action', paper to the Prison Reform Trust Conference, Church House, Westminster, 18 July 1991.

Bottomley, A. K. and Hay, W. (eds) (1991) *Special Units for Difficult Prisoners*, Hull: Centre for Criminology and Criminal Justice, University of Hull.

Bottoms, A. E. (1990) 'The aims of imprisonment', in D. Garland (ed.), *Justice, Guilt and Forgiveness in the Penal System*, Edinburgh: Edinburgh University, Centre for Theology and Public Issues, Paper No. 18.

—— (1991) 'The control of long term prisoners in England: beyond the Control Review Committee Report', in A. K. Bottomley, and W. Hay (eds) *Special Units for Difficult Prisoners*, Hull: Centre for Criminology and Criminal Justice, University of Hull.

Bottoms, A. E. and Light, R. (1987) *Problems of Long-Term Imprisonment*, Aldershot: Gower.

Bouloc, B. (1991) *Penologie*, Paris: Dalloz.

Boyle, J. (1977) *A Sense of Freedom*, Edinburgh: Canongate.

—— (1984) *The Pain of Confinement*, Edinburgh: Canongate.

Brody, S. (1976) *The Effectiveness of Sentencing: A Review of the Literature*, Home Office Research Study No. 35, London: HMSO.

Brookes, S. (1991) *The Effect of Re-Offending on Bail on Crime in Avon and Somerset*, Bristol: Avon and Somerset Police.

Butler, D. and Kavanagh, D. (1980) *The British General Election of 1979*, London: Macmillan.

Campbell, T.D. (1983) *The Left and Rights*, London: Routledge & Kegan Paul.

Carlen, P. (1983) *Women's Imprisonment*, London: Routledge & Kegan Paul.

Carlen, P., Hicks, J., O'Dwyer, J., Christina, D. and Tchaikovsky, C. (1985) *Criminal Women*, Cambridge: Polity Press.

Casale, S. (1984) *Minimum Standards for Prison Establishments*, London: NACRO.

Casale, S. and Plotnikoff, J. (1989) *Minimum Standards in Prisons: A Programme of Change*, London: NACRO.

—— (1990) *Regimes for Remand Prisoners*, London: Prison Reform Trust.

Coid, J. W. (1988a) 'Mentally abnormal prisoners on remand: I – rejected or accepted by the NHS', *British Medical Journal* 296, pp. 1779–82.

—— (1988b) 'Mentally abnormal prisoners on remand: II – comparison of services provided by Oxford and Wessex regions', *British Medical Journal* 296, pp. 1783–4.

Commonwealth Human Rights Initiative (1991) *Put Our World to Rights*, a report by a non-government advisory group chaired by the Hon. Flora MacDonald, London: Commonwealth Human Rights Initiative.

Conlon, G. (1990) *Proved Innocent*, London: Hamish Hamilton.

Conservative Party (1979) *The Conservative Manifesto 1979*, London: Conservative Party.

Cooke, D. J. (1989a) 'Containing violent prisoners: an analysis of the Barlinnie Special Unit', *British Journal of Criminology* 29 (2), pp. 129–43.

—— (1989b) 'The Barlinnie Special Unit', in Scottish Prison Service, *Current Issues in Scottish Prisons: Systems of Accountability and Regimes for Difficult Prisoners*, Occasional Paper No. 2, Edinburgh: HMSO.

—— (1991) 'Violence in prisons: the influence of regime factors, *Howard Journal of Criminal Justice*, 30 (2), pp. 95–109.

Corbin, A. L. (1919) 'Legal analysis and terminology', *Yale Law Journal* 29, pp. 163–7.

Council of Europe (1973) *Council of Europe Standard Minimum Rules for the Treatment of Prisoners*, Strasbourg: Council of Europe.

—— (1991) Committee for the Prevention of Torture and Inhuman and Degrading Treatment or Punishment, *Report to the United Kingdom Government on the Visit to the United Kingdom from 29 July to 10 August 1990*, Strasbourg: Council of Europe.

—— (1992) *Report to the Swedish Government on the Visit to Sweden Carried Out by the European Committee for the Prevention of Torture and Inhuman and Degrading Treatment or Punishment from 5 to 14 May 1991*, Strasbourg: Council of Europe.

Cotgreave, C. J. (1989) 'Specialist social work: what do prisoners need?', *Prison Service Journal* 74, pp. 4–5, 43.

Coyle, A. (1989) 'Incidents in the Scottish Prison Service: history and response', in Scottish Prison Service, *Current Issues in Scottish Prisons: Systems of Accountability and Regimes for Difficult Prisoners*, Occasional Paper, No. 2, Edinburgh: HMSO.

Criminal Lunacy (Departmental) Commission (1882) *Report of the Commission to Inquire into the Subject of Criminal Lunacy*, London: HMSO, Cm. 3418.

Cross, R. (1971) *Punishment, Prison and the Public*, London: Stevens.

Crow, I. and Cove, J. (1984) 'Ethnic minorities and the courts', *Criminal Law Review*, pp. 413–17.

Darkins, A. (1991) *The Implications of Changing the Prison Medical Service to a Prison Health Service*, London: Directorate of Prison Medical Services.

Deitch, M. (1990) 'Developing and Enforcing Minimum Standards in Prisons', paper presented at the Centre for Criminology, University of Edinburgh, 6 November 1990.

Dell, S., Grounds, A. T., James, K. and Robertson, G. (1991) *Mentally Disordered Remanded Prisoners*, Report to the Home Office, Cambridge: Institute of Criminology.

Departmental Committee (1895) 'Report from the Departmental Committee on Prisons' (Gladstone Report) C. 7702, Parliamentary Papers (1895), vol. 56.

Department of Health (1989) *Working for Patients*, London: HMSO Cm. 555.

—— (1991a) *Fourth Biennial Report of the Mental Health Act Commission 1989–1991*, London: HMSO.

—— (1991b) *Drug Misuse and Dependence – Guidelines on Clinical Management*, London: HMSO.

—— (1992) *The Health of the Nation – A Strategy for Health in England*, London: HMSO, Cm. 1986.

Department of Health and Social Security (1974) *Revised Report of the Working Party on Security in NHS Psychiatric Hospitals* (Glancy Report), London: Department of Health and Social Security.

Department of Health/Home Office (1991a) *Review of Health and Social Services for Mentally Disordered Offenders and Others Requiring Similar Services: Reports of the Service Advisory Groups; An Overview with Glossary*, London: Department of Health/Home Office.

—— (1991b) *Review of Health and Social Services for Mentally Disordered Offenders and Others Requiring Similar Services: Report of the Prison Advisory Group*, London: Department of Health/Home Office.

—— (1991c) *Review of Health and Social Services for Mentally Disordered Offenders and Others Requiring Similar Services: Report of the Hospital Advisory Group*, London: Department of Health/Home Office.

—— (1991d) *Review of Health and Social Services for Mentally Disordered Offenders and Others Requiring Similar Services: Report of the Community Advisory Group*, London: Department of Health/Home Office.

—— (1992a) *Review of Health and Social Services for Mentally Disordered Offenders and*

Others Requiring Similar Services: Report of the Finance Advisory Group, London: Department of Health/Home Office.

—— (1992b) *Review of Health and Social Services for Mentally Disordered Offenders and Others Requiring Similar Services: Report of the Staffing and Training Advisory Group*, London: Department of Health/Home Office.

—— (1992c) *Review of Health and Social Services for Mentally Disordered Offenders and Others Requiring Similar Services: Final Summary Report*, London: HMSO Cm. 2088.

DiIulio, J. (1987) *Governing Prisons: A Comparative Study of Correctional Management*, New York: Free Press.

Ditchfield, J. (1990) *Control in Prisons: A Review of the Literature*, Home Office Research Study 118, London: HMSO.

Dobash, R., Dobash, R. and Gutteridge, S. (1986) *The Imprisonment of Women*, Oxford: Basil Blackwell.

Downes, D. (ed.) (1992) *Unravelling Criminal Justice: Eleven British Studies*, London: Macmillan.

Dunbar, I. (1989) *Report to the Secretary of State of the Inquiries into a major Disturbance at HM Remand Centre Risley 30 April to 3 May 1989 and the Circumstances surrounding the Disturbance – Summary*, London: Prison Department.

Dworkin, R. (1977) *Taking Rights Seriously*, London: Duckworth.

East, W. N. and Hubert, W. H. de B. (1939) *The Psychological Treatment of Crime*, London: HMSO.

Edgar, D. (1991) 'Are you being served', *Marxism Today* 28 May.

Emery, F. E. (1970) *Freedom and Justice Within Walls: The Bristol Prison Experiment*, London: Tavistock.

Fitzgerald, E. (1985) 'Prison discipline and the courts' in M. Maguire, J. Vagg and R. Morgan (eds) *Accountability and Prisons: Opening Up a Closed World*, London: Tavistock.

Fitzgerald, M. (1977) *Prisoners in Revolt*, Harmondsworth: Penguin.

Fitzgerald, M. and Sim, J. (1979) *British Prisons*, 2nd edn, Oxford: Basil Blackwell, 1982.

—— (1980) 'Legitimating the prison crisis: a critical review of the May Report', *The Howard Journal of Criminal Justice* 19, pp. 73–84.

Fitzpatrick, P. (1984) 'Law and societies', *Osgoode Hall Law Journal* 22, pp. 115–38.

Forsyth, C. F. (1988) 'The provenance and protection of legitimate expectations', *Cambridge Law Journal* 47 (2), pp. 238–60.

Foucault, M. (1980) 'Two lectures', in *Power/Knowledge*, New York: Pantheon.

Fox, L. W. (1952) *The English Prison and Borstal System*, London: Routledge.

Furby, L., Weinrott, M. and Blackshaw, L. (1989) 'Sex offender recidivism: a review', *Psychological Bulletin* 105 (1), pp. 3–30.

Garland, D. (1990) *Punishment and Modern Society*, Oxford: Clarendon Press.

Gearty, C. (1991) 'The prisons and the courts' in J. Muncie and R. Sparks (eds) *Imprisonment: European Perspectives*, London: Harvester.

Genders, E. and Player, E. (1988) 'Women lifers: assessing the experience' in A. Morris and C. Wilkinson (eds) *Women and the Penal System*, Cambridge: Cambridge Cropwood Conference Series 19.

—— (1989) *Race Relations in Prisons*, Oxford: Clarendon Press.

Gerwith, A. (1984) 'The epistemology of human rights', *Social Philosophy and Policy* 1 (2), pp. 1–24.

Gottfredson, S. D. and McConville, S. (eds) (1987) *America's Correctional Crisis: Prison Population and Public Policy*, New York: Greenwood.

Gunn, J., Maden, T. and Swinton, M. (1991) *Mentally Disordered Prisoners*, London: Home Office.

Hall, S. (1988) *The Hard Road to Renewal*, London: Verso.

Hall, S., Critcher, C., Jefferson, T., Clarke, J. and Roberts, B. (1978) *Policing the Crisis*, London: Macmillan.

Harding, S. (1987) *Feminism and Methodology*, Milton Keynes: Open University Press.

Harding, T. (1987) 'Health in prisons', *Council of Europe Prison Information Bulletin* December, pp. 8–11.

—— (1989) 'The application of the European Convention of Human Rights to the field of psychiatry', *International Journal of Law and Psychiatry* 12, pp. 245–62.

—— (1991) 'Can prison medicine be ethical?', *Journal of Irish Colleges of Physicians and Surgeons* 20 (4), pp. 262–5.

Hardy, R. (1990) (ed.) *The Meaning of Imprisonment*, Lincoln: Lincoln Diocese.

Havel, V. (1990) *Letters to Olga*, London: Faber and Faber.

Hay, W., Sparks, R. and Bottoms, A. E. (1990) *Control Problems and the Long-Term Prisoner*, Report to the Home Office, Cambridge Institute of Criminology.

Held, D., Anderson, J., Gieben, B., Hall, S., Harris, L., Lewis, P., Parker, N. and Tirok, B. (eds) (1983) *States and Societies*, Oxford: Martin Robertson.

Hercules, T. (1989) *Labelled a Black Villain*, London: Fourth Estate.

Hill, P. (1990) *Stolen Years*, London: Transworld.

Hillyard, P. and Percy-Smith, J. (1988) *The Coercive State*, London: Fontana.

Hohfeld, W. N. (1919) *Fundamental Legal Conceptions*, New Haven: Yale University Press.

Home Office (1964) *The Organisation of the Prison Medical Service* (Gwynn Report), London: HMSO.

—— (1966) *Report of the Inquiry into Prison Escapes and Security* (Mountbatten Report), London: HMSO Cmnd. 3175.

—— (1969) *People in Prison*, London: HMSO.

—— (1973) *Report on the Work of the Prison Department 1972*, London: HMSO, Cmnd. 5375.

—— (1975) *Report of the Working Party on Adjudication Procedures in Prisons* (Weiler Report), London: HMSO.

—— (1977) *Prisons and the Prisoner*, London: HMSO.

—— (1979) *Committee of Inquiry into the U.K. Prison Services Report* (May Report), London: HMSO, Cmnd. 7673.

—— (1984) *Managing the Long-Term Prison System: The Report of the Control Review Committee*, London: HMSO.

—— (1985a) *New Directions in Prison Design, Report of a Home Office Study of New Generation Prisons in the USA*, London: HMSO.

—— (1985b) *A Sense of Direction*, a report by Ian Dunbar, London: Home Office.

—— (1985c) *Report of Her Majesty's Chief Inspector of Prisons 1984*, London: HMSO.

—— (1985d) *Report of the Committee on the Prison Disciplinary System* (Prior Report), London: HMSO, Cmnd. 9641.

—— (1986a) *Her Majesty's Prison Service News Release*, 29 October.

—— (1986b) *Criminal Justice: A Working Paper*, London: Home Office.

—— (1987a) *Report of an Inquiry by Her Majesty's Chief Inspector of Prisons for England and Wales into the Disturbances in Prison Service Establishments in England between 29 April–2 May 1986*, London: HMSO.

—— (1987b) *Special Units for Long Term Prisoners: Regimes, Management and Research. A Report by the Research and Advisory Group on the Long Term Prison System*, London: HMSO.

—— (1987c) *A Review of Prisoners' Complaints*, a Report by HM Chief Inspector of Prisons, London: HMSO.

—— (1988a) *Report on the Work of the Prison Service April 1987–March 1988*, London: HMSO, Cm. 516.

—— (1988b) *Bail Accommodation and Secure Bail Hostels*, Consultation Paper, London: Home Office.

—— (1988c) *Report by Her Majesty's Chief Inspector of Prisons on H.M. Remand Centre Risley*, London: Home Office.
—— (1988d) *Report by Her Majesty's Chief Inspector of Prisons on H.M. Prison Parkhurst*, London: Home Office.
—— (1988e) *The Parole System in England and Wales*, Report of the Review Committee (Carlisle Report), London: HMSO, Cm. 532.
—— (1988f) *Punishment, Custody and the Community*, London: HMSO, Cm. 424.
—— (1989a) *Report of Her Majesty's Chief Inspector of Prisons 1988*, London: HMSO.
—— (1989b) *Report by Her Majesty's Chief Inspector of Prisons on H.M. Prison Cookham Wood*, London: Home Office.
—— (1989c) *Report by Her Majesty's Chief Inspector of Prisons on H.M. Prison Styal*, London: Home Office.
—— (1989d) *Report by Her Majesty's Chief Inspector of Prisons on H.M. Prison East Sutton Park*, London: Home Office.
—— (1989e) *Management of Vulnerable Prisoners Working Group Report*, Internal document.
—— (1989f) *Report on the Work of the Prison Service April 1988 – March 1989*, London: HMSO, Cm. 835.
—— (1989g) *Prison Sanitation: Proposals for the Ending of Slopping Out*, Report by HM Chief Inspector of Prisons, London: HMSO.
—— (1990a) *Crime, Justice and Protecting the Public*, London: HMSO, Cm. 965.
—— (1990b) *Report by Her Majesty's Chief Inspector of Prisons on H.M. Prison Brixton*, London: Home Office.
—— (1990c) *Report by Her Majesty's Chief Inspector of Prisons on H.M. Prison Leeds*, London: Home Office.
—— (1990d) *The Practice of Young Offender Throughcare by the Probation Service in Four Young Offender Institutions and Six Probation Areas*, London: HM Inspectorate of Probation.
—— (1990e) *Report on an Efficiency Scrutiny of the Prison Medical Service*, (Efficiency Scrutiny Report) London: Home Office.
—— (1990f) *The Prison Medical Service in England and Wales – Recruitment and Training of Doctors: A Report of a Working Party of the Royal College of Physicians to the Chief Medical Officer March 1989*, (Hoffenberg Report), London: HMSO.
—— (1990g) *Report of Her Majesty's Chief Inspector of Prisons 1989*, London: HMSO.
—— (1990h) *Report of the Parole Board 1989*, London: HMSO.
—— (1991a) *Custody, Care and Justice: The Way Ahead for the Prison Service in England and Wales*, London: HMSO, Cm. 1647.
—— (1991b) *Report on the Work of the Prison Service April 1990–March 1991*, London: HMSO, Cm. 1724.
—— (1991c) *Model Regime for Local Prisons and Remand Centres*, London: HM Prison Department.
—— (1991d) *The Control Review Committee, 1984: Implementation of the Committee's Recommendations*, London: Directorate of Custody, Prison Service Headquarters.
—— (1991e) 'Projections of long term trends in the prison population to 1999', *Home Office Statistical Bulletin*, 19/91, London: Home Office.
—— (1991f) *Tender Documents for the Operating Contract of Wolds Remand Prison*, Schedule 2 and 3, London: Home Office.
—— (1991g) *Report by Her Majesty's Chief Inspector of Prisons on H.M. Prison Coldingley*, London: Home Office.
—— (1991h) *Report by Her Majesty's Chief Inspector of Prisons on H.M. Prison Blundeston*, London: Home Office.
—— (1991i) *Treatment Programmes for Sex Offenders in Custody: A Strategy*, London: Home Office.

—— (1991j) *Regimes for Women*, London: HM Prison Service.
—— (1991k) *Caring for Drug Users – A Multidisciplinary Resource Pack for People Working with Drug Users*, London: Directorate of Prison Medical Services.
—— (1991l) *HIV/AIDS A Multidisciplinary Approach in the Prison Environment*, London: Directorate of Prison Medical Services.
—— (1991m) *Contracting for Prison Health Services: A Consultation Paper*, London: Directorate of Prison Medical Services.
—— (1991n) *Prison Service Briefing*, No. 36, London: Home Office.
—— (1991o) *Management of the Prison Service: Report by Admiral Sir Raymond Lygo KCB*, London: Home Office.
—— (1991p) 'Prison Broad Priority 1991/1992 – hygeine in prisons', Prison Service Briefing No. 30, London: Prison Department.
—— (1992a) *Prison Statistics England and Wales*, London: HMSO Cm. 1800.
—— (1992b) *Statistics of Offences Against Prison Discipline and Punishments England and Wales 1991*, London: HMSO, Cm. 2066.
—— (1992c) *Report of Her Majesty's Chief Inspector of Prisons, April 1991–March 1992*, London: HMSO, Cm. 203.
—— (1992d) *Report of an Unannounced Short Inspection by Her Majesty's Chief Inspector of Prisons, H.M. Prison Manchester*, London: Home Office.
—— (1992e) *Community Prisons: A Consultation Paper*, London: H.M. Prison Service.
—— (1992f) 'Projection of Long-Term Trends in the Prison Population to 2000', *Home Office Statistical Bulletin* 10/92, London: Home Office.
—— (1993) *Vision and Values*, London: Prison Department.
Home Office/Department of Health and Social Security (1974) *Interim Report of the Committee on Mentally Abnormal Offenders*, London: HMSO Cmnd. 5678.
—— (1975) *The Report of the Committee on Mentally Abnormal Offenders* (Butler Report), London: HMSO, Cmnd, 6244.
—— (1987) *Report of the Inter-Departmental Working Group of Home Office and DHSS Officials on Mentally Disturbed Offenders in the Prison System in England and Wales*, London: Home Office.
Hood, R. (1992) *Race and Sentencing: A Study in the Crown Court*, a Report for the Commission for Racial Equality, Oxford: Oxford University Press.
Hood, R. and Sparks, R. (1970) *Key Issues in Criminology*, London: Weidenfeld and Nicolson.
House of Commons (1981) *Fourth Report from the Home Affairs Committee: The Prison Service*, Vol. 1, London: HMSO.
—— (1986) *Third Report from the Social Services Committee: Prison Medical Service*, Paper 72–1, London: HMSO.
—— (1987) *The Government Reply to the Third Social Services Committee Report*, London: HMSO, Cm. 115.
House of Lords (1989) *Select Committee on Murder and Life Imprisonment*, Vol. 1, Part 8, Paper 78–1, London: HMSO.
Howard, J. (1929) *The State of Prisons in England and Wales*, London: Everyman.
Hudson, B. (1989) 'Discrimination and disparity: the influence of race on sentencing', *New Community* 16(1), pp. 23–34.
Ilbert, R. and Ralli, R. A. (1989) *Introduction to the Prison Medical Services*, London: Directorate of Prison Medical Services.
Jacobs, J. (1980) 'The Prisoners' Rights Movement and its impacts 1960–1980', in N. Morris and N. Tonry (eds) *Crime and Justice: An Annual Review of Research* 2, pp. 429–70.
—— (1983) *New Perspectives on Prisons and Imprisonment*, Ithaca: Cornell University Press.
Jessop, B. (1990) *State Theory*, Cambridge: Polity.

Justice (1983) *Justice in Prison,* London: Justice.

Kean, J. (ed) *Civil Society and the State,* London: Verso.

Keat, R. (1991) 'Introduction ' in R. Keat and N. Abercrombie (eds) *Enterprise Culture,* London: Routledge.

Keat, R. and Abercrombie, N. (eds) (1991) *Enterprise Culture,* London: Routledge.

King, R. D. (1985) 'Control in prisons' in M. Maguire, J. Vagg and R. Morgan (eds) *Accountability and Prisons: Opening Up a Closed World,* London: Tavistock.

—— (1991) 'The Woolf Report: an agenda for action', paper to the Prison Reform Trust Conference, Church House, Westminster, 18 July 1991.

King, R. D. and Elliott, K. (1977) *Albany: Birth of a Prison – End of an Era,* London: Routledge.

King, R. D. and McDermott, K. (1989) 'British prisons 1970–1987: the ever deepening crisis', *British Journal of Criminology* 29 (2), pp. 107–28.

—— (1990a) 'My geranium is subversive: some notes on the management of trouble in prisons', *British Journal of Sociology* 41 (4), pp. 445–71.

—— (1990b) 'As full a life' (The Perrie Lectures, 1989), *Prison Service Journal* 77, pp. 30–40.

—— (1991) 'A fresh start: managing the prison service' in R. Reiner and M. Cross (eds) *Beyond Law and Order: Criminal Justice Policy and Politics into the 1990s,* London: Macmillan.

—— (1992) 'Security, control and humane containment in the prison system', in D. Downes (ed) *Unravelling Criminal Justice: Eleven British Studies,* London: Macmillan.

King, R. D. and Morgan, R. (1976) *A Taste of Prison: Custodial Conditions for Trial and Remand Prisoners,* London: Routledge.

King, R. D. and Morgan, R. (1980) *The Future of the Prison System,* with Martin, J. P. and Thomas, J. E. London: Gower.

Kritzman, L. (ed.) (1988) *Michael Foucault: Politics, Philosophy and Culture,* London: Routledge.

Lefebvre, H. (1969) *The Sociology of Marx,* New York: Vintage.

Lewis, H. and Mair, G. (1989) *Bail and Probation Work II: The Use of London Probation Bail Hostels for Bailees,* Home Office Research and Planning Unit Paper No. 50, London: Home Office.

Light, R. (ed.) (1989) *Prisoners' Families,* Bristol: Bristol and Bath Centre for Criminal Justice.

Light, R. and Mattfield, K. (1988) 'Prison disciplinary hearings: the failure of reform', *Howard Journal of Criminal Justice* 27, pp. 266–82.

Livingstone, S. (1988) 'Prisoners have rights, but what rights', *Modern Law Review* 51, pp. 525–30.

Logan, C. H. (1990) *Private Prisons: Cons and Pros,* New York: Oxford University Press.

McConville, S. (1987) 'Aid from industry? Private corrections and prison crowding', in S. D. Gottfredson, and S. McConville (eds) *America's Correctional Crisis: Prison Populations and Public Policy,* New York: Greenwood.

McDermott, K. and King, R. D. (1989) 'A fresh start: the enhancement of prison regimes', *Howard Journal of Criminal Justice* 28 (3), pp. 161–76.

—— (1992) 'Prison Rule 102: "stand by your man": the impact of penal policy on the families of prisoners', in R. Shaw (ed.) *Prisoners' Children: What Are the Issues?,* London: Routledge.

Maclaughlin, R. (1987) *Inside an English Jail,* Dublin: Borderline.

Maden, A., Swinton, M. and Gunn, J. (1992) 'The ethnic origin of women serving a prison sentence', *British Journal of Criminology* 32 (2), pp. 218–21.

Maguire, M. (1985) 'Prisoners' grievances: the role of the board of visitors', in M.

Maguire, J. Vagg and R. Morgan (eds) *Accountability and Prisons: Opening Up a Closed World*, London: Tavistock.
Maguire, M., Vagg, J. and Morgan, R. (eds) (1985) *Accountability and Prisons: Opening Up a Closed World*, London: Tavistock.
Mair, G. and Nee, C. (1990) *Electronic Monitoring: The Trials and Their Results*, Home Office Research Study 100, London: HMSO.
Manderaka-Sheppard, A. (1986) *The Dynamics of Aggression in Women's Prisons*, London: Gower.
Martin, J. P. (1975) *Boards of Visitors of Penal Institutions* (Jellicoe Report), London: Barry Rose.
Miliband, R. (1982) *Capitalist Democracy in Britain*, Oxford: Oxford University Press.
Monger, M. and Pendleton, J. (1980) *Throughcare with Prisoners' Families*, Nottingham: Social Work Studies No. 3, University of Nottingham.
Morgan, P. (1992) *Offending While on Bail: A Survey of Recent Studies*, Home Office Research and Planning Unit Paper No. 65, London: HMSO.
Morgan, R. (1983) 'How resources are used in the prison system', in *A Prison System for the 80s and Beyond: The Noel Buxton Lectures*, London: NACRO.
—— (1987) 'More prisoners denied lawyers help', *New Society* 91, p. 1283.
—— (1989) 'Remands in custody: problems and prospects' *Criminal Law Review*, pp. 481–93.
—— (1991) 'Woolf: in retrospect and prospect', *Modern Law Review* 54, pp. 713–25.
Morgan, R. and Barclay, A. (1989) 'Remands in custody: problems and prospects for change' (The Perrie Lectures, 1988), *Prison Service Journal* 74, pp. 13–36.
Morgan, R. and Bronstein, A. J. (1985) 'Prisoners and the courts: the U.S. experience' in M. Maguire, J. Vagg and R. Morgan (eds) *Accountability and Prisons: Opening Up a Closed World*, London: Tavistock.
Morgan, R. and Jones, S. (1992) 'Bail or Jail?' in E. Stockdale and S. Casale (eds) *Criminal Justice Under Stress*, London: Blackstone.
Morgan, R., Maguire, M. and Vagg, J. (1985) 'Overhauling the prison disciplinary system: notes for readers of the Prior Committee's Report', in M. Maguire, R. Morgan and J. Vagg (eds) *Accountability and Prisons: Opening Up a Closed World*, London: Tavistock.
Morris, A. and Wilkinson, C. (eds) (1988) *Women and the Penal System*, Cropwood Conference Series 19, Cambridge: University of Cambridge, Institute of Criminology.
Morris, N. (1973) 'Minimum standards for medical services in prisons and jails' in G. E. W. Wolstenholme and M. O'Connor (eds) *Medical Care of Prisoners and Detainees*, Amsterdam: Elsevier.
Morris, N. (1990) Untitled paper given at Lincoln Conference, in R. Hardy (ed.) *The Meaning of Imprisonment*, Lincoln: Lincoln Diocese.
Morris, N. and Tonry, N. (eds) (1980) *Crime and Justice: An Annual Review of Research*, 2, Chicago: University of Chicago Press.
Morris, P. (1965) *Prisoners and their Families*, London; George Allen and Unwin.
Moxon, D. (1988) *Sentencing Practice in the Crown Courts*, Home Office Research Study 103, London: HMSO.
Muncie, J. and Sparks, R. (eds) (1991) *Imprisonment: European Perspectives*, London: Harvester.
Murphy, E. (1992) 'The effects of NHS reorganisation on forensic psychiatric services', *Journal of Forensic Psychiatry* 3 (1), pp. 13–30.
NACRO (1991a) *A Fresh Start for Women Prisoners: The Implications of the Woolf Report for Women*, London: NACRO.
—— (1991b) *A Really Fresh Start: NACRO's 'White Paper' in Response to the Woolf Report*, London: NACRO.

—— (1991c) *Seizing the Initiative*, London: NACRO.
—— (1991d) *Prison Overcrowding – Some Facts and Figures*, London: NACRO Briefing.
Nozick, R. (1974) *Anarchy, State and Utopia*, New York: Basic Books.
Office of Population Censuses and Surveys (1992) *The National Prison Survey 1991: A Report to the Home Office of a Study of Prisoners in England and Wales Carried out by the Social Survey Division of OPCS*, by T. Dodd and P. Hunter, London: HMSO.
Owen, T. (1991) 'Prisoners Rights', *New Law Journal* 141, p. 1328.
Padel, U. and Stevenson, P. (1988) *Insiders*, London: Virago.
Parker, D. (1992) 'Agency status, privatisation and improved performance: some evidence from the U.K.', *Journal of Public Sector Management*, 5 (1), pp. 30–8.
Pateman, C. (1988) 'The fraternal social contract', in J. Keane (ed.) *Civil Society and the State*, London: Verso.
Peay, J. (1989) *Tribunals on Trial*, Oxford: Oxford University Press.
Pennock, J. R. and Chapman, J. W. (1981) *Human Rights – Nomos 23*, New York: New York University Press.
Perrie, W. (1981) 'The prison dilemma, explosion of human frustration or explosion of human ideas', *Prison Service Journal* 44 (new series), pp. 10–12.
Pilling, J. (1992) 'Back to basics: relationships in the Prison Service', in *Perspectives on Prison: A Collection of Views on Prison Life and Running Prisons*, London: HMSO.
Posen, I. (1986) 'Holloway Reception Survey', unpublished.
Power, D. J. (1990) 'Prison riots', *Justice of the Peace*, 154, pp. 654–59.
Prison Reform Trust (1990) *Sex Offenders in Prison*, London: Prison Reform Trust.
—— (1991a) *The Identikit Prisoner: Characteristics of the Prison Population*, London: Prison Reform Trust.
—— (1991b) *The Woolf Report: A Summary of the Main Findings and Recommendations of the Inquiry into Prison Disturbances*, London: Prison Reform Trust.
—— (ed.) (1992a) *Beyond Containment: The Treatment of Sex Offenders in the Criminal Justice System*, London: Prison Reform Trust.
—— (1992b) *Implementing Woolf: The Prison System One Year On*, London: Prison Reform Trust.
Prison Reform Trust/Howard League (1991) *Who's Afraid of Implementing Woolf?*, London: Prison Reform Trust/Howard League.
Procek, E. (1981) 'Psychiatry and the social control of women' in A. Morris (ed.) *Women and Crime*, Cambridge: Cropwood Conference Series 13.
PROP (n.d.) *Don't Mark His Face*, London: PROP.
Quinn, P. (1985) 'Prison management and prison discipline: a case study of change', in M. Maguire, M. Morgan and J. Vagg (eds) *Accountability and Prisons: Opening Up a Closed World*, London: Tavistock.
Reich, R. (1972) 'Bargaining in correctional institutions: restructuring the relationship between the inmate and the prison authority', *Yale Law Journal* 81 (4), pp. 726–57.
Reiner, R. and Cross, M. (eds) (1991) *Beyond Law and Order: Criminal Justice Policy and Politics into the 1990s*, London: Macmillan.
Richards, M. (1992) 'The separation of children and parents: some issues and problems', in R. Shaw (ed.) *Prisoners' Children: What are the Issues?*, London: Routledge.
Richardson, G. (1985a) 'Judicial intervention in prison life', in M. Maguire, J. Vagg and R. Morgan (eds) *Accountability and Prisons: Opening Up A Closed World*, London: Tavistock.
—— (1985b) 'The case for prisoners' rights' in M. Maguire, J. Vagg and R. Morgan (eds) *Accountability and Prisons: Opening Up a Closed World*, London: Tavistock.
—— (1986) 'The duty to give reasons: potential and practice', *Public Law*, pp. 437–69.

—— (1991) 'Discretionary life sentences and the European Convention on Human Rights', *Public Law*, pp. 33–40.

—— (1993) *Law, Process and Custody: Prisoners and Patients*, London: Weidenfeld & Nicholson.

Robertson, G., Dell, S., Grounds, A. and James, K. (1992) *Mentally Disordered Remand Prisoners, Home Office Research Bulletin.*

Royal College of Psychiatrists (1992) *Ethical Issues Concerning Psychiatric Care in Prison: Report from the Special Committee on Unethical Psychiatric Practices*, London: Royal College of Psychiatrists.

Rutherford, A. (1983) *Prisons and the Process of Justice*, London: Heinemann.

—— (1993) *Criminal Justice and the Pursuit of Decency*, Oxford: Oxford University Press.

Ryan, M. (1992) 'The Woolf Report: on the treadmill of prison reform?', *Political Quarterly* 63 (1), pp. 50–6.

Ryan, M. and Ward, T. (1989) *Privatisation and the Penal System*, Milton Keynes: Open University Press.

Sampson, A. (1991) 'Private prisons: fight is fixed', *Prison Report* 16, p. 16.

Scottish Office (1988a) *Custody and Care: Policy and Plans for the Scottish Prison Service*, Edinburgh: Scottish Prison Service.

—— (1988b) *Assessment and Control: The Management of Violent and Disruptive Prisoners*, A Scottish Prison Service Discussion Paper, Edinburgh: Scottish Prison Service.

——(1990) *Opportunity and Responsibility: Developing New Approaches to the Management of the Long Term Prison System in Scotland.* Edinburgh: Scottish Prison Service.

—— (1991) *Prisons in Scotland, Report for 1990–91*, Edinburgh, HMSO, Cm. 1663.

Scraton, P. (ed.) (1987) *Law, Order and the Authoritarian State*, Milton Keynes: Open University Press.

Scraton, P., Sim, J. and Skidmore, P. (1991) *Prisons Under Protest*, Milton Keynes: Open University Press.

Shaw, R. (1987) *Children of Imprisoned Fathers*, London: Hodder and Stoughton.

—— (ed.) (1992) *Prisoners' Children: What Are the Issues?*, London: Routledge.

Sim, J. (1987) 'Working for the clampdown: prisons and politics in England and Wales', in P. Scraton (ed.) *Law, Order and the Authoritarian State*, Milton Keynes: Open University.

—— (1990) *Medical Power in Prisons: The Prison Medical Service in England 1774–1989*, Milton Keynes: Open University Press.

—— (1991a) 'We are not animals, we are human beings: prisons, protest and politics in England and Wales 1969–1990', *Social Justice* 18(3), pp. 107–29 (Attica 1971–1991: A Commemorative Issue', edited by R. Weiss).

—— (1991b) '"When you aint got nothing you got nothing to lose": the Peterhead rebellion, the state and the case for prison abolition', paper presented at the British Criminology Conference, University of York, July 1991.

Simon, J. (1974) 'Michael Foucault on Attica: an interview', *Telos* 19, pp. 154–61.

Smart, C. (1977) *Women, Crime and Criminology: A Feminist Critique*, London: Routledge and Kegan Paul.

—— (1984) *The Ties That Bind*, London: Routledge.

Smith, D. (1987) *The Everyday World as Problematic*, Milton Keynes: Open University Press.

Smith, R. (1984) *Prison Health Care*, London: British Medical Association.

—— (1992) 'Prison medicine: beginning again', *British Medical Journal*, 304, pp. 134–5.

Sparks, R. F. (1971) *Local Prisons: The Crisis in the English Penal System*, London: Heinemann.

Squires, P. (1990) *Anti-Social Policy*, London: Harvester.

Stern, V. (1987) *Bricks of Shame: Britain's Prisons*, 2nd edn, Harmondsworth: Penguin, 1989.
Sunkin, M. (1991) 'The judicial review caseload 1987–9', *Public Law*, pp. 490–9.
Sykes, G. M. (1958) *Society of Captives: The Study of a Maximum Security Prison*, Princeton, N.J.: Princeton University Press.
Tchaikovsky, C. (1991) 'Mixed prisons: misogynistic and misguided', *Prison Report*, 16, pp. 12–13.
Teggin, V. (1992) 'New prison rules and offences', *Legal Action* May: 13–15.
Thornton, D. (1987) 'Sex offenders segregated for their own protection under Rule 43', in B. McGurk, D. Thornton and M. Williams (eds) *Applying Psychology to Imprisonment*, London: HMSO.
Tuck, M. (1991) 'Some reflections on the Woolf Inquiry into prison disturbances', paper presented at the British Criminology Conference, University of York, July 1991.
Twinn, S. (1992) 'Littlehey Prison: a new approach', in Prison Reform Trust (ed.) *Beyond Containment: The Treatment of Sex Offenders in the Criminal Justice System*, London: Prison Reform Trust.
Unger, R. (1983) 'The Critical Legal Studies Movement', *Harvard Law Review* 96, pp. 561–675.
United Nations (1955) *United Nations General Assembly Standard Minimum Rules for the Treatment of Prisoners*, New York: United Nations.
—— (1985) *United Nations Congress on the Prevention of Crime and the Treatment of Offenders*, Milan: United Nations.
Vagg, J. (n.d.) 'Scottish Prison Regimes 1988' (unpublished first draft interim Report to the Scottish Office.
von Hirsch, A. (1990) 'The ethics of community penalties', *Crime and Delinquency* 36, pp. 162–73.
Walby, S. (1990) *Theorising Patriarchy*, London: Macmillan.
Walmsley, G. R. (ed.) (1991) *Managing Difficult Prisoners: The Parkhurst Special Unit*, Home Office Research Study 122, London: HMSO.
Walmsley, G. R., Howard, L. and White, S. (1992) *The National Prison Survey 1991: Main Findings*, Home Office Research Study 128, London: HMSO.
Walker, N. (1991) *Why Punish?*, Oxford: Oxford University Press.
Weiss, R. (ed.) (1991) 'Attica 1971–1991: A Commemorative Issue' *Social Justice* 18(3), pp. 107–29.
Woltenholme, G. E. W. and O'Connor, M.(eds) (1973) *Medical Care of Prisoners and Detainees*, Amsterdam: Elsevier.
Women's National Commission (1991) *Women and Prison: Report of an Ad Hoc Working Group*, London: Cabinet Office.
Woolf, Lord Justice (1991) *Prison Disturbances April 1990: Report of an Inquiry by the Rt. Hon Lord Justice Woolf (Parts I and II) and His Honour Judge Stephen Tumim (Part II)*, London: HMSO, Cm. 1456.
World Health Organisation (1990) *Drug Abusers in Prison: Managing their Health Problems*, Report on a WHO meeting, The Hague 16–18 May 1988, WHO Regional European Service No. 27.
Wozniak, E. and McAllister, D. (1991) 'Facilities, Standards and Change in the Scottish Prison Service: The Prison Survey 1990/91', paper presented at the British Criminology Conference, York University, July 1990.

NAME INDEX

SUBJECT INDEX